Handbook of Clinical Techniques in Pediatric Dentistry

Handbook of Clinical Techniques in Pediatric Dentistry

Second Edition

Edited By

Jane A. Soxman, DDS
Allison Park, Pennsylvania, USA

WILEY Blackwell

Registered Office
John Wiley & Sons, Inc., 111 River Street, Hoboken, NJ 07030, USA

Editorial Office
111 River Street, Hoboken, NJ 07030, USA

For details of our global editorial offices, customer services, and more information about Wiley products visit us at www.wiley.com.

Wiley also publishes its books in a variety of electronic formats and by print-on-demand. Some content that appears in standard print versions of this book may not be available in other formats.

Library of Congress Cataloging-in-Publication Data

Names: Soxman, Jane A., editor.
Title: Handbook of clinical techniques in pediatric dentistry / edited by
    Jane A. Soxman.
Description: Second edition. | Hoboken, NJ : Wiley-Blackwell, 2022. |
    Preceded by The handbook of clinical techniques in pediatric dentistry /
    edited by Jane A. Soxman. 2015. | Includes bibliographical references
    and index.
Identifiers: LCCN 2021028073 (print) | LCCN 2021028074 (ebook) | ISBN
    9781119661047 (paperback) | ISBN 9781119661078 (adobe pdf) | ISBN
    9781119661108 (epub)
Subjects: MESH: Dental Care for Children – methods | Pediatric
    Dentistry – methods | Tooth Diseases – therapy
Classification: LCC RK63 (print) | LCC RK63 (ebook) | NLM WU 480 | DDC
    617.6/45 – dc23
LC record available at https://lccn.loc.gov/2021028073
LC ebook record available at https://lccn.loc.gov/2021028074

Cover Design: Wiley
Cover Images: © Jane A. Soxman

Set in 9.5/12.5pt STIXTwoText by Straive, Chennai, India

Printed in Singapore
M104365_050721

Contents

Foreword

As a dentist for over 40 years, my career has been a blend of teaching and research pursuits and the private practice of pediatric dentistry. The integration of sound scientific and evidence-based information with everyday clinical practice has immeasurable value to the clinician. The two must go hand in hand. The practicing dentist must be able to deliver care based on sound scientific principles, while maintaining the practicality of delivering that care in a busy private practice.

Dr. Soxman is ideally suited for this task. As a practicing pediatric dentist for nearly 38 years, she has numerous publications, presented countless continuing education courses throughout the United States, as well as contributing to pediatric dental and general practice residency programs for many years. This love of education and translating scientific evidence into clinical know-how is what makes this second edition of *The Handbook of Clinical Techniques in Pediatric Dentistry* so valuable.

It often seems that not much changes in the world of pediatric dentistry, but the addition of several new chapters in this edition of the book tells a different story. Since the publication of the first edition there have been several significant trends in dentistry for children, and the addition of these chapters reflects those trends. Issues such as caries risk assessment, the noninvasive management of caries, an increased desire for more esthetic restorative options for children, and sleep disordered breathing in children are all clinical concerns

that have increased in importance, hence their inclusion in this edition.

Dr. Soxman has chosen 19 others to contribute to this textbook, and like the blend of her own professional career, her collaborators are a blend of many well-known pediatric dentists in private practice, as well as several accomplished academicians and researchers. I have had the pleasure of knowing, working with, and collaborating with several of these individuals. The result of Dr. Soxman's collaboration is a well-illustrated, simplified, step-by-step approach to most common clinical challenges that a practitioner who treats children needs to know. While the book is scientifically solid, its strength, as in the first edition, is the clinical relevance and presentation of techniques that have been practiced with proficiency by those writing about them.

it is a pleasure to endorse a book of this caliber. It can serve not only as a textbook for those still learning, but as a reference manual for those who have been practicing for several years. Congratulations to Dr. Soxman and her collaborators on producing this updated, comprehensive textbook. I am confident that those clinicians who put into practice what they read in this text will be well served. But more importantly, so will the children who are treated by those clinicians be well served!

William F. Waggoner, DDS, MS, FAAPD, FACD
Las Vegas, NV

Preface to the Second Edition

The second edition of *The Handbook of Clinical Techniques in Pediatric Dentistry* offers dental students, postgraduate dental residents in both pediatrics and general practice, along with practicing dentists and hygienists, succinct evidence-based guidance with supporting photographs, for treatment in the primary and young permanent dentitions. This second edition aims to provide the most recent advances and modifications, along with new methodologies for dental treatment.

Since publication of the first edition, treatment of dental caries at the lesion level has shifted from invasive to less invasive or non-invasive methods. This more conservative approach is a major development in clinical dentistry. The purpose of providing less invasive or noninvasive techniques for dental care is to arrest, reverse, or curtail caries progression without use of local anesthesia, the rubber dam, or the dental drill, and/or to preserve tooth structure. These modalities also may avoid sedation in order to provide quality care for a fearful, special healthcare needs, or uncooperative patient. Pediatric patients, who are too young to cooperate for definitive treatment, can be safely treated, while protecting the developing psyche, without the possible risks with sedation or general anesthesia. This second edition begins with a new chapter, "Non-Invasive and Minimally Invasive Treatment of Dental Caries."

Another new chapter, "Caries Risk Assessment," is included too. The aim of this chapter is to provide a guideline for hygienists and dentists to identify caries risk, enabling the structure of an individualized preventive care plan, along with appropriate management of both noncavitated and cavitated carious lesions.

Other new chapters are "Management of Esthetic Concerns," "Traumatic Injury to the Primary Incisors," "Interceptive Orthodontic Treatment in the Mixed Dentition," "Clinical Examination of the Infant," "Clinical Examination of the Patient with Special Healthcare Needs," "Sleep Disordered Breathing in Children," and, finally, "Pediatric Oral Medicine." Most of these chapters were written by contributors with particular expertise and interest in the subject matter.

Other chapter additions and revisions for the most up-to-date clinical guidelines are included for molar–incisor hypomineralization and the latest research findings on stainless-steel crowns. Behavior guidance and local anesthesia chapters are enhanced by an educator who is known and published with a focus in those two topics. New findings from a systematic review and meta-analysis on nonvital pulp therapy are included in the chapter on nonvital pulp therapy for primary teeth. Indirect pulp therapy for primary teeth has gained popularity as a less invasive vital pulp treatment and is described in the chapter on vital pulp therapy. Finally, the indications and procedures for both indirect and direct pulp therapy in the young permanent dentition complete the mission to provide the most recent evidence-based treatment at the time of this second edition's publication.

Jane A. Soxman, DDS

Preface to the First Edition

While speaking at an annual session of the American Dental Association, Wiley Blackwell publications requested that I meet with a commissioning editor. He inquired whether I had ever considered writing a book and if so, on what subject. My response was without hesitation. Over the past 20 plus years as a national speaker in continuing education and as a seminar instructor for general practice residents, I recalled the myriad of questions asked. I had often thought that a book on clinical techniques would provide much needed guidelines and directions for dental students, general dentists, and graduate general practice and pediatric dental residents. This book would include step-by-step descriptions, augmented with clinical photographs of routinely performed procedures and evidence-based recommendations.

The Handbook of Clinical Techniques in Pediatric Dentistry provides the clinician with an increased level of expertise and skills for timely identification and intervention for various presentations in the developing dentition. It also clearly describes procedures for treatment in the primary and young permanent dentitions. The most commonly encountered treatment needs are discussed, with the goal of increasing clinician and staff confidence, while decreasing chair time and stress. What you will learn and incorporate into your practice will be of tremendous benefit to you, your staff, and the children for whom you care.

Jane A. Soxman, RN, DDS
Allison Park, Pennsylvania, USA

Acknowledgments

My vision for this second edition was to expand the content, including timely topics of relevance written by educators with particular interest and expertise in their chapter topics. Fortunately, every invited contributor joined this endeavor. I am honored and grateful for the contribution of each that fulfilled my intentions for this second edition. The first edition contributors also deserve recognition with updates to the majority of the chapters. This book is embellished with photographs to significantly enhance each chapter, providing a better comprehension of the written text. I sincerely thank each contributor for his or her time and effort to create this second edition, which will surely enhance confidence and the quality of care provided to our youngest patients. I would like also to acknowledge two of my staff members, Karen Evans and Denise Cafeo, who were immediately available to assist with any problem, complying with our guidelines and downloading the exceptional photographs. Finally, once again, for her attentiveness to the quality of the photographs, her patience, her steadfast devotion to me, and her gentle nature in caring for our patients, I dedicate this second edition of *The Handbook of Clinical Techniques in Pediatric Dentistry* to my assistant of 28 years, Beth Ann Sutter.

Jane A. Soxman, DDS

List of Contributors

Editor

Jane A. Soxman, DDS

Diplomate American Board of Pediatric Dentistry

Fellow American Board of Pediatric Dentistry

Private Practice Pediatric Dentistry

Allison Park, PA, USA

Division of Dental Medicine, Allegheny General Hospital

General Practice Dental Residency Seminar Instructor

Pittsburgh, PA, USA

Veterans Affairs Pittsburgh Health Care System

General Practice Dental Residency Educational Consultant

Pittsburgh, PA, USA

Adjunct Assistant Professor of Pediatric Dentistry

Department of Pediatric Dentistry

University of Pittsburgh School of Dental Medicine

Pittsburgh, PA, USA

Contributors

Ehsan N. Azadani, DDS, MS

Diplomate American Board of Pediatric Dentistry

Assistant Professor Division of Pediatric Dentistry

The Ohio State University College of Dentistry and Nationwide Children's Hospital

Columbus, OH, USA

Joe H. Camp, DDS, MSD

Retired

Adjunct Professor, University of North Carolina School of Dentistry

Chapel Hill, NC, USA

Paul S. Casamassimo, DDS, MS

Diplomate American Board of Pediatric Dentistry

Fellow American Board of Pediatric Dentistry

Professor Emeritus

Division of Pediatric Dentistry, The Ohio State University College of Dentistry

Columbus, OH, USA

Giulia M. Castrigano, DMD, MS

Diplomate American Board of Pediatric Dentistry

Fellow American Board of Pediatric Dentistry

Assistant Professor

Division of Dentistry, Cincinnati Children's Hospital

University of Cincinnati Affiliate

Cincinnati, OH, USA

James A. Coll, DMD, MS

Diplomate American Board of Pediatric Dentistry

Fellow American Board of Pediatric Dentistry

Private Practice Pediatric Dentistry 1974–2013

York, PA, USA

Clinical Professor, Department of Pediatric Dentistry

University of Maryland Dental School

Baltimore, MD, USA

Theodore P. Croll, DDS
Diplomate American Board of Pediatric
  Dentistry
Fellow American Board of Pediatric Dentistry
Private Practice Pediatric Dentistry
Doylestown, PA, USA
Adjunct Professor Pediatric Dentistry
University of Texas Health Science Center at
  San Antonio Dental School
San Antonio, TX, USA
Clinical Professor, Pediatric Dentistry, Case
  Western Reserve School of Dental Medicine
Cleveland, OH, USA

Elizabeth S. Gosnell, DMD, MS
Diplomate American Board of Pediatric
  Dentistry
Fellow American Board of Pediatric Dentistry
Department of Pediatrics
University of Cincinnati College of Medicine
Associate Professor Division of Pediatric Den-
  tistry
Cincinnati Children's Hospital Medical Center
Cincinnati, OH, USA

Christel M. Haberland, DDS, MS, FAAPD
Diplomate American Board of Pediatric
  Dentistry
Diplomate American Board of Oral and Max-
  illofacial Pathology
Chair, Department of Pediatric Dentistry
James B. Edwards College of Dental Medicine
Medical University of South Carolina
Charleston, SC, USA

Constance M. Killian, DMD
Diplomate American Board of Pediatric
  Dentistry
Fellow American Board of Pediatric Dentistry
Private Practice Pediatric Dentistry
Doylestown, PA, USA
Adjunct Associate Professor of Pediatric Den-
  tistry
University of Pennsylvania School of Dental
  Medicine
Philadelphia, PA, USA

Ari Kupietzky, DMD, MSc
Diplomate American Board of Pediatric
  Dentistry
Clinical Instructor Department of Pediatric
  Dentistry
The Hebrew University–Hadassah School of
  Dental Medicine
Jerusalem, Israel

Jeanette MacLean, DDS
Diplomate American Board of Pediatric
  Dentistry
Fellow American Board of Pediatric Dentistry
Private Practice, Pediatric Dentistry
Glendale, AZ, USA

Stanley F. Malamed, DDS
Dentist Anesthesiologist
Emeritus Professor of Dentistry
Ostrow School of Dentistry of USC
Los Angeles, CA, USA

AnnMarie Matusak, DDS, MS
Diplomate American Board of Pediatric
  Dentistry
Fellow American Board of Pediatric Dentistry
Assistant Professor, University of Cincinnati
Director, Pediatric Dentistry Residency Pro-
  gram Division of Dentistry
Cincinnati Children's Hospital Medical Center
Cincinnati, OH, USA

Roshan V. Patel, DMD
Private Practice Pediatric
  Dentistry
Fort Worth, TX, USA

Cristina Perez, DDS, MS
Diplomate American Board of Pediatric
  Dentistry
Fellow American Board of Pediatric Dentistry
Diplomate American Board of Orofacial Pain
Associate Professor and Chief, Division of
  Pediatric Dentistry
Director, Pediatric Dental Residency Program
University of Kentucky
Lexington, KY, USA

S. Thikkurissy, DDS, MS
Diplomate American Board of Pediatric
   Dentistry
Fellow American Board of Pediatric Dentistry
Professor & Robert Creedon Chair
Division of Dentistry
Cincinnati Children's Hospital
University of Cincinnati Affiliate
Cincinnati, OH, USA

Janice A. Townsend, DDS, MS
Diplomate American Board of Pediatric
   Dentistry
Fellow American Board of Pediatric Dentistry
Chief, Department Dentistry
Nationwide Children's Hospital
Columbus, OH, USA
Chair, Division of Pediatric Dentistry
The Ohio State University College of Dentistry
Columbus, OH, USA

J. Timothy Wright, DDS, MS
Diplomate American Board of Pediatric
   Dentistry
Bawden Distinguished Professor and Chair
Division of Pediatric and Public Health
Adams School of Dentistry
University of North Carolina
Chapel Hill, NC, USA

Patrice B. Wunsch, DDS, MS
Diplomate American Board of Pediatric
   Dentistry
Fellow American Board of Pediatric Dentistry
Vice Chair, Department of Pediatric Dentistry
Professor, School of Dentistry
Virginia Commonwealth University
Richmond, VA, USA

1

Noninvasive and Minimally Invasive Treatment of Dental Caries

Jane A. Soxman, Jeanette MacLean, and Christel Haberland

Noninvasive clinical techniques for the pediatric dental patient provide alternative standard of care treatment with therapeutic interventions that offer methods to arrest or slow caries progression until definitive treatment can be safely performed with pharmacologic modalities or the child can cooperate for treatment. These techniques typically require no rubber dam isolation or local anesthesia, both of which often incite fearful or avoidance behavior. Soft tissue trauma, with cheek/lip or tongue chewing, the most common adverse event reported by members of the American Academy of Pediatric Dentistry, is no longer a postoperative issue (Calvo *et al.*, 2019). Parents/guardians are often reluctant to accept sedation or general anesthesia for treatment, particularly if other options are presented. Deep sedation or general anesthesia poses increased risks for toddlers and should be reserved for instances where dental disease outweighs the benefits of active surveillance or noninvasive or minimally invasive treatment with interim therapeutic restoration or medicaments to slow or arrest caries progression (Lee *et al.*, 2013, 2017; Stratmann *et al.*, 2014; Orser *et al.*, 2018; AAPD, 2019–2020a). The incidence of recurrent caries, reported to be as high as 79% after general anesthesia, also supports the cost-effective alternative of noninvasive or minimally invasive treatment (Almeida *et al.*, 2000; Amin *et al.*, 2010; Lin & Lin, 2016; Oubenyahya & Bouhabba, 2019;

AAPD, 2019–2020d). Noninvasive or minimally invasive treatment for early childhood caries, prior to the need for emergency care, would not only enhance quality of life for a child, but significantly reduce treatment costs with hospitalizations and emergency room visits (AAPD, 2019–2020e). Additionally, medical circumstances may prohibit pharmacologic modalities.

Nonrestorative, noninvasive, or minimally invasive treatment is defined as the management of caries at the lesion level and with minimal loss of sound tooth structure. These interventions can be used in both cavitated and noncavitated carious lesions and for both the primary and permanent dentitions. The decision to use a particular modality of treatment should be determined by considering the type of carious lesion (noncavitated or cavitated), the dentition (primary or permanent), and the tooth surface involved (occlusal, facial/lingual, or interproximal). Other factors to be considered are patient centered and include caries risk analysis (CRA; discussed in Chapter 24). In October 2018, the American Dental Association (ADA) published evidence-based guidelines on nonrestorative treatments for carious lesions that included the following: 38% silver diamine fluoride (SDF), 5% sodium fluoride varnish, 1.23% acidulated phosphate fluoride gel, 5000 ppm fluoride (1.1% sodium fluoride) toothpaste or gel, casein phosphopeptide and amorphous calcium

Handbook of Clinical Techniques in Pediatric Dentistry, Second Edition. Edited by Jane A. Soxman.
© 2022 John Wiley & Sons, Inc. Published 2022 by John Wiley & Sons, Inc.

phosphate (CPP-ACP), and resin infiltration (Slayton *et al.*, 2018). Other treatments for caries that atraumatically remove minimal or no tooth structure offer evidence-based alternatives for uncooperative children or those with special healthcare needs. These techniques include interim therapeutic restoration (ITR) and the Hall technique (HT) for stainless-steel crowns (AAPD, 2019–2020b, c).

38% Silver Diamine Fluoride

38% SDF is a topical antimicrobial and remineralizing agent used for desensitization and caries arrest. Systematic reviews and meta-analyses have demonstrated that SDF is capable of arresting an average of 80% of cavitated caries lesions, with the highest rates of arrest occurring with biannual application (Slayton *et al.*, 2018). The procedure is quick, simple, painless, inexpensive, and well tolerated by young, phobic, and medically frail patients, making it particularly advantageous for pediatric and geriatric patients, and those without access to dental care (Horst *et al.*, 2016). Parents tend to prefer SDF treatment in posterior teeth; however, 70–76% prefer SDF even for anterior teeth when it presents an alternative to sedation and general anesthesia (Figure 1.1a, b) (Crystal *et al.*, 2017).

A 38% SDF solution is 25% silver, 8% ammonia, and 5% fluoride. One drop (0.05 mL) of Advantage Arrest™ 38% SDF (Elevate Oral Care, Palm Beach, Florida, USA) contains 2.24 mg of fluoride and 4.74 mg silver (Crystal & Niederman, 2016). A study on the short-term serum pharmacokinetics of SDF found fluoride exposure was below the US Environmental Protection Agency (EPA) oral reference dose, and while the silver exposure exceeded the dose for cumulative daily exposure over a lifetime, its occasional use (typically biannual application) was well below the concentrations associated with toxicity (Vasquez *et al.*, 2012). One drop per 10 kg of body weight is

considered a safe dose and, depending on the size of the lesion(s), may treat as many as 5–6 teeth (Horst *et al.*, 2016). There are no reports of adverse outcomes or known side effects, other than the trade-mark black stain of active caries, transient metallic taste, and potential gingival irritation, similar to a bleach burn, which resolves on its own in a few days.

Indications for SDF treatment:

- High caries risk.
- Patients who cannot tolerate surgical restorations due to age (pediatric, geriatric), behavior, special needs, medical condition, dental phobia, anxiety, or psychologic condition.
- Need to delay or avoid the use of sedation or anesthesia.
- More lesions than can be treated in one appointment.
- Financial barriers.
- Poor access to care.
- Salivary dysfunction (xerostomia, polypharmacy, salivary dysfunction).
- Difficult-to-treat lesions (root caries, furcations, molar incisor hypomineralization).
- Recurrent caries at a restoration margin.
- Carious primary teeth that will soon exfoliate.
- Carious lesions that are either asymptomatic or have reversible pulpitis.
- Hypersensitivity.

Contraindications for SDF treatment:

- Silver allergy (rare).
- Irreversible pulpitis.
- Carious lesions extending to the pulp.
- Mouth sores, ulcerative gingivitis (or coat soft tissue lesion(s) with petroleum jelly).

Procedure

- Protective eyewear and a plastic-lined bib are placed on the patient.
- Petroleum jelly is applied to the lips and peri-oral area to prevent inadvertently staining the lips or face with SDF.

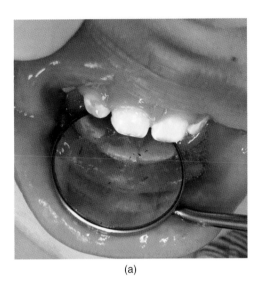

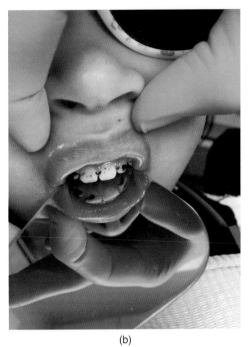

(a)   (b)

Figure 1.1 (a) Carious lesions on maxillary primary incisors. (b) Maxillary primary incisors post application of silver diamine fluoride.

- The tooth should be clean and free from food or debris. No caries removal is necessary.
- Isolate with Dri-Aids™ (Microbrush International, Grafton, WI, USA) and/or cotton rolls.
- Thoroughly dry the tooth with compressed air or, if air is not tolerated, gauze.
- Place one drop of SDF on a plastic dappen dish or open a unit-dose vial.
- Dip a microbrush into the SDF and then apply to the tooth for 1–3 minutes. Fully saturate the lesion and then allow the SDF to absorb via capillary action. Carefully apply only to the desired tooth surface(s) to minimize risk of accidental staining of unintended surfaces.
- For proximal lesions, place woven floss into the contact, and apply SDF to the lingual, buccal, and occlusal aspect of the contact, saturating the floss, using caution to not allow the floss to contact the patient's lips (Figure 1.2) (Hammersmith *et al.*, 2020).
- Do not light-cure, rinse, or blow compressed air onto the SDF while it is absorbing.
- After it has absorbed via capillary action for at least 1–3 minutes, you may blot the excess SDF with gauze and/or coat the treated site(s) with fluoride varnish. Varnish is optional; however, it helps improve the patient experience by masking the poor taste and preventing SDF from staining other teeth.
- No eating or drinking restrictions.

Topical Fluoride

Fluoride's role in the protection from dental caries is well recognized, and it is considered the first line of defense for caries prevention. More recently, evidence suggests that

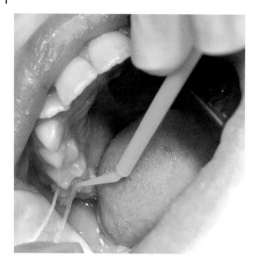

Figure 1.2 Application of silver diamine fluoride to woven floss for interproximal caries.

fluoride can also be used for the treatment of incipient or noncavitated carious lesions. In 2018, the ADA published evidence-based recommendations for nonrestorative treatments for dental caries (Slayton *et al.* 2018). Those recommendations include the use of sealants plus 5% sodium fluoride (NaF) varnish (application every 3–6 months) for noncavitated occlusal caries in both primary and permanent teeth. The research suggests that this application is more effective than sealants or varnish alone (Honkala *et al.* 2015). Application every 3–6 months of 1.23% acidulated phosphate fluoride (APF) gel on noncavitated carious occlusal surfaces of both primary and permanent teeth was also recommended (Agrawal & Pushpanjali, 2011). Additionally, the use of a once-a-week, 0.2% NaF mouth rinse for incipient carious lesions in permanent teeth has been recommended (Florio *et al.*, 2001). For facial or lingual noncavitated lesions on primary and permanent teeth, the ADA recommends 1.23% APF gel (application every 3–6 months) or 5% NaF varnish with application every 3–6 months (Autio-Gold & Courts, 2001) (Figure 1.3).

Casein Phosphopeptide and Amorphous Calcium Phosphate

CPP-ACP is a topical cream for tooth remineralization and desensitization. Recaldent™ (CPP-ACP) is derived from milk protein and releases bioavailable calcium and phosphate, commercially available as MI Paste® and MI Paste Plus (with 900 ppm fluoride; GC Corporation, Tokyo, Japan) (Reynolds *et al.*, 2008). It is contraindicated in individuals with a true casein allergy, but is tolerated by those with lactose sensitivity. There is limited evidence that CPP-ACP can reverse active white spot lesions (Fernández-Ferrer *et al.*, 2018). After brushing and flossing, the paste can be applied 1–2 times a day, directly or in custom trays.

Concentrated fluoride agents, such as 5000 ppm fluoride toothpaste, can help prevent and arrest demineralization. However, the surface hypermineralization by fluoride can block diffusion pathways, preventing the subsequent natural remineralization by salivary calcium and phosphate. Arrested lesions may stay the same size, but can also become unsightly and stained by organic debris. One method of reversing this is to acid-etch the fluoride-treated lesions to facilitate remineralization of the lesion by CPP-ACP (Lopatiene *et al.*, 2016). This is known as the Etch and MI Paste Technique. Total treatment time is 15 minutes, in 4–6 sessions, 10–14 days apart, with MI Paste applied daily at home. The technique can also be effective in certain congenital enamel defects (Figures 1.4–1.6, and 1.7).

Procedure

- Clean teeth with plain pumice.
- Protect soft tissue with cotton isolation.
- Apply 37% phosphoric acid-etch for 2 minutes.
- Rinse.
- Apply/burnish MI Paste for 5 minutes.

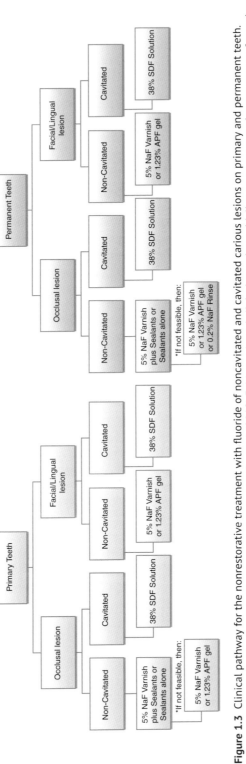

Figure 1.3 Clinical pathway for the nonrestorative treatment with fluoride of noncavitated and cavitated carious lesions on primary and permanent teeth.
Source: Adapted from Slayton, R.L., Urquhart, O., Araujo, M.W.B., *et al.* (2018) Evidence-based clinical practice guideline on nonrestorative treatments for carious lesions: A report from the American Dental Association. *Journal of the American Dental Association*, **149** (10), 845–846.

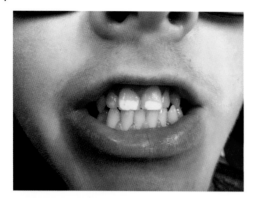

Figure 1.4 Maxillary permanent incisors with congenital enamel defects.

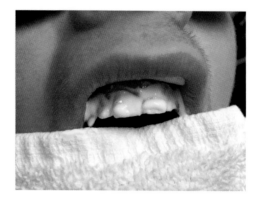

Figure 1.6 CPP-ACP paste applied/burnished to maxillary permanent incisors for 5 minutes.

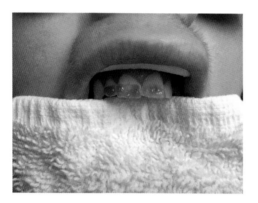

Figure 1.5 Maxillary permanent incisors with 37% phosphoric acid applied for 2 minutes.

- For stubborn lesions, use a rubber cup to apply pumice and MI Paste.
- Rinse.
- Patient applies paste 1–2 times daily at home.

Resin Infiltration

Resin infiltration is a noninvasive method to reduce or arrest the progression of non-cavitated interproximal caries limited to the inner half of enamel or outer third of dentin (Figures 1.8a, b and 1.9a, b). Resin infiltration may be also used to treat white spot lesions; however, this method is not discussed in this chapter. A low-viscosity resin penetrates the

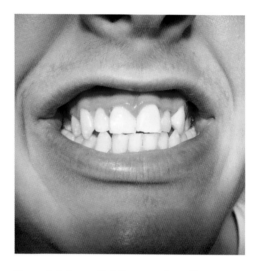

Figure 1.7 6-month follow-up of maxillary permanent incisors post treatment with 5 rounds of etch and MI Paste technique.

porous enamel lesion body, creating a diffusion barrier, blocking pathways for cariogenic acids (AAPD, 2019–2020c; Meyer-Lueckel *et al.*, 2012). Resin infiltration of noncavitated interproximal carious lesions in primary molars requires less patient/parent or legal guardian cooperation than flossing and has been shown to be more efficacious than flossing or use of fluoride toothpaste alone (Ammari *et al.*, 2018). The difference between topical application of fluoride and resin infiltration is that the diffusion barrier is created inside the lesion and not on the surface. This intervention bridges

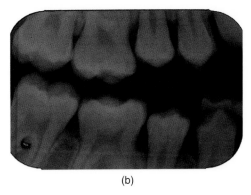
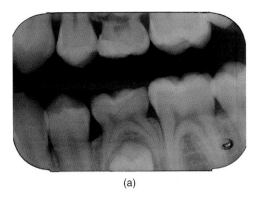

(a)   (b)

Figure 1.8 (a) Bitewing radiograph showing caries limited to outer half of enamel in maxillary left first permanent molar. (b) Bitewing radiograph showing lesion in outer third of dentin in maxillary right first permanent molar.

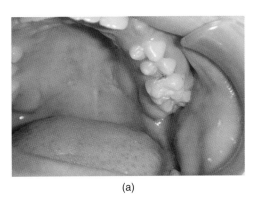
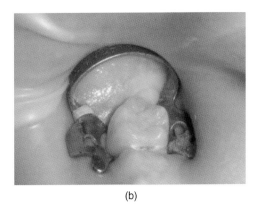

(a)   (b)

Figure 1.9 (a) Clinical photograph of noncavitated carious lesion mesial of maxillary left first permanent molar. (b) Clinical photograph of noncavitated carious lesion mesial of mandibular right first permanent molar.

the gap between nonoperative and operative treatment choices, as well as postpones the first restoration placement (Soxman, 2010). Additionally, this concept supports a conviction that caries can be controlled and arrested prior to cavitation (Kabakchieva *et al.*, 2014). Operator adherence to the protocol is essential. Cost may also be a factor for use, although the procedure maybe covered by some insurance plans.

The ADA clinical practice guideline reported low to very low certainty for efficacy of arresting noncavitated interproximal carious lesions in primary and permanent dentitions with resin infiltration (Slayton *et al.*, 2018). More recent studies reported that the available

evidence provided high confidence that interproximal carious lesion progression may be slowed or arrested with resin infiltration when compared to other noninvasive or preventive modalities (Elrashid *et al.*, 2019; Jorge *et al.*, 2019; Sarti *et al.*, 2020).

Infiltrant resin (triethylene-glycol-dimethacrylate-based resin) is manufactured by DMG (Hamburg, Germany) as the Icon system. Icon is not radiopaque. Filler materials necessary to make the resin radiopaque would negatively affect the infiltrant's flow properties and ability to penetrate the lesion. The kit contains a wedge, 15% hydrochloric acid, 95% ethanol, and the resin infiltrant in applicator syringes.

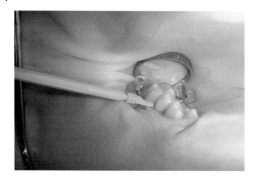

Figure 1.10 Wedge to open interproximal area.

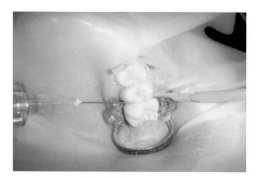

Figure 1.13 Icon-Dry applied.

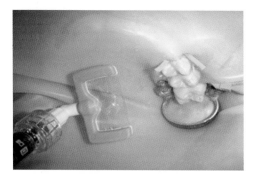

Figure 1.11 Icon applicator.

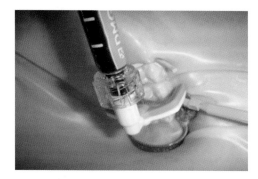

Figure 1.14 Icon infiltrant resin applied.

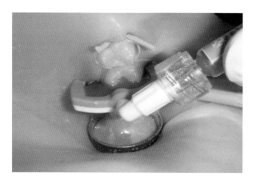

Figure 1.12 Hydrochloric acid gel placed with application aid.

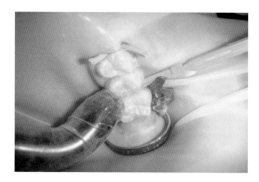

Figure 1.15 Light curing infiltrant.

Total treatment time per lesion is about 15 minutes (Figures 1.10–1.15).

Procedure

- Clean proximal surface with floss.
- Local anesthesia may be administered if deemed necessary, but typically not needed.
- Rubber dam is applied.
- The dental wedge is inserted to open the proximal area (an orthodontic separator may be placed a week prior to the treatment to open the contact).
- 15% hydrochloric acid (HCL) gel to erode the lesion and open the pores is applied for

120 seconds with applicator perforations toward the lesion.

- The surface is rinsed and dried for 30 seconds.
- The pore system is dehydrated with Icon-Dry, 95% ethanol, and air-dried for 30 seconds.
- Chair light may be turned off.
- Lesion body is flooded with Icon infiltrant resin, penetrating the lesion pores, for 180 seconds and dispersed with oil-free air.
- Excess resin is removed with floss and the area is light-cured for 40 seconds.
- Icon infiltrant is applied again for 60 seconds with the same protocol as the initial application.
- The area is light-cured for 40 seconds.
- The wedge is removed and the area is rinsed with water before removing the rubber dam.

Interim Therapeutic Restoration

ITR may be the procedure of choice for restoration in uncooperative children, young children, or children with special needs when definitive restorative treatment cannot be performed. ITR avoids the use of sedation or general anesthesia until a child is old enough to cooperate, or curtails caries progression and/or emergency care while awaiting for the availability of sedation or general anesthesia services (Kateeb *et al.*, 2013; AAPD, 2019–2020b, c).

Indication

Alterative/atraumatic restorative technique (ART) is performed with similar indications and techniques as ITR; however, ART restorations have been traditionally placed where people have limited ability to obtain dental treatment and without a plan for future replacement. ART is endorsed by the World Health Organization and the International Association of Dental Research (AAPD, 2019–2020b, c). ART was first introduced 26 years ago in Tanzania and has developed into

an accepted protocol for caries management to improve quality and access to dental treatment over the world (Frencken *et al.*, 2012). Mahoney *et al.* (2008) state that ART should be used only when the restoration can be periodically evaluated to insure the integrity of the restoration.

ITR is minimally invasive and includes only asymptomatic primary incisors or molars with lesions confined to dentin with sound enamel margins, along with a plan for future follow-up and final restoration (Amini & Casamassimo, 2012). ITR with glass ionomer is preferable to SDF for cavitated lesions. Food particles impacted in a cavitation could decrease the efficacy of SDF. Superficial carious lesions are removed and form and function are more closely achieved compared to SDF. This method of restoration is more successful in children with moderate caries experience compared to those with high caries experience, and is considered to have a good prognosis in young children (da Silva *et al.*, 2020). Two surfaces may be treated, but the use of a matrix and rubber dam increases the complexity of the procedure, and the longevity of a multisurface glass ionomer restoration is reduced compared to a one-surface restoration. Survival rates over the first 2 years of 93% for single-surface and 62% for multiple-surface primary molar restorations are reported (de Amorim *et al.*, 2012). Tedesco *et al.* (2017) recommended cementing an orthodontic or space maintainer band to hold the glass ionomer. They found no statistical difference in success between two surface composite and glass ionomer restorations over 2–3 years (Tedesco *et al.*, 2017). Carious lesions ideal for ITR are mesial caries on maxillary incisors, facial caries, cervical caries, and occlusal caries in the primary dentition (Figures 1.16–1.19).

Stepwise excavation of open carious lesions is another indication for ITR (AAPD, 2019b-2020b, c). Partial removal of carious dentin avoids pulpotomy. Microbial counts of bacteria are reduced under the restoration with or without complete removal of the carious dentin

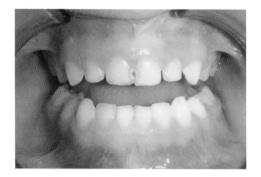

Figure 1.16 Mesial caries maxillary primary central incisors.

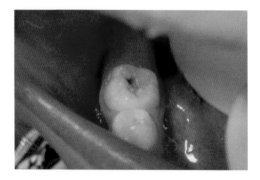

Figure 1.19 Occlusal caries mandibular right second primary molar.

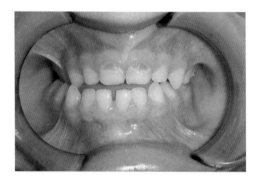

Figure 1.17 Facial caries maxillary primary central incisors.

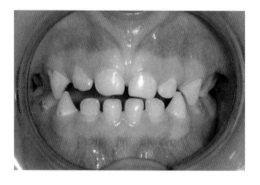

Figure 1.18 Cervical caries primary canines and first primary molars.

(Lula *et al.*, 2009). Varying levels of biodegradation may occur on resin-based restorative materials by esterase activity of *Streptococcus mutans*. A study by Gautam *et al.* (2017) showed restoration with a resin-modified glass ionomer (RMGI) was more resistant to degradation.

Procedure

The procedure can be performed in 5 minutes or less without the use of local anesthesia or a rubber dam. The nonpainful carious dentin is removed with a large round bur in a slow-speed rotary instrument or with a SmartBur® II (SS White Dental, Lakewood, NJ, USA) (Figure 1.20a, b). The single-use SmartBur is used for caries removal to avoid pulp exposure and permit a more comfortable procedure without the use of local anesthesia. This bur cannot cut healthy dentin or enamel, and is an ideal bur for ITR. Using the same size bur as the cavitation will simultaneously remove the peripheral carious dentin during excavation of the infected carious dentin on the base of the preparation. A spoon excavator may also be used, but cautiously, due to the risk of unroofing the pulp chamber with a large mass of carious dentin (Figure 1.21a, b). A Dri-Angle or Dri-Aid is used to cover Stensen's duct and provide cheek retraction for a posterior restoration. When restoring a mandibular primary molar, a second Dri-Angle/Dri-Aid may be placed on the lingual to retract the tongue, while placing the glass ionomer restoration (Figure 1.22). A NeoDry on the buccal and 2 × 2 gauze placed under the Dri-Angle on the lingual improve comfort (Figure 1.23).

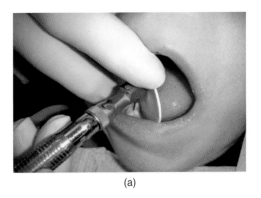

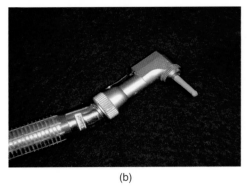

(a)

(b)

Figure 1.20 (a) Slow speed with round carbide bur to remover superficial nonpainful carious dentin. (b) Smart bur to remove superficial nonpainful carious dentin.

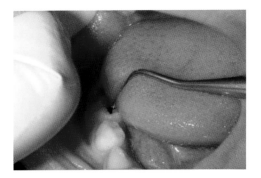

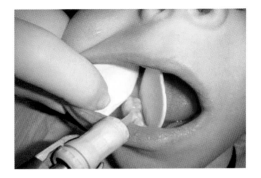

Figure 1.21 Spoon excavator to remove superficial nonpainful carious dentin.

Figure 1.22 Dri-Angles to retract cheek and tongue while placing glass ionomer.

Materials

A high-viscosity glass ionomer or RMGI are the materials of choice for restoration owing to the ease of use and physical properties. Glass ionomer is fluoride releasing, esthetically acceptable, tolerates some moisture contamination, chemically bonds to the tooth, and chemically cures. Recurrent caries are the primary reason for replacement of restorations in primary teeth. Raggio *et al.* (2016) found glass ionomer cements to be significantly associated with a reduction in the incidence of secondary caries. ITR with RMGI instead of the traditional more invasive method and a resin-based restorative material may decrease the need for additional restorative care in children with high caries risk (Gautam *et al.*, 2017). Application with the use of preloaded capsules in a capsule applier or gun significantly reduces working time. After placement in the preparation, finger pressure may be used to compress the material, removing occlusal contacts to increase the longevity of the restoration (Figure 1.24). Finishing is not necessary. Select a glass ionomer with a fast setting time to insure the procedure is completed in the shortest possible chair time. An RMGI will increase working and setting time. Mouth props are available in various sizes for pediatrics and may be used if necessary. A strand of dental floss should be placed to insure easy retrieval should the prop be dislodged, avoiding choking or aspiration (Figure 1.25).

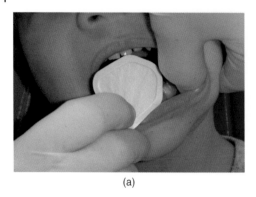 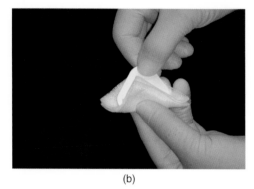

(a) (b)

Figure 1.23 (a) NeoDry. (b) 2 × 2 gauze placed under Dri-Angle.

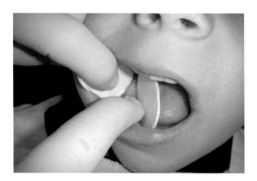

Figure 1.24 Clinician's finger compressing glass ionomer into preparation.

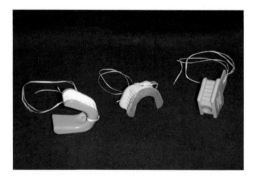

Figure 1.25 Mouth props.

Hall Technique

Stainless-steel crowns (SSCs) are placed on asymptomatic, multisurface carious primary molars without the use of local anesthesia, caries removal, or tooth preparation (Innes *et al.*, 2011). The concept of HT involves caries control by interrupting the activity of the biofilm (AAPD 2019–2020c; Innes *et al.*, 2017). This technique originated, and is well accepted, in the United Kingdom, where general dentists provide the majority of treatment. HT has not been adopted in the United States to the same extent and is typically an alternative when conventional treatment cannot be performed (AAPD, 2019–2020c). A number of evidence-based studies support consideration of HT instead of sedation or general anesthesia to treat early childhood caries whenever feasible, as previously discussed. With the documented instances of recurrent caries, SSCs are less likely to require retreatment (AAPD, 2019–2020d). HT as a nontraditional caries management strategy has been shown to have higher success rates over 2.5 years compared to conventional treatment with complete caries removal and restoration with a compomer (Santamaria *et al.*, 2018).

Contraindications for HT:

- Clinical symptoms of irreversible pulpitis or abscess.
- No clear band of dentin between the lesion and the pulp.
- Radiographic evidence of pulpal involvement, periradicular or furcation involvement.

- Tooth with minimal tooth structure for crown retention.
- Inability to manage the airway.

If a rubber dam is not in place, airway protection must be assured, particularly with an uncooperative child. Inability to assure protection of the airway is a contraindication for HT. Placing an opened 2 × 2 or 4 × 4 in the posterior of the oral cavity, sitting the patient in a more upright position, or attaching the SSC to the gloved finger with medical adhesive or athletic tape assists in guarding against aspiration (MacLean, 2020).

If the interproximal space is closed, an orthodontic separator may be placed a few days before the procedure to open the contact. Orthodontic pliers also may be used to place the separator(s). Alternatively, two strands of floss are threaded through a separator and the separator is stretched in opposite directions and placed into the contact (Chapter 17, Figure 17.8). At the time of the procedure, the separator may be removed with an explorer. Local anesthesia is not necessary, eliminating one of the most common fears, the "shot." Additionally, as noted earlier, a common postoperative adverse event with accidental lip or tongue injury does not occur (Calvo *et al.*, 2019). Food residues are gently removed with a spoon, pumice, or wet applicator. A preformed SSC is crimped if necessary for good marginal adaptation. The distal surface of the preformed SSC must be well adapted to avoid impaction of the tooth distal to the crown during eruption. Size 4 is the most common size for a primary molar, so a size 5 SSC may be selected for HT. Because size will vary, measuring the mesiodistal size of the primary molar with a millimeter ruler or a Boley gauge and matching that to a preformed SSC is an alternative to intraoral attempts to find the correct size SSC (Chapter 8, Figure 8.8). The SSC is filled with glass ionomer cement and seated with finger pressure, followed by the child's own biting force or with or without the use of a bite stick (Seale & Randall, 2015; Schwendicke *et al.*,

2019). Because the occlusal of the primary molar is not reduced, an open bite may occur, but will adjust to a normal occluso-vertical dimension within 15–30 days (van der Zee & van Amerongen, 2010). A more recent study states that alterations in the overbite subside by 6 months after the procedure (Ebrahimi *et al.*, 2020). Postoperative gingival discomfort is minimal, since there is no cutting of gingival tissue with tooth preparation. To obviate concern that lesion progression and bacterial toxins could induce a pulpitis, application of the antimicrobial SDF to inhibit dentin protease, deactivate any remaining nutrients, and remineralize tooth structure may be included in the procedure (Horst *et al.*, 2016).

Primary molars prepared both traditionally and with HT showed success rates of 95% (Velan *et al.*, 2018). Acceptable clinical and radiographic success rates were also reported in other studies (Innes *et al.*, 2011; Ludwig *et al.*, 2014; Clark *et al.*, 2017; Midani *et al.*, 2019; Schwendicke *et al.*, 2019; Ebrahimi *et al.*, 2020). Cost-effectiveness and reduced treatment time for HT versus conventional treatment (CT) were shown with a mean cost per unit to be $7.81 for CT versus $2.45 for HT, along with 33.9 minutes for CT versus 9.1 minutes for HT (Elamin *et al.*, 2019; Schwendicke *et al.*, 2019). Clinical outcomes after 2 years showed much higher success rates with HT than restorations with plastic restorative material (Boyd *et al.*, 2018). Elamin *et al.* (2019) concurred with other studies, but also reported less postoperative anxiety. Similarly, another study reported less treatment time, simplicity of the technique, and a high degree of acceptance by parents and children (Ebrahimi *et al.*, 2020).

Benefits of HT:

- Reduced cost per procedure compared to traditional SSCs.
- Faster procedure.
- No tooth preparation, which is more favorable for pulp.

- No local anesthesia, removing fear of the injection and accidental postoperative injury to the lip/tongue due to anesthesia.
- No cutting of the gingival tissue.
- Avoidance of sedation or general anesthesia, with concomitant reduced costs and risks.
- Less postoperative anxiety for the child.
- Decreased stress for the child, staff, dentist, and parent.
- Ability to be performed by any dentist without advanced training.
- Proven efficacy with randomized control trials.

Silver Modified Alternative Restorative Technique

SDF-arrested lesions can be restored using the principles of minimal intervention dentistry, often without the need for local anesthetic or sedation, known as silver modified atraumatic restorative treatment (SMART). Hydrophilic biomimetic materials, such as glass ionomer cement, RMGI, and glass hybrid restoratives, can restore and further remineralize lesions by releasing fluoride and chemically sealing at the margins (Gotjamanos, 1996; Mei *et al.*, 2016; Korwar *et al.*, 2015). SDF does not adversely affect bond strength to glass ionomer cements or restoratives (Ng *et al.*, 2020; Puwanawiroj *et al.*, 2018). SDF does not restore form or function, it can remineralize, but it does not regenerate missing tooth structure. In order to improve the function, esthetics, and cleansability of the tooth, as well as to prevent further deterioration, fracture, or abscess, it is advantageous to restore SDF-treated cavitated lesions as time, behavior, and finances allow; however, not every SDF-treated tooth requires a restoration.

Clinical considerations for restoration placement following SDF treatment:

- Age, behavior, and medical status of the patient.
- Risk/benefit of the need for advance behavior guidance.

- Openness of the lesion to remineralization by saliva.
- Accessibility of the lesion for adequate biofilm removal.
- Potential for space loss.
- Existing or imminent fracture of remaining tooth structure.
- Dental age, when will the tooth exfoliate.
- Presence of a food trap.
- Parents'/patient's desires.

Procedure

SDF is applied to arrest caries, desensitize the tooth, and stabilize the patient until age, behavior, time, and finances allow placement of a restoration. If SDF is applied the same day as a glass ionomer restorative, even self-curing materials will stain gray over time. Waiting a minimum of 2 weeks after SDF application to place a SMART restoration will allow time for the SDF to increase the surface micro-hardness of the carious lesion, decrease dentin hypersensitivity, and allow the restorative material to stay white, since there will no longer be free silver ions present at the surface of the lesion (Figure 1.26a–f). High-viscosity glass ionomer cements (HVGIC) and glass hybrid restoratives, such as EQUIA Forte® (GC Corporation, Tokyo, Japan), are the ideal materials for SMART due to their high fluoride release, improved physical properties, flexural strength, and resistance to wear (Gurgan *et al.*, 2020; Grossi *et al.*, 2018).

- Clean the tooth with plain pumice, rinse, and dry.
- Local anesthesia and rubber dam isolation are not necessary, because SDF is an effective desensitizer and HVGIC is hydrophilic.
- Prepare the carious surface following the principles of minimal intervention dentistry and the atraumatic approach, whereby soft caries and unsupported enamel are removed via hand excavation with a spoon excavator and/or slow-speed round bur, conserving as much tooth structure as possible, and using caution not to expose the pulp.

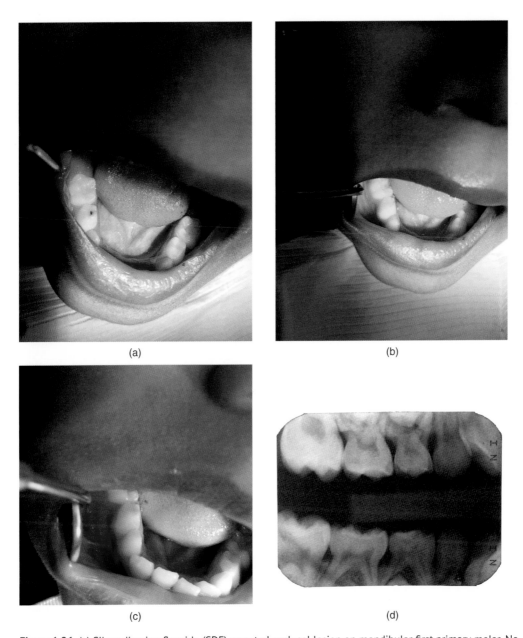

(a) (b)

(c) (d)

Figure 1.26 (a) Silver diamine fluoride (SDF)-arrested occlusal lesion on mandibular first primary molar. No caries were excavated due to the hardness of the lesion. (b) Immediately following placement of an occlusal SMART restoration using EQUIA Forte and Fuji-COAT™ (GC Corporation, Tokyo, Japan). Notice that the opacity of the glass hybrid restorative effectively masks the black scar of the SDF-arrested lesion. (c) Two-year follow-up. Notice the color stability and wear resistance of the SMART restoration and the chemically sealed, sound margins. (d) Two-year follow-up radiograph. Notice the unremoved affected dentin sealed under the SMART restoration. (e) Three-year follow-up. The mandibular first primary molar is mobile and near exfoliation, with the SMART restoration intact. (f) Three-year follow-up radiograph.

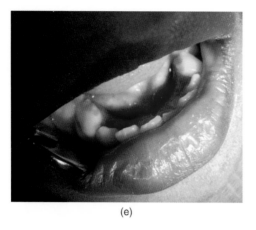

(e)   (f)

Figure 1.26 (*Continued*)

- Apply cavity conditioner (20% polyacrylic acid) for 10 seconds, rinse and dry, but do not desiccate.
- Tap the glass ionomer capsule on its side to loosen the glass particles, push the plunger in to activate the capsule, and then triturate for 10 seconds.
- Immediately apply the HVGIC to the tooth.
- Adapt the glass ionomer restorative to the grooves and/or cavity using a condenser, a microbrush dipped in a self-adhesive resin (coat), or damp Q-tip, and remove excess material.
- Working time is a short 1 minute, 15 seconds; however, this can vary with humidity. Use

caution not to overwork or manipulate the material, as this may disrupt the crosslinking and the material could fail. (Note: In a dry climate, try not to work the material beyond 45 seconds.)
- Wait 2 minutes, 30 seconds for the glass ionomer restorative to set. If a self-adhesive resin is used to coat the material, it must be light-cured for 20 seconds.
- Adjust the occlusion and place anatomy as needed, using finishing burs or polishing stones with copious water spray.
- Instruct the patient to have a soft diet for 48 hours.

References

Agrawal, N. & Pushpanjali, K. (2011) Feasibility of including APF gel application in a school oral health promotion program as a caries-preventive agent: a community intervention trial. *Journal of Oral Science*, 53, 185–191.

Almeida, A.G., Rosemann, M.M., Sheff, M., Huntington, N., & Hughes, C.V. (2000) Future caries susceptibility in children with early childhood caries following treatment under general anesthesia. *Pediatric Dentistry*, 22, 302–306.

American Academy of Pediatric Dentistry. (2019–2020a) Use of anesthesia providers in the administration of office-based deep sedation/general anesthesia to the pediatric dental patient. *The Reference Manual of Pediatric Dentistry*. Chicago, IL: American Academy of Pediatric Dentistry; 327–330.

American Academy of Pediatric Dentistry. (2019–2020b) Policy on interim therapeutic restorations (ITR). *The Reference Manual of Pediatric Dentistry*. Chicago, IL: American Academy of Pediatric Dentistry; 64–65.

American Academy of Pediatric Dentistry. (2019–2020c) Pediatric restorative dentistry. *The Reference Manual of Pediatric Dentistry*. Chicago, IL: American Academy of Pediatric Dentistry; 340–352.

American Academy of Pediatric Dentistry. (2019–2020d) Policy on early childhood caries (ECC): unique challenges and treatment options. *The Reference Manual of Pediatric Dentistry*. Chicago, IL: American Academy of Pediatric Dentistry; 74–75.

American Academy of Pediatric Dentistry. (2019–2020e) Policy on early childhood caries (ECC): classifications, consequences, and preventive strategies. *The Reference Manual of Pediatric Dentistry*. Chicago, IL: American Academy of Pediatric Dentistry; 71–73.

Amin, M.S., Bedard, D., & Gamble, J. (2010) Early childhood caries: recurrence after comprehensive dental treatment under general anesthesia. *European Archives of Paediatric Dentistry*, 11, 269–273.

Amini, H. & Casamassimo, P. (2012) Early childhood caries managed with interim therapeutic restorations. In: Moursi, A.M. (ed.), *Clinical Cases in Pediatric Dentistry*. Oxford: Wiley-Blackwell; 190–197.

Ammari, M.M., Jorge, R.C., Souza, I.P.R., & Soviero, V.M. (2018) Efficacy of resin infiltration of proximal caries in primary molars: 1 year follow-up of a split mouth randomized controlled clinical trial. *Clinical Oral Investigation*, 22, 1355–1362.

Autio-Gold, J.T. & Courts, F. (2001) Assessing the effect of fluoride varnish on early enamel carious lesions in the primary dentition. *Journal of the American Dental Association*, 132, 1247–1253.

Boyd, D.H., Page, L.F., & Thomson, W.M. (2018) The Hall technique and conventional restorative treatment in New Zealand children's primary oral health care – clinical outcomes at two years. *International Journal of Paediatric Dentistry*, 28, 180–188.

Calvo, J.M., Obadan-Udoh, E., Walji, M., & Kalenderian, E. (2019) Adverse events in pediatric dentistry: an exploratory study. *Pediatric Dentistry*, 41, 455–467.

Clark, W., Geneser, M., Owais, A., Kanellis, M., & Qian, F. (2017) Success rates of Hall technique stainless steel crowns in primary molars: a retrospective pilot study. *General Dentistry*, 65, 32–35.

Crystal, Y.O., Janal, M.N., Hamilton, D.S., & Niederman, R. (2017) Parental perceptions and acceptance of silver diamine fluoride staining. *Journal of the American Dental Association*, 148 (7), 510–518.

Crystal, Y.O. & Niederman, R. (2016) Silver diamine fluoride treatment considerations in children's caries management. *Pediatric Dentistry*, 38 (7), 466–471.

da Silva, C.M., Figueiredo, M.C., Casagrande, L., Larissa Lenzi, T. (2020) Survival and associated risk factors of atraumatic restorative treatment restorations in children with early childhood caries. *Journal of Dentistry for Children*, 87, 12–17.

de Amorim, R.G., Leal, S.C., & Frencken, J.E. (2012) Survival of atraumatic restorative treatment (ART) sealants and restorations: a meta-analysis. *Clinical Oral Investigation*, 16, 429–441.

Ebrahimi, M., Shirazi, A.S., & Afshari, E. (2020) Success and behavior during atraumatic restorative treatment, the Hall technique, and the stainless steel crown technique for primary molar teeth. *Pediatric Dentistry*, 42, 187–192.

Elamin, F., Abdelazeem, N., Salah, I., Mirghani, Y., & Wong, F. (2019) A randomized clinical trial comparing Hall vs conventional technique in placing preformed metal crowns from Sudan. *PLoS One*, 14, e0217740.

Elrashid, A.H., Alshaiji, B.S., Saleh, S.A., Zada, K.A., & Baseer, M.A. (2019) Efficacy of resin infiltrate in non-cavitated proximal carious lesions: a systematic review and meta-analysis. *Journal of International Society of Preventive & Community Dentistry*, 9, 211–218.

Fernández-Ferrer, L., Vicente-Ruíz, M., García-Sanz, V., Montiel-Company, J.M.,

Paredes-Gallardo, V., *et al.* (2018) Enamel remineralization therapies for treating postorthodontic white-spot lesions: A systematic review. *Journal of the American Dental Association*, 149 (9), 778–786.e2. doi:10.1016/j.adaj.2018.05.010.

Florio, F.M., Pereira, A.C., Meneghim, Mde. C., & Ramacciato, J.C. (2001) Evaluation of non-invasive treatment applied to occlusal surfaces. *American Society of Dentistry for Children*, 68, 326–331.

Frencken, J.E., Leal, S.C., & Navarro, M.F. (2012) Twenty-five year atraumatic restorative treatment (ART) approach: a comprehensive overview. *Clinical Oral Investigation*, 16, 1337–1346.

Gautam, A.K., Thakur, R., Shashikiram, N.D., Shilpy, S., Agarwal, N., & Tiwari, S. (2017) Degradation of resin restorative materials by Streptococcus mutans: a pilot study. *Journal of Clinical Pediatric Dentistry*, 41, 225–227.

Gotjamanos, T. (1996) Pulp response in primary teeth with deep residual caries treated with silver fluoride and glass ionomer cement ("atraumatic" technique). *Australian Dental Journal*, 41 (5), 328–334. doi:10.1111/j.1834-7819.1996.tb03142.x.

Grossi, J.A., Cabral, R.N., Ribeiro, A.P.D., & Leal, S.C. (2018) Glass hybrid restorations as an alternative for restoring hypomineralized molars in the ART model. *BMC Oral Health*, 18 (1), 65. doi:10.1186/s12903-018-0528-0.

Gurgan, S., Kutuk, Z.B., Cakir, F.Y., & Ergin, E. (2020) A randomized controlled 10 years follow up of a glass ionomer restorative material in class I and class II cavities. *Journal of Dentistry*, 94, 103175. doi:10.1016/j.jdent.2019.07.013.

Hammersmith, K.J., DePalo J.R., Casamassimo, P.S., MacLean, J.K., & Peng, J. (2020) Silver diamine fluoride and fluoride varnish may halt interproximal caries progression in the primary dentition. *Journal of Clinical Pediatric Dentistry*, 44 (2), 79–83. doi:10.17796/1053-4625-44.2.2.

Honkala, S., ElSalhy, M., Shyama, M., Al-Mutawa, S.A., Boodai, H., & Honkala, E.

(2015) Sealant versus fluoride in primary molars of kindergarten children regularly receiving fluoride varnish: one-year randomized clinical trial follow-up. *Caries Research*, 49, 458–466.

Horst, J.A., Ellenikiotis, H., & Milgrom, P.L. (2016) UCSF protocol for caries arrest using silver diamine fluoride: rationale, indications and consent. *Journal of the California Dental Association*, 44 (1), 16–28.

Horst, J., Frachella, J.C., & Duffin, S. (2016) Response to letter to the editor. *Pediatric Dentistry*, 38, 462–463.

Innes, N.P., Evans D.J., Bonifacio, C.C., Geneser, M., Hesse, D., *et al.* (2017) The Hall technique 10 years on: questions and answers. *British Dental Journal*, 222, 478–483.

Innes, N.P., Evans, D.J., & Stirrups, D.R. (2011) Sealing caries in primary molars: randomized control trial, 5-year results. *Journal of Dental Research*, 90, 1405–1410.

Jorge, R.C., Ammari, M.M., Soviero, V.M., & Souza, I.P.R. (2019) Randomized controlled clinical trial of resin infiltration in primary molars: 2 years follow-up. *Journal of Dentistry*, 90, 103184.

Kabakchieva, R.I., Gateva, N.H., & Mihaylova, H.D. (2014) Non-operative treatment of non-cavitated approximal carious lesions of permanent children's teeth. *Journal of IMAB*, 20, 626–630.

Kateeb, E., Warren, J., Damiano, P., Momany, E., Kanellis, M., *et al.* (2013) Atraumatic restorative treatment (ART) in pediatric dentistry residency programs: a survey of program directors. *Pediatric Dentistry*, 35, 500–505.

Korwar, A., Sharma, S., Logani, A., & Shah, N. (2015) Pulp response to high fluoride releasing glass ionomer, silver diamine fluoride, and calcium hydroxide used for indirect pulp treatment: an in-vivo comparative study. *Contemporary Clinical Dentistry*, 6 (3), 288–292. doi:10.4103/0976-237X.161855.

Lee, H., Milgrom, P., Huebner, C.E., Weinstein, P., Burke, W., *et al.* (2017) Ethics rounds: death after pediatric dental anesthesia: an avoidable tragedy? *Pediatrics*, 140 (6), e20172370. doi:10.1542/peds.2017-2370.

Lee, H.H., Milgrom, P., Starks, W., & Burke, W. (2013) Trends in death associated with pediatric dental sedation and general anesthesia. *Pediatric Anesthesiology*, 23, 741–746.

Lin, Y-T. & Lin, Y-T.J. (2016) Factors associated with the risk of caries development after comprehensive dental rehabilitation under general anesthesia. *Journal of Dental Science*, 11, 164–169.

Lopatiene, K., Borisovaite, M., & Lapenaite, E. (2016) Prevention and treatment of white spot lesions during and after treatment with fixed orthodontic appliances: a systematic literature review. *Journal of Oral & Maxillofacial Research*, 7 (2), e1. doi:10.5037/jomr.2016 .7201.

Ludwig, K.H., Fontana, M., Vinson, L.A., Platt, J.A., & Dean, J.A. (2014) The success of stainless steel crowns placed with Hall technique: a retrospective study. *Journal of the American Dental Association*, 145, 1248–1253.

Lula, E.C., Monteiro-Neto, V., Alves, C.M., & Ribeiro, C.C. (2009) Microbiological analysis after complete or partial removal of carious dentin in primary teeth: a randomized clinical trial. *Caries Research*, 43, 354–358.

MacLean, J. (2020) The Hall technique. *Dentaltown*, 21, 82–87.

Mahoney, E., Kilpatrick, N., & Johnston, T. (2008) Restorative paediatric dentistry. In: Cameron, A.C. & Widmer, R.P. (eds.), *Handbook of Pediatric Dentistry*, 3rd edn. London: Mosby; 71–93.

Mei, M.L., Zhao, I.S., Ito, L., Lo, E.C.-M., & Chu, C.-H. (2016) Prevention of secondary caries by silver diamine fluoride. *International Dental Journal*, 66 (2), 71–77. doi:10.1111/idj.12207.

Meyer-Lueckel, H., Bitter, K., & Paris, S. (2012) Randomized controlled clinical trial on proximal caries infiltration: three-year follow-up. *Caries Research*, 46, 544–548.

Midani, R., Splieth, C.H., Mustafa, A.M., Schmoeckel, J., Mourad, S.M., & Santamaria, R.M. (2019) Success rates of preformed metal crowns placed with the modified and standard Hall technique in a paediatric dentistry setting. *International Journal of Paediatric Dentistry*, 29, 550–556.

Ng, E., Saini, S., Schulze, K.A., Horst, J., Le, T., & Habelitz, S. (2020) Shear bond strength of glass ionomer cement to silver diamine fluoride-treated artificial dentinal caries. *Pediatric Dentistry*, 42 (3), 221–225.

Orser, B.A., Suresh, S., & Evers, A.S. (2018) SmartTots update regarding anesthetic neurotoxicity in the developing brain. *Anesthesia Analog*, 126, 1393–1396.

Oubenyahya, H. & Bouhabba, N. (2019) General anesthesia in the management of early childhood caries: an overview. *Journal of Dental Anesthesia and Pain Medicine*, 19, 313–322.

Puwanawiroj, A., Trairatvorakul, C., Dasanayake, A. P., & Auychai, P. (2018) Microtensile bond strength between glass ionomer cement and silver diamine fluoride-treated carious primary dentin. *Pediatric Dentistry*, 40 (4), 291–295.

Raggio, D.P., Tedesco, T.K., Calvo, A.F., & Braga, M.M. (2016) Do glass ionomer cements prevent caries lesions in margins of restorations in primary teeth? A systemic review and meta-analysis. *Journal of the American Dental Association*, 147, 177–185.

Reynolds, E.C., Cai, F., Cochrane, N.J., Shen, P., Walker, G.D., *et al.*, (2008) Fluoride and casein phosphopeptide-amorphous calcium phosphate, *Journal of Dental Research*, 87 (4), 344–348. doi:10.1177/154405910808700420.

Santamaria, R.M., Innes, N.P.T., Machiulskiene, V., Schmoeckel, J., Alkilzy, M., & Splieth, C.H. (2018) Alternative caries management options for primary molars: 2.5-year-outcomes of a randomized clinical trial. *Caries Research*, 51, 605–614.

Sarti, C.S., Vizzotto, M.B., Filgueiras, L.V., Bonifácio, C.C., & Rodrigues, J.A. (2020) Two-year split mouth randomized controlled clinical trial on the progression of proximal carious lesions on primary molars after resin infiltration. *Journal of Pediatric Dentistry*, 42, 110–115.

Schwendicke, F., Krois, J., Robertson, M., Splieth, C., Santamaria, R., & Innes, N. (2019) Cost effectiveness of the Hall technique in a randomized trial. *Journal of Dental Research*, 98, 61–67.

Seale, N.S. & Randall. R. (2015) The use of stainless steel crowns: a systematic literature review. *Pediatric Dentistry*, 37, 147–162.

Slayton, R.L., Urquhart, O., Araujo, M.W.B., Fontana, M., Guzmán-Armstrong, S., *et al.* (2018) Evidence-based clinical practice guideline on nonrestorative treatments for carious lesions. *Journal of the American Dental Association*, 149, 837–849.

Soxman, J.A. (2010) Improving caries diagnosis and early intervention in the primary and young permanent dentition. *General Dentistry*, 58, 188–193.

Stratmann, G., Lee, J., Sall, J.W., Lee, B.H., Rehan S Alvi, R.S., *et al.* (2014) Effect of general anesthesia in infancy on long-term recognition memory in humans and rats. *Neuropsychopharmacology*, 28, 2275–2287.

Tedesco, T.K., Calvo, A.F., Lenzi, T.L., Hesse, D., Guglielmi, C.A.B., *et al.* (2017) ART is an alternative for restoring occlusoproximal cavities in primary teeth—evidence from an updated systematic review and meta-analysis. *International Journal of Paediatric Dentistry*, 27, 201–209.

van der Zee, V. & van Amerongen, W.E. (2010) Influence of pre-formed metal crowns (Hall technique) on the occlusal vertical dimension in the primary dentition. *European Archives of Paediatric Dentistry*, 11, 225–227.

Vasquez, E., Zegarra, G. Chirinos, E., Castillo, J.L., Taves, D.R., *et al.* (2012) Short term serum pharmacokinetics of diammine silver fluoride after oral application. *BMC Oral Health*, 12, 60.

Velan, E., Mitchell, S., & O'Connell, A.C. (2018) Restorative dentistry and dental materials. In: Nowak, A.J. & Casamassimo, P.S. (eds.), *The Handbook of Pediatric Dentistry*, 5th edn. Chicago, IL: American Academy of Pediatric Dentistry; 157–176.

2

Sealants

Jane A. Soxman and Patrice B. Wunsch

According to the 2019–2020 American Association of Pediatric Dentistry (AAPD) Evidence-based Clinical Practice Guideline for Use of Pit-and-Fissure Sealants, even with documented evidence of success and clinical guidelines for use, dental sealants are underutilized (Wright *et al.*, 2016). The teeth at highest risk by far are the permanent first and second molars, where fluoride has its least preventive effect on the pits and fissures. The incidence of caries in permanent teeth increases with age, such that children 9–10 years of age have a higher carious lesion incidence than children 6–8 years of age, and children 16–19 years of age have a higher carious lesion incidence than children 12–15 years of age (Wright *et al.*, 2016). The eruption time for first and second permanent molars is 1.5 years, but premolars take only 1–2 months (Antonson *et al.*, 2012). With consideration of all of these factors, sealants provide the best method to prevent occlusal caries in young permanent molars. Sealants on the occlusal surfaces of primary molars are retained at a rate of 74.0–96.3% at 1 year and 70.6–76.5% at 2.8 years (Beauchamp *et al.*, 2008).

In 2016, the AAPD Council on Scientific Affairs addressed a number of questions regarding the use of pit-and-fissure sealants. After conducting systematic searches of the literature, they were able to provide recommendations with measures of the quality of evidence and strength of recommendation.

For the question on whether sealants should be used as compared to not being used for primary and permanent molars with clinically sound and noncavitated occlusal surfaces, the panel did recommend their use, with the quality of evidence moderate, and the strength of recommendation strong (Wright *et al.*, 2016).

Permanent molars are highly porous at eruption and susceptible to caries. Complete maturation of the enamel does not occur until 62 months after eruption. Placing a sealant as soon as the tooth can be adequately isolated is highly efficacious in reducing the incidence of pit-and-fissure caries (Kataoka *et al.*, 2007). The risk for caries is the highest during the first few years after eruption.

When restoring the primary dentition, consideration may be given to sealing the occlusal surfaces of the primary molars in high caries-risk children. This may be a goodwill gesture, as insurance may not cover this procedure, but sealant use in the primary molars is beneficial since it protects the occlusal surfaces from future colonization of mutans streptococci.

Caries Detection

Forceful probing of occlusal surfaces with an explorer pierces immature, porous enamel, creating enamel defects and possibly converting incipient caries to frank cavitation

(Kuhnisch *et al.*, 2007). An explorer may be gently run through the fissures to check for any changes or breaks in the enamel surface, followed by forcefully rinsing with water to remove plaque and debris. Sealant integrity and retention can also be evaluated with the explorer (Fontana *et al.*, 2010). Strassler *et al.* (2005) found laser fluorescence to be 90% accurate for caries detection. Laser fluorescence caries detection devices use a laser light to scan below the enamel surface, detecting demineralized tooth structure. Prophylaxis pastes with blue or green dye cause an inaccurate reading in the caries detection device. Staff can be taught to use the device, saving time for the dentist.

Moisture Control

Inadequate moisture control is the primary reason for sealant loss. Resin-based sealants are hydrophobic and require isolation that assures no salivary contamination. Isolation may be accomplished with a number of methods. The rubber dam provides ideal isolation, but may not be tolerated by some children without the use of local anesthesia. Alternatives such as cotton rolls ligated with dental floss or Dri-Aids/Dri-Angles may control salivary contamination, but retracting the tongue in the mandible may elicit a gag reflex. Use of a NeoDry to absorb parotid saliva on the buccal mucosa instead of the cardboard Dri-Aid/Dry-Angle provides a softer means for salivary control (Figure 2.1a). Placing a 2 × 2 gauze under the Dri-Aid/Dri-Angle on the floor of the mouth provides relief from the cardboard and a significant improvement in the child's acceptance (Figure 2.1b, c). Use of a mouth prop is helpful for the child who cannot maintain an open mouth. The Parkell dry-field mouth prop (Edgewood, NY, USA) is inexpensive and can be sterilized (Figure 2.2).

The Isolite 3 (Zyris, Goleta, CA, USA) provides illumination for improved field of vision (Figure 2.3a). Zyris Isodry and DryShield (DryShield, Fountain Valley, CA, USA) are nonlatex, integrate continuous high-volume suction, a flexible bite block, airway protection, and cheek and tongue retraction (Figure 2.3b). Upper and lower quadrants are simultaneously isolated, saving time. Isolite 3, Isodry, and DryShield require a manufacturer's attachment to high-volume suction. Another method for isolation is Mr. Thirsty® One-Step (Zirc Dental Products, Buffalo, MN, USA) with similar features (Figure 2.3c), but it is not as flexible and can be directly attached to high-volume suction. Mouthpieces for the Isolite 3, Isodry, and Mr. Thirsty One-Step are single use, whereas the DryShield is autoclavable.

The Blue Boa® (Blue Boa, Mediran, ID, USA) is flexible, light-weight, directly attaches to high-volume suction and can be sterilized (Figure 2.4a). The hydroformic saliva ejector attached to the Blue Boa assists in tongue retraction (Figure 2.4b). With difficulty in moisture control, the Adper Prompt L-Pop™ (3M-ESPE, St. Paul, MN, USA), a self-etch adhesive, provides improved bonding. Fluoride varnish may also offer a moisture-tolerant alternative for a patient with a strong gag reflex or inability to cooperate. Fluoride varnish was equally effective in caries reduction on occlusal surfaces of first permanent molars of high-risk children when applied over 30 months (Chestnutt *et al.*, 2017). Glass ionomer cements offer an effective alternative with difficulty in maintaining ideal isolation, but are not as retentive as a resin-based sealant (Alirezaei *et al.*, 2018).

Etching/primer

The occlusal surface should have a chalky-white, opaque appearance after adequate etching and thoroughly air-drying. Salivary contamination will eradicate the etched enamel (Figure 2.5). An ethyl alcohol primer may be applied to insure dry enamel before placing the sealant. Self-etch systems are not

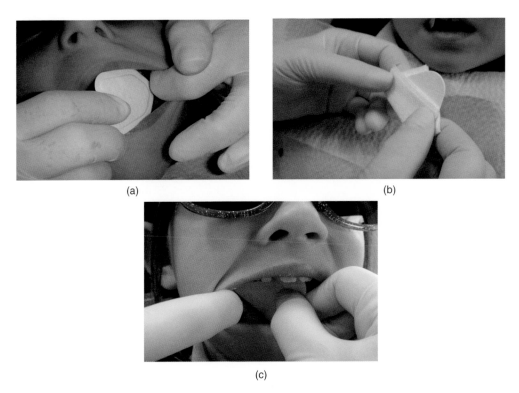

(a)

(b)

(c)

Figure 2.1 **(a)** NeoDrys placed on buccal. **(b)** Placing 2 × 2 gauze under Dri-Angle for comfort on lingual. (c) Dri-Angle with 2 × 2 gauze on lingual to retract tongue.

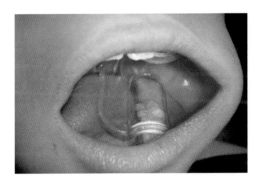

Figure 2.2 Parkell dry-field mouth prop.

as retentive as traditional acid etching (Botton *et al.*, 2016).

Bonding Agent

The use of a dentin bonding agent has been suggested if there is difficulty maintaining a dry field. If the enamel is contaminated with saliva, the intermediate bonding agent layer and the resin sealant may be light-cured individually or simultaneously. If the tooth is dry, the bonding agent layer should be light-cured separately from the resin sealant (Torres *et al.*, 2005).

For added retention, some dentists advocate the use of a bonding agent between the sealant and the etched enamel. Etchant is placed, rinsed, and dried. A thin layer of bonding agent is then applied and lightly air-dried, followed by a light layer of sealant. The two are cured together so that the bonding agent and sealant are one.

Etch and bonding agent may contribute to antimicrobial activity below the sealant, and their application may aid in preventing the survival of any viable bacteria left deep in the grooves (Paddick *et al.*, 2005).

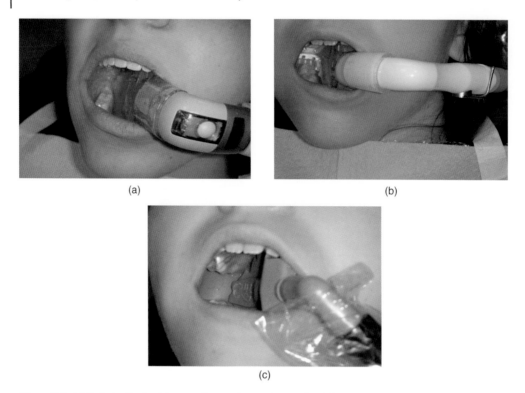

(a)

(b)

(c)

Figure 2.3 (a) Zyris Isolite 3 with manufacturer's attachment for light and suction. (b) DryShield. (c) Mr. Thirsty One-Step.

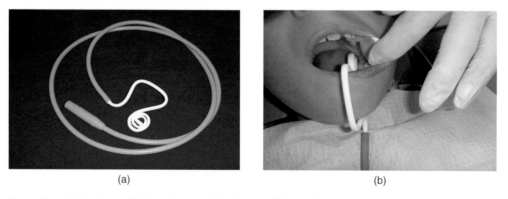

(a)

(b)

Figure 2.4 (a) Blue Boa with hydroformic saliva ejector. (b) Hydroformic saliva ejector attached to Blue Boa for tongue retraction and salivary control during sealant procedure.

A number of bonding agents work well in providing additional retentiveness for the sealant. Some are based on ease of use and provider preference.

- OptiBond™ Solo Plus (Kerr Corp., Brea, CA, USA) comes in either a bottle or unit dose.

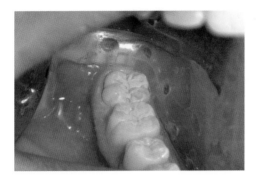

Figure 2.5 Chalky-white appearance of thoroughly dried enamel.

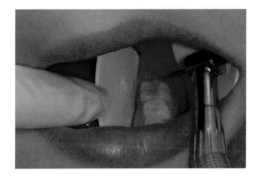

Figure 2.6 Enameloplasty with small round diamond bur.

- ExciTE® F (Ivoclar Vivodent, Schaan, Liechtenstein) comes in an easy-to-use click-and-bond dispenser tip.

Partially Erupted Teeth

Sealant placement in partially erupted teeth is difficult due to isolation challenges; therefore, it is recommended to use a material that is hydrophilic, such as a glass ionomer type of sealant or glass ionomer cement. Something as easy as the placement of a glass ionomer liner cement, such as Vitrebond™ (3M-ESPE), in the grooves of an erupting permanent molar can help to prevent bacterial invasion in the depths of the grooves. The tooth is then monitored until it is fully erupted, at which time the glass ionomer cement is removed and replaced with either a resin-based sealant or glass ionomer–based sealant. A low-viscosity, flowable, high fluoride-releasing glass ionomer sealant (GC Fugi TRIAGE® White, GC America, Alsip, IL, USA) provides another option for partially erupted molars in a high caries-risk patient (Antonson *et al.*, 2012).

Surface Preparation

Enameloplasty with a size 2 round diamond bur, 330 bur, or fissurotomy bur to open fissures before placing a sealant is sometimes recommended to identify or remove incipient caries and increase the bonding surface (Bagherian & Shirazi, 2016) (Figure 2.6). Feigal and Donly (2006) found that marginal leakage was less in prepared fissures, but minimal application of sealant material rather than overfilling the fissure is probably more beneficial than enameloplasty. Sealant loss may predispose a tooth to caries, particularly if enameloplasty was performed before sealant placement (Dhar & Chen, 2012). Handpiece pumice prophylaxis does not increase sealant bond strength or retention. Retention was as high with a toothbrush prophylaxis as with a handpiece (Farsai *et al.*, 2010). In-office topical fluoride treatment does not interfere with the etching pattern and sealant retention (Feigal & Donly, 2006). This study was performed before the use of fluoride varnish for in-office topical fluoride treatment. Pretreatment with silver diamine fluoride in the fissures of noncarious permanent molars improved retention properties. Acid-etch was not used in this protocol (Perez-Hernandez *et al.*, 2018).

Light-curing

Insufficient curing affects sealant retention. Clear sealant cures deeper than opaque (Yu *et al.*, 2009). Cusp tips place more distance

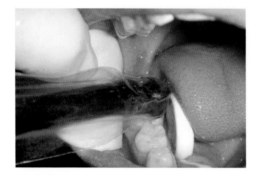

Figure 2.7 Curing light on cusp tips of molar.

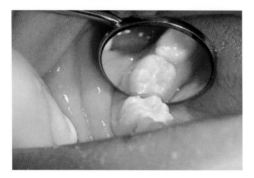

Figure 2.8 Sealant limited to fissures.

between the polymerization light and the sealant. The curing depth should be 1.5 mm due to tags within the fissures. The curing light should touch the cusp tips to assure a deep enough cure (Figure 2.7).

The curing light is routinely checked for light intensity with a curing radiometer. The tip of the light should be checked for material buildup and should fit the radiometer (Maghaireh *et al.*, 2013). Each material will include information on the recommended wavelength range for activation.

Retention and Follow-up

Parents/guardians are informed of the various factors that influence sealant retention. Even under proper application conditions, 5–10% of sealants can be expected to fail annually (Yazici *et al.*, 2006). Sealant retention may be compromised due to behavior, poor oral hygiene, hypoplastic or hypocalcified enamel, severe bruxing, chewing hard candy, and caries susceptibility. Limiting sealant application to the fissures, avoiding the cuspal planes, will enhance retention (Figure 2.8). Compromised marginal integrity can result in caries developing beneath the sealant. Evaluation should include not only carefully checking margins, but also viewing from various angles with a good light source to detect the presence of a shadow, which is typically evidence of caries below the sealant. Sealants require maintenance. The importance of preventive care follow-up visits to monitor marginal leakage, caries beneath the sealant, or sealant loss must be stressed.

References

Alirezaei, M., Bagherian, A., & Shirazi, A.S. (2018) Glass ionomer cements as fissure sealing materials: yes or no? *Journal of the American Dental Association*, 149, 640–649.

Antonson, S.A., Antonson, D.E., Brener, S., Crutchfield, C., Larumbe, J., *et al.* (2012) Twenty-four month clinical evaluation of fissure sealants on partially erupted permanent first molars. *Journal of the American Dental Association*, 143, 115–122.

Bagherian, A. & Shirazi, A. (2016) Preparation before acid etching in fissure sealant therapy: yes or no? *Journal of the American Dental Association*, 147, 943–951.

Beauchamp, J., Caufield, P.W., Crall, J., Donly, K., Feigal, R., *et al.* (2008) Evidence-based clinical recommendations for the use of pit-and-fissure sealants. *Journal of the American Dental Association*, 139, 257–267.

Botton, G., Morgental, C.S., Scherer, M.M., Larissa Lenzi, T, Fernandes Montagner, A., & de Oliveira Rocha, R. (2016) Are self-etch adhesive systems effective in the retention of occlusal sealants? A systematic review and meta-analysis. *International Journal of Paediatric Dentistry*, 26, 402–411.

Chestnutt, I.G., Playle R., Hutchings S., Morgan-Trimmer, S., Fitzsimmons, D., *et al.* (2017) Fissure seal or fluoride varnish? A randomized trial of relative effectiveness. *Journal of Dental Research*, 96, 754–761.

Dhar, V. & Chen, H. (2012) Evaluation of resin-based and glass ionomer based sealants placed with or without tooth preparation—a two year clinical trial. *Pediatric Dentistry*, 34, 46–50.

Farsai, P.S., Uribe, S., & Vig, K.W.L. (2010) How to clean the tooth surface before sealant application. *Journal of the American Dental Association*, 141, 696–698.

Feigal, R.J. & Donly, K.J. (2006) The use of pit and fissure sealants. *Pediatric Dentistry*, 28, 143–150.

Fontana, M., Zero, D.T., Beltran-Aguilar, E.D., & Gray, S.K. (2010) Techniques for assessing tooth surfaces in school-based sealant programs. *Journal of the American Dental Association*, 141, 854–860.

Kataoka, S., Sakuma, S., Wang, J., Yoshihara, A., & Miyazaki, H. (2007) Changes in electrical resistance of sound fissure enamel in first permanent molars for 66 months from eruption. *Caries Research*, 41, 161–164.

Kuhnisch, J., Dietz, W., Stosser, L., Hickel, R., & Heinrich-Weltzien, R. (2007) Effects of dental probing on occlusal surfaces: a scanning electron microscopy evaluation. *Caries Research*, 41, 43–48.

Maghaireh, G.A., Alzraikat, H., & Taha, N.A. (2013) Assessing the irradiance delivered from light-curing units in private dental offices in Jordan. *Journal of the American Dental Association*, 144, 922–927.

Paddick, J.S., Brailsford, S.R., & Kidd, E.A.M. (2005) Phenotypic & genotype selection of microbiota surviving under dental restorations. *Applied and Environmental Microbiology*, 71, 2467–2472.

Perez-Hernandez, J., Aguilar-Diaz, F.C., Venegas-Lancon R.D., Gayosso, C.A.A., Villanueva-Vilchis, M.C., & de la Fuente-Hernández, J. (2018) Effect of silver diamine fluoride on adhesion and microleakage of a pit and fissure sealant to tooth enamel: in vitro trial. *European Archives of Paediatric Dentistry,* 19, 411–416.

Strassler, H.E., Grebosky, M., Porter, J., & Arroyo, J. (2005) Success with pit and fissure sealants. *Dentistry Today*, 24, 124–133.

Torres, C.P., Balbo, P., Gomes-Silva, J.M., Pereira Ramos, R., Palma-Dibb, R.G., & Borsatto, M.C. (2005) Effect of individual or simultaneous curing on sealant bond strength. *Journal of Dentistry for Children*, 72, 31–35.

Wright, J.T., Crall, J.J., Fontana, M., Gillette, E.J., Nový, B.B., *et al.* (2016) Evidence-based clinical practice guideline for the use of pit-and-fissure sealants, American Academy of Pediatric Dentistry, *American Dental Association. Pediatric Dentistry*, 38 (5), E120–E36.

Yazici, A.R., Kiremitci, A., Celik, C., Ozgünaltay, G., & Dayangaç, B. (2006) A two-year clinical evaluation of pit and fissure sealants placed with and without air abrasion pretreatment in teenagers. *Journal of the American Dental Association*, 137, 1401–1405.

Yu, C., Tantbirojn, D., Grothe, R.L., Versluis, A., Hodges, J.S., & Feigal, R.J. (2009) The depth of cure of clear versus opaque sealants as influenced by curing regime. *Journal of the American Dental Association*, 140, 331–338.

3

Local Anesthesia for the Pediatric Patient

Janice A. Townsend, Jane A. Soxman, and Stanley F. Malamed

Fear of the injection is the primary reason children give for being afraid of going to the dentist (AlShareed, 2011). With appropriate preparation, the use of topical anesthetic, distraction, and good injection technique, most children are unaware of receiving the injection.

Communication

Parents/guardians should be told not to discuss the injection before an appointment for restoration or extraction with the child. The injection is described by the dental team with age-appropriate terms, such as calling the local anesthetic "sleepy juice." The child is told that his/her tooth will go to sleep for a little while but will "awaken" later, just as the child awakens each morning. The rubber dam is referred to as a blanket to cover the sleeping tooth. After the rubber dam is removed, the child is told that the tooth, lip, and/or tongue will soon awaken. A time frame described in hours for a return to normal sensation, when the tooth will feel exactly the same as before taking the nap, is meaningless to a child. A concrete time, such as lunchtime or dinnertime, may be a better word choice for the child to understand.

Infiltration in the mandible results in lip anesthesia, which can be distressing and compounds the anesthetic sensation. If possible, begin with buccal infiltration in the maxilla for a primary molar to desensitize the child. This approach will help him/her to become accustomed to the sensation created by the local anesthesia before introducing more profound mandibular anesthesia, including the lower lip and/or tongue. Parents/guardians are informed before administering the local anesthetic that the feeling of being numb after the procedure is completed is often more distressing for the child than the injection or procedure itself. This exaggerated response is usually seen immediately after the rubber dam is removed (Figure 3.1). The young child complains that "it hurts." Informing the parents prior to the appointment of this normal behavior can help alleviate anxiety.

Agents

Topical Anesthetic

Needle penetration is related to the discomfort of intraoral injections (Meechan *et al.*, 2005). Topical anesthetic reduces needle insertion and injection pain during infiltration, as well as reducing the increasing anxiety during the injection (Cho *et al.*, 2017). Lidocaine-based (amide) topical anesthetics are rapidly absorbed into the systemic circulation and can contribute to drug overdose. Topical anesthetics should be applied sparingly to tissue dried with gauze and limited to the area of needle penetration (Figure 3.2a). Benzocaine-based ester topical, with concentration up to 20%, is poorly absorbed into the circulatory system with minimal chance of overdose, but also is for use only in small amounts (Kohli *et al.*, 2000). Topical anesthetic should remain in place for at least 2 minutes, is more effective on mucosa than attached gingiva, and should provide temporary loss of soft tissue sensation 2–3 mm in depth (Priyatham & Nuvvula, 2016). A small piece of gauze ligated with floss is placed over the topical to avoid spreading or swallowing of the anesthetic; the gauze should always be visible to provide easy removal if necessary (Figure 3.2b). Note that benzocaine can induce methemoglobinemia, but most reported cases are the result of application of large amounts of over-the-counter products for toothache or teething. However, even small quantities of 20% topical benzocaine on disrupted gingival tissues can result in extensive absorption, and caution should be used with children under 2 years of age (Wilburn-Goo & Lloyd, 1999).

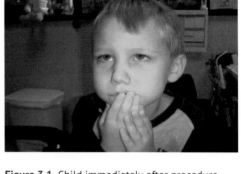

Figure 3.1 Child immediately after procedure distressed by the numb sensation.

Injectable Local Anesthetics

The dosage for all local anesthetics should be calculated based on the child's weight and should never exceed the listed maximum dosage. The amount of local anesthetic in a cartridge is dependent on the concentration of the anesthetic and the size of the cartridge. The volume of the typical local anesthetic cartridge in the United States is 1.76 mL and using 1.8 mL for calculations will give a conservative dosage. The concentration of solution can by calculated by adding 10 mg for every cc of solution multiplied by the percentage. For example, 4% solutions will have 40 mg/mL of drug and 2% solutions will have 20 mg/mL of drug.

Local anesthetic overdoses were found in 41% of malpractice insurance claims involving anesthesia for pediatric dental patients. Of those claims, 43% occurred when local anesthetic was the only drug administered (Chicka *et al.*, 2012). A study by Townsend *et al.* (2020) used the National Poison Data System to identify cases of local anesthetic adverse events in pediatric patients. The most common clinical effects reported were seizure, tachycardia, and drowsiness/lethargy. Management therapies included observation

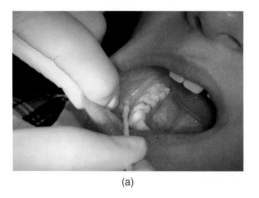

(a)

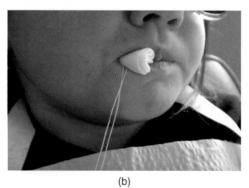

(b)

Figure 3.2 (a) Placing topical anesthetic for buccal infiltration. (b) 2 × 2 gauze ligated with floss after placement of topical anesthetic.

and administration of oxygen. Seizure after injection was attributed to high blood levels in the brain, caused by an excessive amount of local anesthesia and/or intravenous injection Townsend *et al.*, 2020). Adverse events have been reported with dosages below the maximum recommended dosage. With an average dose of a given drug, Malamed (2020) identified 15% of patients as hyper-responders. Within this group, another 15% were deemed to be extreme hyper-responders (Malamed, 2020).

The cortical plate of bone is thin, and the bone is more vascular, with rapid uptake of local anesthesia in the pediatric patient. The use of a vasoconstrictor, epinephrine, reduces the risk of rapid systemic absorption and overdose. A vasopressor-containing local anesthetic is recommended for use when more than one quadrant is being restored in the same visit (American Academy of Pediatric Dentistry, 2020). Calculations can be simplified by the "rule of 25," which states that for healthy patients a dentist may safely use 1 cartridge of any marketed local anesthetic for every 25 lb of patient weight (Moore & Hersh, 2010).

Lidocaine is the amide with the longest use in dentistry and is most commonly used in North America (Moore & Hersh, 2010). The maximum dosage of 2% lidocaine with 1 : 100,000 epinephrine is 4.4 mg/kg or 2.0 mg/lb (Webb *et al.*, 2012; American Academy of Pediatric Dentistry, 2020).

Articaine has a long history of use in Europe and Canada and is gaining popularity in the United States. The low pH of the epinephrine in both articaine and lidocaine may cause a burning sensation. The maximum recommended dosage of 4% articaine with 1 : 100,000 epinephrine is 7.0 mg/kg or 3.2 mg/lb (Webb *et al.*, 2012; Widmer *et al.*, 2008; American Academy of Pediatric Dentistry, 2020). There is 40 mg/mL of drug in 4% solutions, and 2% solutions contain 20 mg/mL. Articaine has been shown to be safe and effective in children as young as 2 years of age (Adewumi *et al.*, 2008), but is not approved by the US Food and Drug Administration (FDA) for children younger than 4 years. Articaine with 1 : 200,000 epinephrine has been associated with significantly longer duration of soft tissue numbness compared to 2% lidocaine with 1 : 100,000 epinephrine (Ram & Amir, 2006). The use of 1 : 200,000 epinephrine instead of the 1 : 100,000 concentration with the 4% articaine should not change the efficacy and may be preferable for the pediatric patient. A study by Meechan (2011) did not find effectiveness of buccal infiltration in the mandibular first molar region to be influenced by the epinephrine concentration. Articaine 4% has been reported to be more effective in obtaining profound anesthesia in infected sites, and may be the local anesthetic of choice for extraction of an abscessed tooth (Kurtzman, 2014). Taneja *et al.* (2020) reported the effectiveness of articaine to be better than lidocaine, along with leading to less postprocedural pain in pediatric patients.

Prilocaine is not a potent vasodilator and can provide anesthesia without a vasoconstrictor. A significant concern associated with the use of prilocaine is its ability to induce methemoglobin, which interferes with oxygen transportation (American Academy of Pediatric Dentistry, 2020; Trapp & Will, 2010). Prilocaine should be avoided in children with oxygen transport diseases such as sickle cell disorder, anemia, respiratory disease, cardiovascular disease, or abnormal hemoglobin. Gutenberg *et al.* (2013) found that administration of 4% prilocaine without a vasoconstrictor with a dose of 5 mg/kg resulted in significantly elevated levels of methemoglobin. Because peak methemoglobin blood levels are reached 1 hour after injection, children should be observed for at least 1 hour after a procedure using 4% prilocaine as the local anesthetic. Gutenberg *et al.* (2013) did not find increased methemoglobin levels using 2% lidocaine with 1 : 100,000 epinephrine.

Mepivacaine 3%, pH 4.5–6.8, does not contain epinephrine and may reduce injection discomfort (Friedman, 2000). Mepivacaine has more rapid systemic uptake with or without a vasoconstrictor than lidocaine, even when lidocaine with no vasoconstrictor is used. The maximum dosage of 3% plain mepivacaine, 4.4 mg/kg or 2.0 mg/lb, should be carefully calculated (American Academy of Pediatric Dentistry, 2020). Despite the lack of vasoconstrictor, the soft tissue durations of mepivacaine with no vasoconstrictor and lidocaine with epinephrine are nearly identical (Moore & Hersh, 2010).

Bupivacaine is not recommended for a young child or for some patients with special health-care needs with mental or physical disabilities, because of prolonged anesthesia with risks of self-inflicted soft tissue injury.

Most procedures for primary molars are performed with infiltration of one-third to two-thirds of a cartridge of 2% lidocaine with 1 : 100,000 epinephrine. Vital pulp therapy and extractions in the mandible may require inferior alveolar nerve (IAN) block, along with buccal infiltration using two-thirds to a full cartridge of 2% lidocaine with 1 : 100,000 epinephrine or 4% articaine with 1 : 200,000 epinephrine.

All local anesthetic solutions are acidic in nature. The pH of a "plain" drug is approximately 6.5, while that of a local anesthetic containing a vasoconstrictor (e.g., epinephrine, levonordefrin) is in the range of 3.3–4.5. Administration of such a highly acidic solution is associated with an uncomfortable burning sensation, as well as increased postinjection soreness.

The low pH between 2.9 and 4.4 may contribute to pain during injection and delay onset of anesthesia. The ability to quickly and easily change the pH (buffer) the local anesthetic solution to a higher, more physiologic pH of about 7.35 is associated with several clinical advantages: (i) a more comfortable injection experience for the patient, (ii) a significantly more rapid onset of pulpal anesthesia, (iii) more profound anesthesia, and (iv) less postinjection soreness (Malamed *et al.*, 2013). Kattan *et al.* (2019) agree that

buffered local anesthetics are more effective than nonbuffered, with 2.29 times more successful achievement of pulpal anesthesia. A buffered local anesthetic solution can be prepared in the office by purchasing a multidose vial of sodium bicarbonate. Two buffering systems are also available on the market: Anutra Local Anesthetic Delivery System (Anutra Medical, Morrisville, NC, USA); and Onset® (OnPharma, Los Gatos, CA, USA). To the contrary, another study concluded that routine alkalinization or buffering decreased onset time by only 1.5 minutes and did not decrease pain with injection. These findings were considered to be significant considering the time and expense of buffering local anesthesia (Aulestia-Viera *et al.*, 2018).

Warming local anesthetic solution from room temperature to body temperature before injection has not been shown to decrease discomfort (Ram *et al.*, 2002).

Armamentarium and Techniques

Needles for dental injection are manufactured as follows: long (32 mm), short (22 mm), and extra-short (10 mm), with gauges that range from 23 to 30. There is no significant difference in pain experienced during tissue penetration with 25-, 27-, or 30-gauge needles for maxillary injections, or with a 25- or 27-gauge needle for mandibular injections (Flanagan *et al.*, 2007). The benefits of a larger-gauge needle are reduced likelihood of breakage or deflection and less pressure necessary for aspiration. More pressure is necessary to inject local anesthetic through a 30-gauge needle, possibly causing hydrostatic damage and increasing discomfort during injection (Kurtzman, 2014). Injection may be performed with a short needle if the thickness of the soft tissue is less than 20 mm (American Academy of Pediatric Dentistry, 2020). A 27-gauge short needle is preferable to a 30-gauge needle for inferior alveolar block in a child. The orientation of the bevel of the 27-gauge needle either toward

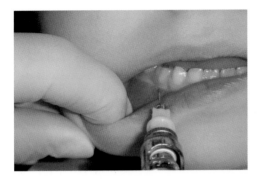

Figure 3.3 Infiltration at mucogingival junction.

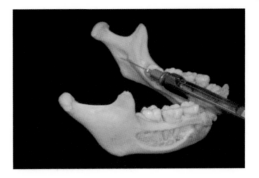

Figure 3.5 Mandible of 8-year-old child showing level of inferior alveolar foramen with syringe level to occlusal plane.

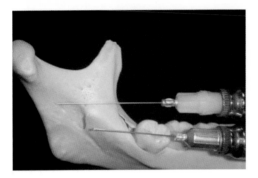

Figure 3.4 Comparison of 27-gauge long needle and 27-gauge short needle for inferior alveolar nerve block to demonstrate preferable short length in mandible of 8-year-old child.

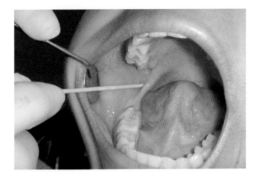

Figure 3.6 Mouth stretched wide open for visualizing the pterygomandibular raphe and pterygotemporal depression, noted with cotton-tipped applicator stick.

or away from the mandibular ramus does not affect achievement of pulpal anesthesia (Steinkruger *et al.*, 2006).

For infiltration, a 27-gauge extra-short needle is typically adequate. The tip of the needle should penetrate the mucosa by no more than 1 mm before anesthetic is slowly expressed and the needle is advanced steadily (Figure 3.3).

A 27-gauge short needle is recommended for IAN block in the pediatric patient (Figure 3.4). In general, the length of the needle is dependent on soft tissue thickness. The highest incidence of intravascular injection has been reported to occur with the IAN block. Aspiration should be performed before and repeatedly during the injection to avoid injecting too rapidly and intravascular injection (Malamed, 2011). The most influential factor to prevent overdose from intravascular injection is the rate of anesthetic administration: 60 seconds to inject a full cartridge is consistently recommended in the literature (Webb *et al.*, 2012). The mandibular foramen is below the occlusal plane in the primary dentition and level with the occlusal plane by 8.5 years of age (Figure 3.5). With growth, the vertical height of the ramus increases, so the needle is moved upward for insertion. For patients with a short face or for older patients, the needle insertion is further from the occlusal plane than in long-face or younger patients. The anteroposterior position of the mandibular foramen is one-half to two-thirds the width of the ramus, measured from the anterior border (Epars *et al.*, 2013). Injecting anesthetic below the mandibular foramen is the most common

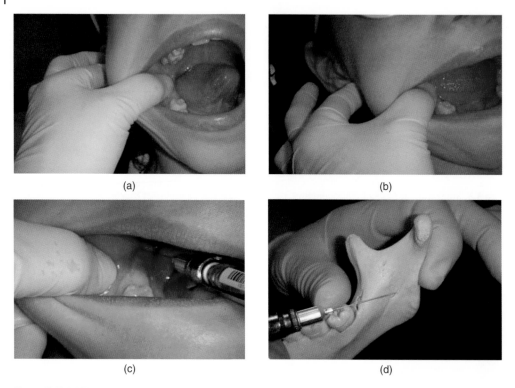

(a)

(b)

(c)

(d)

Figure 3.7 (a) Technique for administering inferior alveolar nerve block anesthesia with operator's thumb on the coronoid notch. (b) Operator's index finger on posterior border of ramus. (c) Inferior alveolar nerve block with syringe level to occlusal plane for 8-year-old child. (d) Photograph showing operator's approximate thumb position, accounting for soft tissue with inferior alveolar foramen two-thirds of the distance between thumb and index finger.

cause of inadequate anesthesia (Malamed, 2011).

For IAN block, the operator places his or her thumb intraorally on the coronoid notch, which is the deepest depression on the anterior border of the ramus, and the index finger on the posterior border of the ramus. The thumb and index finger may be reversed according to operator preference. The barrel of the syringe is at the opposite corner of the mouth, and the syringe is parallel with the occlusal plane at an appropriate level for the patient's age. The pterygomandibular raphe, a tendinous band of the buccopharyngeal fascia that is attached superiorly to the pterygoid hamulus and inferiorly to the posterior end of the mylohyoid line of the mandible, is an important landmark for administration of local anesthesia. This band of tissue becomes taunt and is more readily identified with the patient opening his or her mouth as wide as possible (Figure 3.6). The needle is inserted in the pterygotemporal depression, a triangular depression lateral to the raphe. The local anesthetic is injected upon reaching two-thirds of the distance between the thumb and index finger (Figure 3.7a–d).

Behavior Guidance/distraction

Anxiety is the biggest predictor of poor pain control (Nakai *et al.*, 2000). The clinician should talk to the child and keep the syringe out of his/her sight. Distraction with audiovisual glasses is an effective means to reduce pain with the injection of local anesthesia (El-Sharkawi *et al.*, 2012) (Figure 3.8). Telling

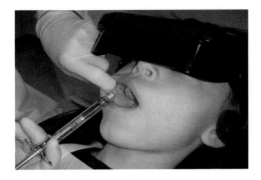

Figure 3.8 Audiovisual glasses for distraction during injection of local anesthesia.

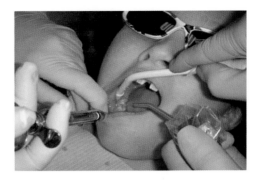

Figure 3.11 Water and suction at injection site while performing buccal infiltration in mandible.

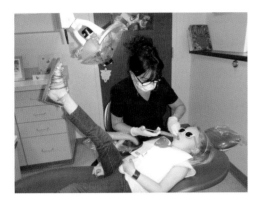

Figure 3.9 Patient raising a leg during injection of local anesthesia.

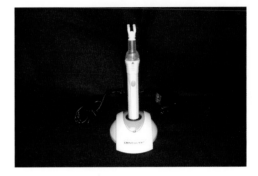

Figure 3.12 DentalVibe™ device.

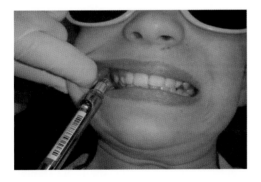

Figure 3.10 Child biting down hard during buccal infiltration in maxilla.

the child to raise his/her leg during the injection, or bite down hard during infiltration, or using the air/water syringe to spray water while suctioning at the injection site also provides excellent distraction (Figures 3.9–3.11).

The DentalVibe™ (Bing Innovations, Boca Raton, FL, USA) may significantly decrease fear of the "shot" and provide a more comfortable or pain-free injection by overriding the discomfort of tissue distension with vibration. Features include being cordless, rechargeable, illumination with fiber-optic LED light, and disposable nonlatex tips to provide retraction with pulsed vibration, blocking the neural pain pathway (Figure 3.12).

The first question parents/guardians often ask, after being informed of the need for a restoration, is whether a "shot" will be necessary for the procedure. Explanation and demonstration regarding the use of the DentalVibe™ ease the parent/guardian's concern, which typically transfers to the child, resulting in less apprehension or fear at the outset for both. In the author's experience, the device is not well accepted in children

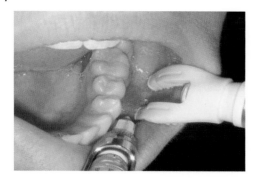

Figure 3.13 DentalVibe™ for buccal infiltration.

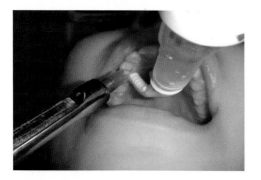

Figure 3.14 DentalVibe™ for palatal injection.

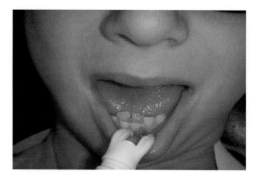

Figure 3.15 DentalVibe™ to augment topical anesthetic for extraction of extremely mobile coronal fragments.

may reduce injection pain and improve behavior (Libonati *et al.*, 2018). Children and adolescents with previous negative experiences benefit from the less threatening appearance of the CCLAD compared to a conventional syringe. Use of these devices minimizes the pain associated with intraligamentary (periodontal ligament or PDL) and palatal injections.

Postoperative Instructions and Documentation

Postoperative instructions warning about soft tissue injury after local anesthesia should be given with the parent/guardian present. A sticker, reminding the child not to bite or suck on his/her lip, cheek, or tongue, should be placed on the child's shirt on the same side as the anesthetized lip and/or tongue. Hot beverages should be avoided. A photograph of the appearance of a lip after chewing or biting during lip anesthesia can be shown to the parent/guardian and, if he/she is old enough to understand, also the child (Figure 3.16).

The patient's chart should include the dosage of local anesthetic administered in milligrams, the site of injection, and the type of injection(s), such as infiltration, intraosseous, or block, along with needle gauge and length (extra-short or short). The patient's reaction to the injection and postinjection instructions

younger than 4 years, but is very effective to reduce injection anxiety in adolescent patients. In two separate studies, adolescent patients and patients 6–12 years of age reported less pain during injections performed using the DentalVibe™ (Ching *et al.*, 2014; Shilpapriya *et al.*, 2015). Discomfort with palatal injection is significantly reduced with all ages. Tell–show–do, as discussed in Chapter 23, precedes the injection. Topical anesthetic is necessary to diminish the discomfort of the needle piercing the tissue. The needle is inserted next to one of the comfort tip prongs (Figures 3.13 and 3.14). Extraction of over-retained, extremely mobile primary incisor or primary molar coronal fragments can be performed quickly and virtually painlessly using topical anesthetic, augmented with the DentalVibe™ placed next to the coronal fragment (Figure 3.15).

Evidence also suggests that computer-controlled local anesthetic delivery (CCLAD)

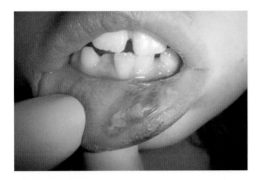

Figure 3.16 Lip swelling and ecchymosis due to lip chewing.

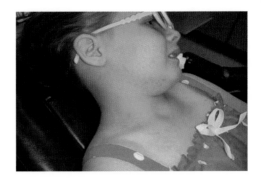

Figure 3.18 Rash due to suspected allergic reaction to penicillin.

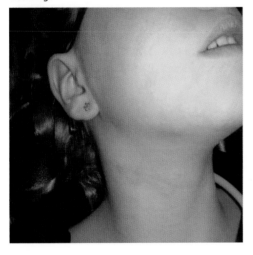

Figure 3.17 Diffuse splotching of skin due to anxiety.

given to the parent/guardian and the patient should also be included in the chart (American Academy of Pediatric Dentistry, 2020).

Adverse Events

The most common adverse event is soft tissue damage (Calvo *et al.*, 2019). The dentist or a staff member should monitor the child after the injection, while awaiting effective anesthesia. The possibility of soft tissue damage from accidental self-inflicted soft tissue damage, along with damage to the tissues during preparation of the tooth, should be included in the consent. If damage to the lip or oral mucosa occurs, vitamin E applied to the area may soothe and hasten healing.

The incidence of a true allergic reaction to local anesthesia is extremely rare and may be confused with other etiologies. Before beginning any procedure, note red splotches, rash, or evidence of trauma to rule out allergic reaction to the local anesthetic, or point it out to the parent to avoid the practice taking responsibility for an injury that previously occurred. Any unusual finding is immediately shown to the parent/guardian and documented in the chart. Anxiety may cause a diffuse rash (Figure 3.17). An allergic reaction to medication being taken may also present as a rash (Figure 3.18).

References

Adewumi, A., Hall, M., Guelmann, & Riley, J. (2008) The incidence of adverse reactions following 4% septocaine (Articaine) in children. *Pediatric Dentistry*, 30, 424–428.

AlShareed, M. (2011) Children's perception of their dentists. *European Journal of Dentistry*, 5, 186–190.

American Academy of Pediatric Dentistry. (2020) Use of local anesthesia for pediatric dental patients. *The Reference Manual of Pediatric Dentistry*. Chicago, IL: American Academy of Pediatric Dentistry; 286–292.

Aulestia-Viera, P.V., Braga, M.M., & Borsatti, M.A. (2018) The effect of adjusting the pH of local anaesthetics in dentistry: a systematic review and meta-analysis. *International Endodontic Journal*, 51, 862–876.

Calvo, J.M., Obadan-Udoh, E., Walji, M., & Kalenderian, E. (2019) Adverse events in pediatric dentistry: an exploratory study. *Pediatric Dentistry*, 41, 455–467.

Chicka, M.C., Dembo, J.B., Mathu-Muju, K.R., Nash, D.A., & Bush, H.M. (2012) Adverse events during pediatric dental anesthesia and sedation: a review of closed malpractice insurance claims. *Pediatric Dentistry*, 34, 231–238.

Ching, D., Finkelman, M., & Loo, C.Y. (2014) Effect of the DentalVibe injection system on pain during local anesthesia in adolescent patients. *Pediatric Dentistry*, 36, 51–55.

Cho, S.-Y., Kim, E., Park, S.-H., Roh, B.-D., Lee, C.-Y., *et al.* (2017) Effect of topical anesthesia on pain from needle insertion and injection and its relationship with anxiety in patients awaiting apical surgery: a randomized double-blind clinical trial. *Journal of Endodontics*, 43, 364–369.

El-Sharkawi, H.F.A., Housseiny, A.A., & Aly, A.M. (2012) Effectiveness of new distraction technique on pain associated with injection of local anesthesia for children. *Pediatric Dentistry*, 34, 142–145.

Epars, J.-F., Mavropoulos, A., & Kiliaridis, S. (2013) Influence of age and vertical facial type on the location of the mandibular foramen. *Pediatric Dentistry*, 35, 369–373.

Flanagan, T., Wahl, M.J., Schmitt, M.M., & Wahl, J.A. (2007) Size doesn't matter: needle gauge and injection pain. *General Dentistry*, 55, 216–217.

Friedman, M.J. (2000) New advances in local anesthesia. *Compendium of Continuing Education in Dentistry*, 21, 432–440.

Gutenberg, L.L., Chen, J.W., & Trapp, L. (2013) Methemoglobin levels in generally anesthetized pediatric dental patients receiving prilocaine versus lidocaine. *Anesthesia Progress*, 60, 99–108.

Kattan, S., Lee, S.-M., Hersh, E.V., & Karabucak, B. (2019) Do buffered local anesthetics provide more successful anesthesia than nonbuffered solutions in patients with pulpally involved teeth requiring dental therapy? *Journal of the American Dental Association,* 150, 165–177.

Kohli, K., Ngan, P., Crout, R., & Linscott, C.C. (2000) A survey of local and topical anesthesia use by pediatric dentists in the United States. *Pediatric Dentistry*, 23, 265–269.

Kurtzman, G.M. (2014) Improving the local anesthesia experience for our patients. *Dentistry Today*, 33, 120–126.

Libonati A., Nardi, R., Gallusi G., Angotti, V., Caruso, S., *et al.* (2018) Pain and anxiety associated with Computer-Controlled Local Anaesthesia: systematic review and meta-analysis of cross-over studies. *European Journal of Paediatric Dentistry*, 19, 324–332.

Malamed, S.F. (2011) Is the mandibular nerve block passé? *Journal of the American Dental Association Special Supplement*, 142, 3S–7S.

Malamed, S. (2020) *Handbook of Local Anesthesia*, 7th edn. St. Louis, MO: Elsevier; 102, 104, 186.

Malamed, S.F., Hersh E., Poorsattar S., & Falkel M. (2013) Faster onset and more comfortable injection with alkalinized 2% lidocaine with epinephrine 1:100,000. *Compendium of Continuing Education in Dentistry*, 34 (special issue 1), 11.

Meechan, J.G., Howlett, P.C., & Smith, B.D. (2005) Factors influencing the discomfort of intraoral needle penetration. *Anesthesia Progress*, 52, 91–94.

Meechan, J.G. (2011) The use of the mandibular infiltration anesthetic technique in adults. *Journal of the American Dental Association Special Supplement*, 142, 19S–24S.

Moore, P.A. & Hersh, E.V. (2010) Local anesthetics: pharmacology and toxicity. *Dental Clinics of North America*, 54, 587–599.

Nakai, Y., Milgrom, P., Mancl, L., Coldwell, S.E., Domoto, P.K., & Ramsay, D.S. (2000)

Effectiveness of local anesthesia in pediatric dental practice. *Journal of the American Dental Association*, 131, 1699–1705.

Priyatham, S. & Nuvvula, S. (2016) Intraoral topical anaesthesia in pediatric dentistry: review. *International Journal of Pharma and Bio Sciences*, 7, 346–353.

Ram, D. & Amir E. (2006) Comparison of Articaine 4% and lidocaine 2% in paediatric dental patients. *International Journal of Paediatric Dentistry*, 16, 262–256.

Ram, D., Hermida, L., & Peretz, B. (2002) A comparison of warmed and room-temperature anesthetic for local anesthesia in children. *Pediatric Dentistry*, 24, 333–336.

Shilpapriya, M., Jayanthi, M., Reddy, V.N., Sakthivel, R., Selvaraju, G., & Vijayakumar, P. (2015) Effectiveness of new vibration system on pain associated with injection of local anesthesia in children. *Journal of Indian Society of Pedodontics and Preventive Dentistry*, 33, 173–176.

Steinkruger, G., Nusstein, J., Reader, A., Beck, M., & Weaver, J. (2006) The significance of needle bevel orientation in achieving a successful inferior alveolar nerve block. *Journal of the American Dental Association*, 137, 1685–1691.

Taneja S., Singh, A., & Jain A. (2020) Anesthetic effectiveness of Articaine and Lidocaine in pediatric patients during dental procedures: a systematic review and meta-analysis. *Pediatric Dentistry*, 42, 273–279.

Townsend, J.A., Spiller, H., Hammersmith, K., & Casamassimo, P.S. (2020) Dental local anesthesia-related pediatric cases reported to U.S. poison control centers. *Pediatric Dentistry*, 42,116–122.

Trapp, L. & Will J. (2010) Acquired methemoglobinemia revisited. *Dental Clinics of North America*, 54, 665–675.

Webb, M.D., Howell, D.L., & Moursi, A.M. (2012) Intraoperative pain management. In: Moursi, A.M. (ed.), *Clinical Cases in Pediatric Dentistry*. Oxford: Wiley Blackwell; 245–248.

Widmer, R., McNeil, D.W., McNeil, C.B., McDonald, J., Alcaino, E.A., & Cooper, M.G. (2008) Child management. In: Cameron, A.C. & Widmer, R.P. (eds.), *Handbook of Pediatric Dentistry*, 3rd edn. London: Mosby; 9–37.

Wilburn-Goo, D. & Lloyd, L.M. (1999) When patients become cyanotic: acquired methemoglobinemia. *Journal of the American Dental Association*, 130, 826–831.

4

Primary Incisor Restoration

Ari Kupietzky

Early childhood caries (ECC) is usually seen in 18–36-month-old children, although it can present even younger. Initially, the maxillary incisors develop a band of dull white demineralization along the gum line that goes undetected by the parents. As the condition progresses, the white lesions develop into cavities that girdle the necks of the teeth in a brown or black collar. Frequently, by the time the child is brought to the dentist, much of the anterior clinical crowns is decayed or lost. In advanced cases, the crowns of the four maxillary incisors may be destroyed completely, leaving decayed brownish-black root stumps (Ripa, 1988). The premature loss or unsightly appearance of grossly decayed primary anterior teeth may be initially of concern to parents; however, as the child matures, it may also affect the patient's self-image. Treatment of these badly decayed teeth remains a challenge for the dentist. The toddler and preschooler, due to their young age and lack of cognitive abilities, are usually very uncooperative for dental treatment, and their behavior plays a big factor in the choice of restoration. Many appear with poor oral hygiene practices, presenting swollen, inflamed, and bleeding gingiva.

Treatment plans advocated for grossly decayed primary anterior teeth include restorations, crowns, or extractions followed by partial dentures. This chapter presents step-by-step procedures for the placement of bonded resin composite strip crowns, full-coverage prefabricated crowns, and the anterior esthetic fixed appliance (modified Nance or Groper appliance).

Pretreatment

When a toddler presents to the dental clinic and is diagnosed with ECC, specific counseling and patient preparation must be implemented before any definitive restorative treatment may be commenced. Changing the feeding practices and implementing tooth brushing with fluoridated toothpaste are the first steps in controlling the disease. Once these are accomplished, definitive restorative treatment modalities can then be mandated.

Oral Hygiene

It is advantageous to obtain ideal oral hygiene before commencement of treatment. Parents should be instructed and convinced that they bear partial responsibility for the success of treatment by preparing their child's gingiva for the procedure. Inflamed gingiva (Figure 4.1a) may interfere with proper curing of the restorations, resulting in discolored crowns as a result of excessive bleeding during the curing process. Two to three weeks of proper home care is usually enough to achieve healthy, pink, nonbleeding gingiva that will facilitate restorative treatment (Figure 4.1b).

Handbook of Clinical Techniques in Pediatric Dentistry, Second Edition. Edited by Jane A. Soxman.
© 2022 John Wiley & Sons, Inc. Published 2022 by John Wiley & Sons, Inc.

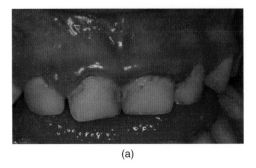
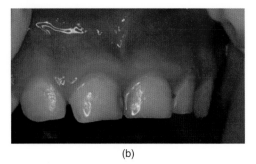

(a)   (b)

Figure 4.1 (a) The gingival tissue of patients with early childhood caries tends to be inflamed, leading to hemorrhage and compromised esthetics. Inflamed gingiva may interfere with proper curing of the restorations, resulting in discolored crowns due to excessive bleeding. (b) Three weeks of proper tooth brushing resulted in pink, healthy gingiva, which was necessary to facilitate an aesthetic result.

Indications

Full coronal restoration of carious primary incisors may be indicated when (i) caries is present on multiple surfaces; (ii) the incisal edge is involved; (iii) there is extensive cervical decalcification; (iv) pulpal therapy is indicated; (v) caries may be minor, but oral hygiene is very poor (high-risk patients); or (vi) the child's behavior makes moisture control very difficult, creating difficulties in placing Class III restorations (Waggoner, 2002). In addition, the clinician may opt for full coverage in lieu of large Class III restorations: due to the small clinical crown, the relatively large size of the pulp chamber, the close proximity of the pulp horns to the interproximal surfaces, and the thinness of the enamel, repairing interproximal decay in these teeth requires preparations that are conservative in depth with close attention to detail, both to the preparation itself and to the material placement. The technique sensitivity of placing Class III esthetic restorations is very high. Moisture control, hemorrhage control from the gingiva, and retention of the rubber dam are challenges to be overcome to obtain a successful result (Waggoner, 2002); the placement of a full-coverage crown will likely be more successful and longer lasting.

Bonded Resin Composite Strip Crown

The bonded resin composite strip crown (Figure 4.2) is perhaps the most esthetic of all the restorations available to the clinician for the treatment of severely decayed primary incisors (Webber *et al.*, 1979). However, strip crowns are also the most technique sensitive and may be difficult to place (Croll, 1995). Some simple clinical tips may assist the clinician in achieving an esthetic and superior outcome.

Strip Crown Preparation

Preparation of the strip crown may be accomplished before the treatment visit. The crown is pierced with a sharp explorer at the mesial or distal incisal angle to create a core vent for the escape of any air bubbles entrapped in the crown (Figure 4.3a). Care must be taken not to damage the proximal seams of the crown. After vent preparation, sharp, curved scissors should be used to trim the crown gingival margins (Figure 4.3b). To ensure sharpness, only task-designated scissors are recommended for this purpose. If there is any doubt of proximal seam integrity, the crown should be discarded.

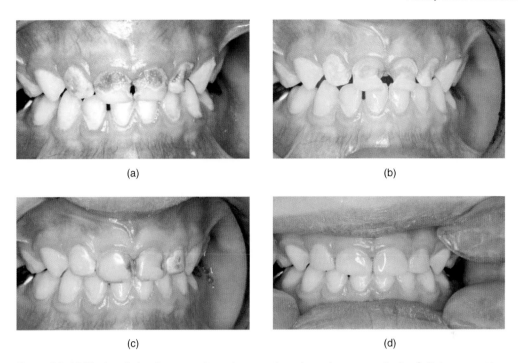

(a) (b)

(c) (d)

Figure 4.2 (a) The bonded resin composite strip crown is perhaps the most esthetic of all the restorations available to the clinician for the treatment of severely decayed primary incisors. Preoperative view. (b) Caries removal followed by placement of resin-modified glass ionomer cement. Note healthy ginigiva. (c) Try-in of crown formers. (d) Postoperative view.

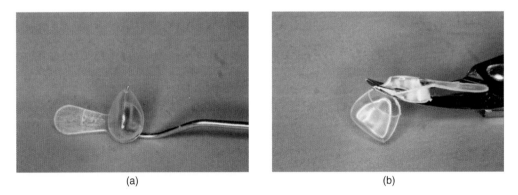

(a) (b)

Figure 4.3 (a) The crown is pierced with a sharp explorer at the mesial or distal incisal angle to create a core vent for the escape of any air bubbles entrapped in the crown. (b) Following vent preparation, sharp, curved scissors should be used to trim the crown gingival margins.

All crowns may be trimmed to an approximate level and can be fine-tuned chairside during treatment.

Isolation and Rubber Dam Placement

The routine use of ligature ties to deflect gingival tissue and retain the rubber dam in place

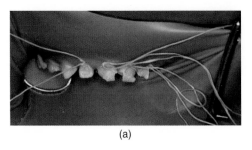

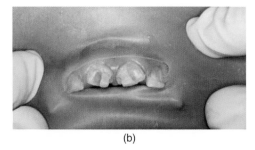

(a)   (b)

Figure 4.4 (a) The routine use of ligature ties to deflect gingival tissue and retain the rubber dam in place is not suggested, although this is a valid technique used routinely by many dentists with success. (b) It is suggested to use the slit-dam method.

is not suggested, although this is a valid technique used routinely by many dentists with success (Figure 4.4a). Ligature ties at many times may be the cause of bleeding and discomfort for the patient. Their use may inhibit rapid removal and replacement of the rubber dam during treatment. After curing, the removal of the ligatures, which are situated under the hardened restoration, is often difficult and necessitates the otherwise unnecessary subgingival bur finishing for their complete removal. Therefore, with the exception of a case involving severe subgingival carious incisors, it is suggested to use the slit-dam method (Croll, 1985). The application is rapid, and the desired teeth are completely available for restorative treatment. Two large holes are punched out 1–2 cm apart and are joined by a scissors cut. The rubber dam may be held in place with digital pressure (Figure 4.4b) or with the use of an elastic band extending between the rubber dam frame and wrapped around the patient's head (Reid *et al.*, 1991). Note that the rubber dam is kept in place only during caries removal; during crown placement the rubber dam may be removed.

In cases involving severe subgingival carious incisors, it is suggested to use the elastomer method introduced by Psaltis and Kupietzky. Orthodontic elastomeric ligatures are used in place of those for the specific purposes of rubber dam retraction and virtual elimination of the problems of blood and saliva contamination of the operative areas. The success of the technique depends on three key steps, as follows:

1. Use a rubber dam punched with four holes of the smallest possible size. This allows the tightest fit, eliminates leakage, and enables the elastomers to retract the dam more effectively around the teeth. It is recommended to space the four holes over the center of each maxillary incisor. Placement too close together will result in stretching of the rubber dam between the teeth and subsequent leakage around the teeth.

2. Place orthodontic elastomers over each incisor after placement of the rubber dam. This is accomplished by threading two strands of floss through each elastomer (Figure 4.5a) and then stretching it over the tooth (Figure 4.5b). If the interproximal areas are sharp or jagged due to caries, the elastomers may tear during this process. If so, slice through the jagged areas with a thin fissure bur (no. 169 or 1169) to eliminate them. In many cases, the elastomers can be flossed into place by pulling them simultaneously from each tooth's labial and lingual surfaces. It is also sometimes necessary to facilitate this procedure by using a Hollenback carver or a similar hand instrument that can tuck the elastomer well into the gingival sulcus around each tooth (Figure 4.5c). When the elastomers have been properly placed over a well-punched rubber dam, they will almost immediately begin to contract. Consequently, they will

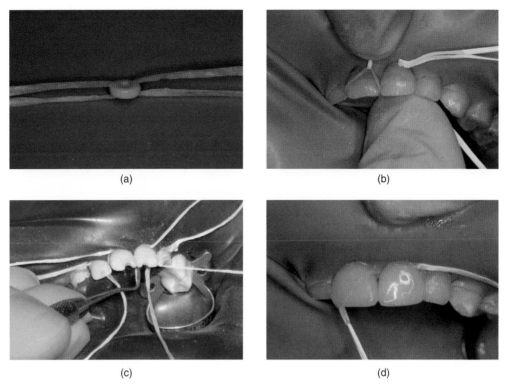

(a)   (b)

(c)   (d)

Figure 4.5 (a) Thread two strands of floss through each elastomer. (b) The elastomer is stretched and eased over the tooth with the labial and palatal floss strands. (c) A Hollenback carver or a similar hand instrument may be used to guide the elastomer in place. (d) The elastomers are removed from the facial by using the floss that was left in place.

also retract the dam and gingival tissues. If any treatment is to be completed in the posterior segments, it is best to proceed and complete them first to give the elastomers more time to continue this retraction process. Once the elastomers are in place, remove the piece of floss from the lingual side, but leave the labial floss in place.

3. Remove the elastomers with the labial floss after the preparation and restoration of the incisors have been completed (Figure 4.5d). It is critical to remove the elastomers, as they will continuously migrate up the conical-shaped root on any of the incisors and, if left in place, can atraumatically and asymptomatically "extract" the tooth. Hence, the facial floss provides an easy way to remove the elastomer and serves as a reminder. The proper use of these

elastomers eliminates the tedious tying (and removal) of floss ligatures and virtually eliminates any hemorrhaging to ensure a clean field for placement of the strip crowns.

Caries Removal and Crown Placement—curing and Finishing

During caries excavation and removal, extra care should be taken not to damage any gingiva. A stainless-steel, round, medium to large bur should be used in a low-speed handpiece for this purpose (Figure 4.6a, b) following initial high-speed tooth reduction. After the application of a resin-modified glass ionomer liner/base for dentin protection (Figure 4.6c, d), all crowns should be fitted and placed (Figure 4.6e). It is suggested to fill and cure

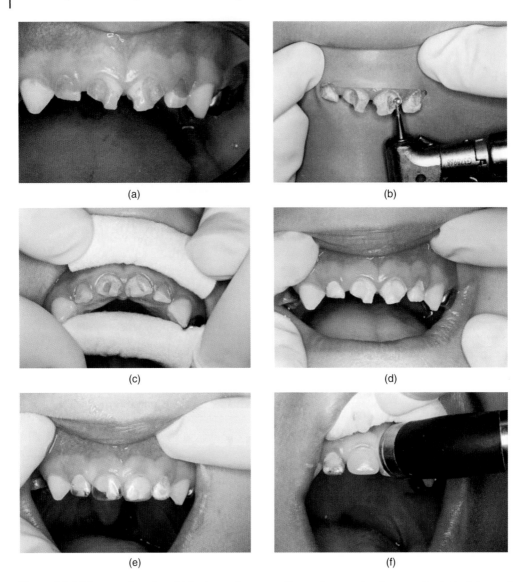

(a)   (b)

(c)   (d)

(e)   (f)

Figure 4.6 (a) Preoperative view. (b) During caries excavation and removal, extra care should be taken not to damage any gingiva. A stainless-steel, round, medium to large bur should be used in a low-speed handpiece for this purpose. Indirect pulp capping is favorable over pulpal exposure; only infected dentin should be removed. (c) Large cotton rolls are used in place of rubber dam once high-speed and subsequent water spray are not needed anymore. (d) A resin-modified glass ionomer liner/base is applied for dentin protection. (e) All crowns should be fitted and placed to ensure proper spacing. (f) It is suggested to fill and cure each crown individually with unfilled crown forms in place on their respective teeth to ensure proper spacing between restorations. (g) Special care should be taken to carefully remove (before filled crown placement) a collar of cured bonding agent, which will interfere with proper seating of the crown form if it is left in place. (h) A sharp, handheld instrument such as a cleoid/discoid carver is recommended to peel off the strip crown shell. Care should be taken to apply contra-digital pressure for the patient's benefit. (i) An excellent result was obtained following the use of the above-described method. Labial view. (j) Palatal view.

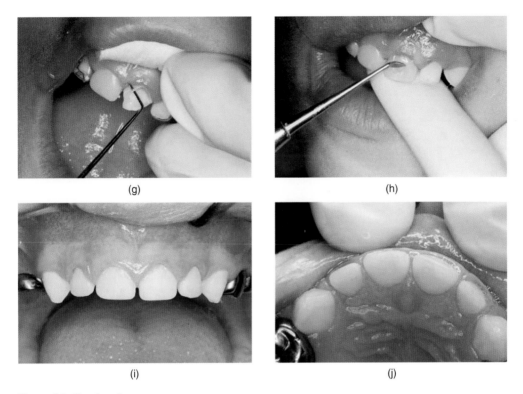

(g)   (h)

(i)   (j)

Figure 4.6 (*Continued*)

each crown individually with unfilled crown forms in place on their respective teeth to ensure proper spacing between restorations (Figure 4.6f). Special care should be taken to carefully remove (before filled crown placement) a collar of cured bonding agent, which will interfere with proper seating of the crown form if it is left in place (Figure 4.6g). Another cause of failure is overfilling the crown with composite material, resulting in the tearing of the mesial and distal seams of the crown. Minimal filling is highly recommended. Instead of using a rotary instrument to remove the crown form, a sharp, handheld instrument such as a cleoid/discoid carver is recommended to peel off the strip crown shell (Figure 4.6h). This results in only minimal damage to the cured restoration and, consequently, little if any polishing is necessary, and the luster of the labial crown surface is preserved. Care should be taken to apply contra-digital pressure for the patient's benefit.

An excellent result was obtained after the use of the above-described method and is presented in Figure 4.6i and j.

The preoperative and postoperative radiographic views are presented in Figure 4.7a and b.

Full-coverage Prefabricated Crowns

In extreme cases (e.g., severely inflamed gingival tissue, advanced coronal decay, and poor parental compliance), hemorrhage and compromise of the composite aesthetic restoration may be a concern. In these cases, restoration of anterior teeth can be accomplished with preformed anterior crowns (PACs). These restorations can be placed in a single, relatively short appointment, and their aesthetics are not affected by saliva or hemorrhage. There are disadvantages, including relative inflexibility,

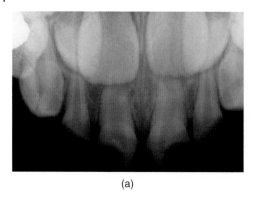
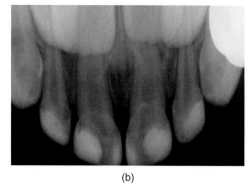

(a)   (b)

Figure 4.7 (a) Preoperative radiograph. (b) Postoperative radiograph.

breakage risk under heavy force, significant removal of tooth structure, expense, limited shade choice, and placement difficulty in crowded spaces.

The most common type of PAC is the pre-veneered anterior stainless-steel crown (SSC). A recent development has been the introduction of the zirconium anterior crown available from various manufacturers, including Cheng Crowns (Exton, PA, USA), Sprig Oral Health Technologies (formerly EZ Pedo; Loomis, CA, USA), Kinder Krowns (St. Louis Park, MN, USA), and NuSmile (Houston, TX, USA). The preparation and placement of the PAC are described in Figures 4.8 and 4.9.

The preparation of a PAC is similar to that of a bonded resin composite strip crown, with a number of modifications as follows:

1. The crown size should be approximated before commencement of tooth reduction.
2. Crown reduction is more extensive compared to that of a bonded resin composite strip crown: reduce the incisal length of the tooth by approximately 2 mm and open the interproximal contacts. The proximal reduction must be adequate to allow the selected crown to fit passively and should be made parallel to slightly converging incisally. The tooth should be reduced circumferentially by approximately 20% or 0.5–1.25 mm as necessary. Adequate reduction of the tooth is extremely important for the crown selected to seat passively.

3. Subgingival reduction: the crown margin should be carefully extended and refined to a feather-edge margin approximately 2 mm subgingivally on all surfaces (Figure 4.10). Avoid excessive tooth reduction in the cervical areas for adequate crown retention. For performing these tooth reductions, thin, tapered diamond, or carbide burs may be used. It is important to separate the preparation steps into two using different burs—supragingival and subgingival—to control hemorrhage and avoid excessive tissue trauma.

4. Try-in: it is very important that the crown sits passively on the prepped tooth. The appropriate-sized crown will extend subgingivally without any distortion of the gingiva. No force should be applied when seating the crown. Care must be taken to cleanse the internal surfaces of the crown of any blood residue, as this will interfere with proper cementation. Note: one brand (NuSmile ZR Try-In Crowns) has a unique system of try-in crowns, which are used only for provisional fit and then replaced with a new crown to be cemented, thus avoiding contamination with saliva or blood from the prepared internal surface.

5. Cementation: a high-quality self-curing glass ionomer cement should be used. The crowns must be firmly held in position until the cement is set.

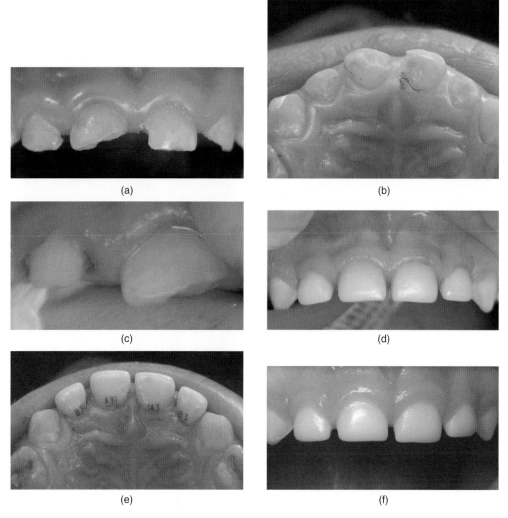

Figure 4.8 (a) Preoperative labial view. Lack of crowding will facilitate placement of preformed anterior crowns: NuSmile ZR crowns were used for restoration of all four maxillary incisors. (b) Preoperative palatal view. (c) Close-up of preparation of lateral incisor: note extensive tooth reduction, including subgingival preparation, which is necessary for proper-size crown. (d) Cemented NuSmile ZR crowns. Immediate postoperative labial view. (e) Immediate postoperative palatal view. (f) Follow-up. Note excellent gingival adaptation and esthetic result. (g) Follow-up view demonstrating functional occlusion and esthetics. (h) Periapical radiograph at recall: no pathologies noted, centrals approaching exfoliation. Source: Courtesy of Dr. Sean R. Whalen, Westminster, CO, USA.

When comparing the two methods—that is, the bonded resin composite strip crown and PAC—it must be emphasized that in the latter technique, tooth reduction is much greater (Clark *et al.*, 2016). Effective anesthesia must be obtained, and in many instances elective pulp therapy may be necessary to allow enough reduction and placement of a well-fitting crown.

Inadequate tooth reduction will result in the placement of an oversized crown and an unesthetic result. In addition to the esthetic concerns, tooth reduction must be made adequately, as zirconia crown retention is closely related to occluso-cervical heights: 2 mm occluso-cervical height is crucial for prefabricated zirconia crown retention (Jing *et al.*, 2019).

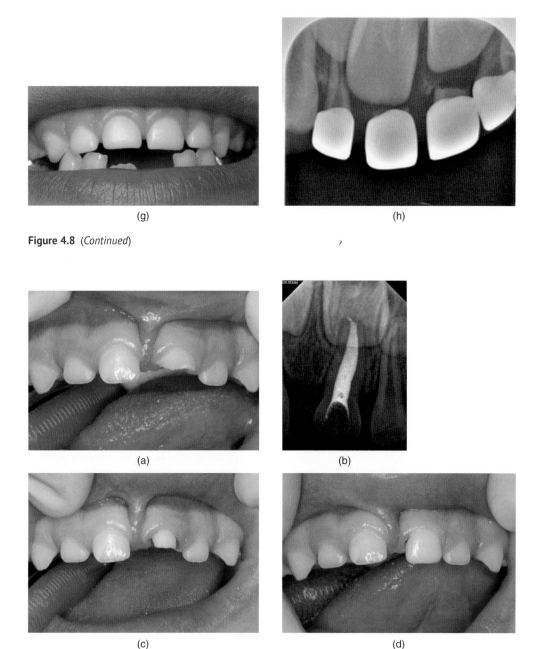

(g) (h)

Figure 4.8 (*Continued*)

(a) (b)

(c) (d)

Figure 4.9 (a) Preoperative view of complicated crown fracture of maxillary left primary central incisor with pulpal exposure. Spaced dentition will facilitate placement of a preformed anterior crown (PAC). (b) Radiograph following root canal therapy. (c) Preparation for NuSmile ZR crown. (d) Immediate postoperative labial view of cemented NuSmile ZR crown. (e) Immediate postoperative palatal view. (f) A discolored bonded resin strip crown following root canal therapy. The translucency of the crown exhibits the underlying change in tooth color. A PAC may be indicated for use in cases involving endodontic treatment of incisors. (g) Six-month follow-up. Note excellent esthetics and no discoloration of restored tooth. Source: Courtesy of Dr. Tania Roloff, Hamburg, Germany.

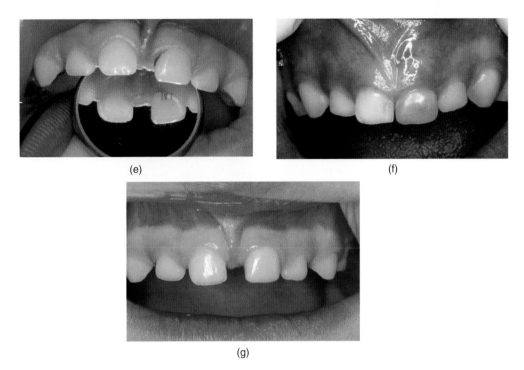

(e)   (f)

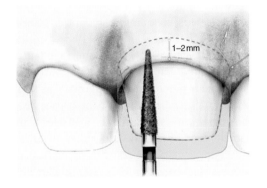

(g)

Figure 4.9 (*Continued*)

Figure 4.10 Subgingival reduction: the crown margin should be carefully extended and refined to a feather-edge margin approximately 2 mm subgingivally on all surfaces.

Anterior Esthetic Fixed Appliances

Considerations

The rehabilitation of a young toddler who has developed multiple tooth loss subsequent to rampant EEC or extensive dental trauma may be achieved with an anterior esthetic fixed appliance. Many parents will seek an esthetic solution to replace the lost teeth. When considering the need for an anterior appliance to replace missing primary incisors, the following points should be discussed with the parents (Waggoner & Kupietzky, 2001). The strongest factor for placing an anterior esthetic appliance is *parental* desire and not physiologic need. While space maintenance, masticatory function, speech development, and tongue habits may be of some consideration, there is no strong evidence that early loss of maxillary incisors will have any significant, long-lasting effect on the growth and development of the child. Parents may express concern about their child's ability to eat without four incisors. They need to be reassured that feeding is generally not a problem (Koroluk & Riekman, 1991). Children who have had all four maxillary incisors extracted as a result of EEC appear to function well without them. Empirically, many appear to have an improved ability to eat and function, likely because the badly decayed or infected incisors inflicted pain on eating.

Another consideration is the child's speech development after extraction of all four incisors. This issue remains somewhat controversial, with conflicting opinions as to the affect, if any, on speech development caused by missing primary incisors. It may be prudent to consider appliances for children younger than 3 years who have not yet developed their speech skills. However, children older than 4 years will usually compensate for the tooth loss and not exhibit any long-term speech disorders.

Although space maintenance in the posterior region is an important consideration when there is early loss of primary molars, the anterior segment, from canine to canine, appears to be stable, even with the early loss of several incisors, with no net loss of space from canine to canine. Occasionally, especially in a crowded dentition, if one or more incisors are lost, there may be some rearrangement of space between the remaining incisors, but no space maintenance is usually required if the loss occurs after the eruption of the primary canines (Ngan & Wei, 1988).

The bottom line is that in most cases, the decision to place an anterior esthetic fixed appliance is individual and personal, to be made by the parent in conjunction with the clinician. If parents do not indicate a desire to replace missing anterior teeth, no treatment is usually required. However, if they do wish to replace the missing teeth, they should not be discouraged (Christensen & Fields, 1994). Indeed, some children may be aware of their edentulous appearance and request treatment. When properly fabricated and fitted, these appliances restore a natural and pleasing appearance and thus provide an opportunity for normal psychologic development.

Contraindications

The contraindications for the placement of an anterior fixed appliance include patients with seizure disorders, intellectual disability, poor

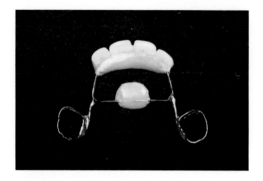

Figure 4.11 The modified Nance holding arch: note palatal acrylic button in the rugae area.

ability to follow up, and very poor hygiene; immune-compromised patients; continuation of inappropriate feeding habits; and significant deep bite, overjet, or anterior crossbite.

Clinical Procedure

Appliance Design

There are many types of appliances that can be fabricated, including a modified Nance holding arch (Figure 4.11) and the Groper appliance (Figure 4.12). The latter appliance is similar to a Nance holding arch, but with plastic teeth processed onto the wire instead of a palatal acrylic button in the rugae area. The round wire should be 0.036–0.040 in. in diameter and is attached to either the first or second primary molars with prefabricated stainless-steel bands or SSCs. First molars are preferred as abutments over second molars due to a shorter wire span and less potential interference with erupting 6-year molars. The plastic or acrylic teeth are attached to metal cleats that have been soldered to the palatal wire bar. The teeth sit directly on the alveolar crest, without any gingival-colored acrylic extending into the vestibule or onto the palate (Figure 4.12).

In instances of asymmetric alveolar ridge deformities, it is suggested to add gingival-colored acrylic to mask the missing height and

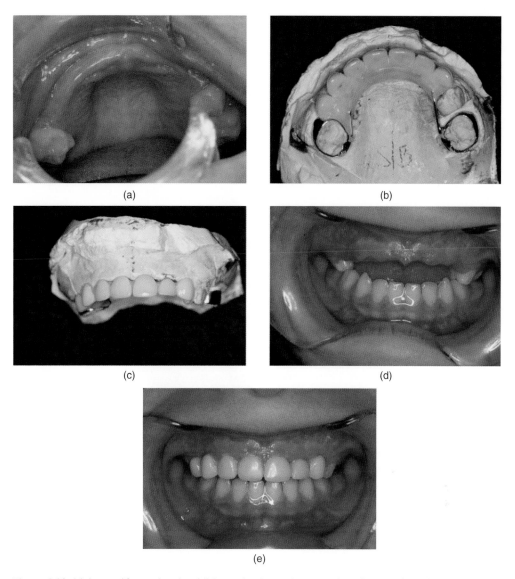

(a)

(b)

(c)

(d)

(e)

Figure 4.12 (a) At age 19 months, the child sustained complete avulsion of all maxillary incisors, canines, and right first primary molar. (b) At age 34 months, a Groper appliance was fabricated. The plastic or acrylic teeth are attached to metal cleats that have been soldered to the palatal wire bar. (c) The teeth sit directly on the alveolar crest without any gingival-colored acrylic extending into the vestibule or onto the palate. (d) Labial view of edentulous anterior region. (e) Intraoral view demonstrating the appliance after 2 years of use.

thus achieve symmetry and better esthetics (Figure 4.13).

In general, it is easier to achieve good esthetic results when replacing all four maxillary incisors. The appliance may be used to replace single, double, or triple incisors, but more detailed attention will need to be paid when choosing color and designing the appliance's tooth morphology to match the remaining natural teeth in these clinical situations.

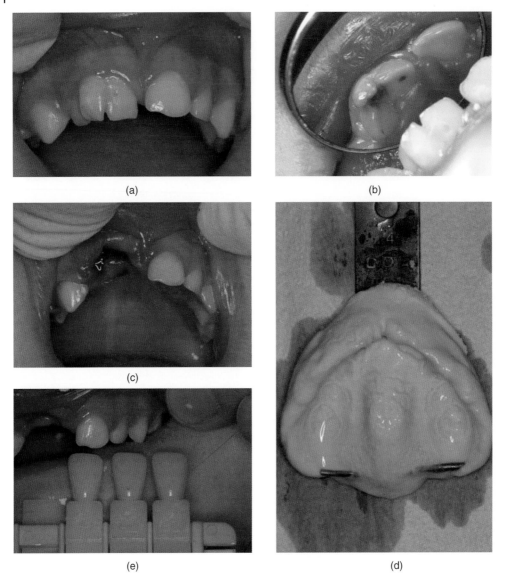

(a)

(b)

(c)

(d)

(e)

Figure 4.13 (a) A 30-month-old patient with fusion and concrescence of upper right primary central, lateral, and supernumerary teeth. (b) Palatal view demonstrating deep caries; extraction was treatment choice to be followed by placement of fixed appliance. (c) After extraction, note resulting alveolar defect. (d) Alginate impression taken without bands. (e) Color selection is important due to asymmetric tooth loss. (f) Upper and lower working models are mandatory. In addition, wax bite registration is required. (g) Groper appliance: note gingival extension to compensate for alveolar bone loss and asymmetric ridge. (h) Anterior view without appliance. (i) Appliance *in situ*. Note morphology of right central incisor constructed to mimic the shape of the natural left incisor.

Steps in Fabrication

First Appointment

1. Fit bands on first or second molars.

2. Take an alginate impression of the maxillary jaw with the bands on the teeth (Figure 4.13d). Remove the impression, place, and secure the bands in the

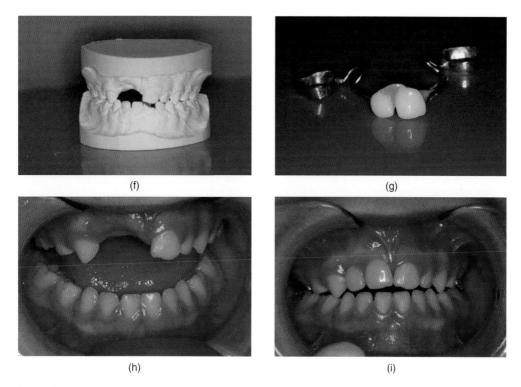

(f)

(g)

(h)

(i)

Figure 4.13 *(Continued)*

impression and pour up with dental stone (Figure 4.13f). Note that some laboratories may request that bands be removed after being fitted and an impression be taken *without* the bands in place. The fitted bands are then sent to the laboratory and placed by the technician into the plaster working model.

3. Take a mandibular alginate impression and wax bite registration.
4. Select the color (Figure 4.13e).

Second Appointment

1. If not performed at the previous appointment, anesthetize and extract the anterior teeth. Small pieces of absorbable gelatin sponge placed into the sockets will aid hemostasis.
2. Try-in the appliance. Adjust as needed with three-prong pliers and crown crimpers.
3. Cement the appliance with glass ionomer cement or resin-modified glass ionomer cement (Figure 4.13g–i).

Timing of Placement: Same Day as Extraction or Delay for Healing

The timing of placement is somewhat controversial. Historically, it was suggested to allow 6–8 weeks after tooth loss before fabrication. This delay was thought to allow a better-fitting, more esthetically pleasing appliance. However, personal experience has found that delay is not necessary and immediate placement is possible. Same-day extraction and appliance placement can result in an excellent clinical outcome. Perhaps one reason to delay treatment is to ascertain whether the parents' concern about esthetics is a real one. Many parents who contemplated an appliance will opt to change their decision and not place it after they observe how well their child adapts to the postextraction situation. They may observe during this waiting period that no negative change in their child's functioning, eating, or speech has occurred. Esthetically, many parents' image of their child improves within the delay period, and their esthetic concern will dissipate.

Summary

Successful restoration of severely decayed primary incisors may be one of the greatest challenges in pediatric dentistry. Patients with ECC have a greater propensity for developing new and recurrent caries. It is critical for the dentist to treat the disease and not only the individual teeth. Restorative treatment should commence contingent on proper home care. Proper technique can be successfully achieved with the right planning and execution.

Note

Selected text and figures have been adapted with permission from Dr. Kupietzky's previous works:

Kupietzky, A. (2001) The treatment and long-term management of severe multiple avulsions of primary teeth in a 19-month-old child. *Pediatric Dentistry*, **23**, 517–521. Figure 4.12.

Kupietzky, A. (2002) Bonded resin composite strip crowns for primary incisors. *Pediatric Dentistry*, **24**, 145–148. Figures 4.3a, b, 4.4a, b, 4.6a, b, e, g, h, i.

Psaltis, G. & Kupietzky, A. (2008) A simplified isolation technique for placement of composite strip crowns. *Pediatric Dentistry*, **30**, 436–438. Figures 4.5a, b, 4.5c, d.

References

Christensen, J.R. & Fields, H.W. (1994) Space maintenance in the primary dentition. In: Pinkham, J.R. (ed.), *Pediatric Dentistry: Infancy through Adolescence*, 2nd edn. Philadelphia, PA: W.B. Saunders; 358–363.

Clark, L., Wells, M.H., Harris, E.F., & Lou, J. (2016) Comparison of amount of primary tooth reduction required for anterior and posterior zirconia and stainless steel crowns. *Pediatric Dentistry*, 38, 42–46.

Croll, T.P. (1985) Alternative methods for use of the rubber dam. *Quintessence International*, 16, 387–392.

Croll, T.P. (1995) Restorative dentistry for preschool children. *Dental Clinics North America.*, 39, 737–770.

Jing, L., Chen, J.W., Roggenkamp, C., & Suprono, M.S. (2019) Effect of crown preparation height on retention of a prefabricated primary posterior zirconia crown. *Pediatric Dentistry*, 15, 229–233.

Koroluk, L.D. & Riekman, G.A. (1991) Parental perceptions of the effects of maxillary incisor extractions in children with nursing caries. *Journal of Dentistry for Children*, 58, 233–236.

Ngan, P. & Wei, S.H.Y. (1988) Management of space in the primary and mixed dentitions. In: Wei, S.H.Y. (ed.), *Pediatric Dentistry: Total Patient Care*. Philadelphia, PA: Lea & Febiger; 462–470.

Reid, J.S., Callis, P.D., & Patterson, C.J.W. (1991) *Rubber Dam in Clinical Practice. London: Quintessence Publishing*; 29–30.

Ripa, L.W. (1988) Nursing caries: a comprehensive review. *Pediatric Dentistry*, 10, 268–282.

Waggoner, W.F. (2002) Restoring primary anterior teeth. *Pediatric Dentistry*, 24, 511–516.

Waggoner, W.F. & Kupietzky, A. (2001) Anterior esthetic fixed appliances for the preschooler: considerations and a technique for placement. *Pediatric Dentistry*, 23, 147–150.

Webber, D., Epstein, N., & Tsamtsouris, A. (1979) A method of restoring primary anterior teeth with the aid of a celluloid crown form and composite resins. *Pediatric Dentistry*, 1, 244–246.

5

Primary Molar Adhesive Tooth Restoration
Constance M. Killian and Theodore P. Croll

Almost 70 years ago, when Hogeboom (1953) offered the sixth edition of his classic pediatric dentistry textbook, *Practical Pedodontia or Juvenile Operative Dentistry and Public Health Dentistry*, the materials used to repair primary teeth were as follows: "gutta-percha," black copper cement, Fleck's Red Copper Cement, silver amalgam, copper amalgam, Kryptex ("a good silicate"), silver nitrate, ammoniated silver nitrate, chromium alloy deciduous crowns, and rapid setting plastic filling materials (requiring "ample pulp protection"). Stainless-steel crowns are still very useful and are known for their durability and reliability. "Plastic" filling materials have made their way to the forefront of direct application restorative dentistry, but today's materials have little resemblance to the original resin products. Silver amalgams are still used by some dentists for repair of primary teeth, but because they do not bond to tooth structure, have a dark color, and suffer from the continuing false controversy over their safety, they are being offered to parents less and less.

An ideal direct application dental restorative material for primary molars would be biocompatible and tooth colored, adhere to tooth structure with no subsequent marginal leakage, have sufficient physical properties so as not degrade in the mouth, have "on-command" hardening after being applied

to the tooth structure, and handle easily for the practitioner.

Decades of progress have brought us advanced direct placement restoratives that come close to meeting all the above-mentioned requirements to be considered ideal. Resin-based composites (RBCs) and the glass polyalkenoate (glass ionomer or GI) systems have been at the forefront of the "adhesive dentistry" revolution that has immeasurably progressed restorative dentistry for children. Berg (1998) succinctly reviewed modern adhesive restorative materials that are useful in clinical pediatric dentistry.

The Ideal Operative Field: Rubber Dam Isolation

The use of adhesive materials for restoring carious, malformed, or fractured primary molars demands careful attention for moisture control. Many adhesive materials, particularly RBCs, are sensitive to moisture and require isolation of teeth to be treated. There is no better way to achieve such isolation and create an ideal operative field than the rubber dam.

Dr. Sanford Barnum first used a "rubber cloth" to isolate a mandibular molar of R.C. Benedict on March 15, 1864 (Christen, 1977). From that time on, that manner of isolating

Handbook of Clinical Techniques in Pediatric Dentistry, Second Edition. Edited by Jane A. Soxman.
© 2022 John Wiley & Sons, Inc. Published 2022 by John Wiley & Sons, Inc.

teeth became the standard protocol in the profession for restorative dentistry (Francis, 1865; Barbakow, 1964). Croll (1985) listed the following benefits of rubber dam use:

- Operating time is reduced.
- Visibility for the dentist is improved.
- Tongue and cheek are protected and out of the way.
- The mouth stays moist and more comfortable for the patient.
- The patient is protected from aspirating or swallowing excess material, water spray, infected tooth substance, or broken instrument fragments.
- Soft tissues in the region of operation are better protected from accidental engagement.
- Risk of pulpal contamination is decreased once pulp space is exposed.
- Superfluous patient conversation is decreased.
- Patients become more relaxed and feel safer.
- A dry operating field is much easier to establish and maintain.

Because of the anatomic form of primary molars, stringent tooth-by-tooth application of a rubber dam, as taught in dental schools, can be quite difficult, frustrating, and time-consuming in restorative dentistry for young patients. The rubber dam procedure does not need to be abandoned, however. The "slit dam" technique is an easier but very effective way to apply rubber dam for the restoration of primary molars (Croll, 1985). The steps for isolation using the slit dam technique are as follows:

1. Select an appropriate rubber dam clamp and secure an 18 in. piece of dental floss to the loop of the clamp.
2. Place the rubber dam on the frame. For pediatric patients, a 5 in. frame is typically sufficient ("nonlatex" dam should be used for patients with sensitivity or allergy to latex).
3. Punch two holes in the dam, one for the most posterior tooth to be isolated and the other for the most anterior tooth to be isolated.

4. Using scissors, cut a slit to connect the two holes in the dam (Figure 5.1a–c).
5. Use rubber dam forceps to seat the selected clamp onto the most posterior tooth being isolated.
6. Carefully stretch the rubber dam over the clamp, extending it to reveal the quadrant being treated. If necessary, a piece of dental floss or a wooden wedge may be used to secure the dam to the mesial aspect of the most anterior tooth.

Figure 5.1 shows the slit dam being used to isolate the teeth to be restored.

Adhesive Primary Molar Tooth Restoration

Because of the availability of preventive and restorative dental materials that can micromechanically or chemically bond to tooth structure, much has changed over the last three decades. The term "adhesive dentistry" applies to certain categories of dental materials, including pit-and-fissure sealants, RBCs, compomers (COs), and GI systems, including resin-modified glass ionomers (RMGIs). Practitioners should be familiar with the indications for the various materials and fully understand the advantages and disadvantages of each. Awareness of the limitations of each class of material and those of specific brands is essential to success with their use. Knowledge of the handling characteristics of each material is also critical to insure that all the advantages of their use will be optimized.

Pit-and-Fissure Sealants

Pediatric dentistry specialists and general dentists treating young children have mixed opinions about pit-and-fissure sealants for primary teeth. The purpose of resin-bonded sealants is to obdurate enamel imperfections so that bacteria and food debris cannot gain

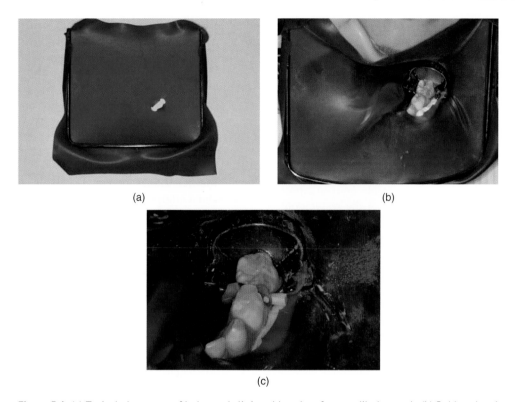

(a)　　　　　　　　　　　　　　　(b)

(c)

Figure 5.1 (a) Typical placement of holes and slit in rubber dam for mandibular teeth. (b) Rubber dam in place, demonstrating "slit dam" technique. Note placement of Molt mouth prop for patient comfort and bite stability. In addition, a cotton roll has been placed in the buccal vestibule for dry isolation. (c) Close-up view of "slit dam" in place creating an ideal operative field.

access to the depths of those imperfections. Bonded resin sealants can succeed in primary molars; however, in very young children, their application requires just as much time and effort as does restoration of those teeth if they develop caries lesions … and often they do not. Many dentists, including these authors, recognize that bonded resin sealants do not adhere as well to properly etched primary tooth enamel, even if an ideal technique is used and the enamel is roughened with a diamond bur. Some practitioners report that they will seal a primary molar with at-risk grooves, for no additional fee, when an adjacent tooth is being restored. For example, if a primary first molar requires disto-occlusal repair, the neighboring primary second molar can be sealed, with the rubber dam already in position. The use of resin-bonded sealants for primary molars

should be considered on a case-by-case basis for children.

Resin-Based Composites

RBC material is used for tooth-colored restorations in primary posterior teeth. When used as indicated and with careful technique in cooperative patients, RBCs have been shown to be effective for Class I, II, and V restorations of primary molars.

RBC materials are classified on the basis of their particle size, ranging from 0.1 μm (microfilled) to 100 μm (macrofilled). Smaller particle size allows for greater polishability and esthetics, whereas larger particle size provides for greater strength. There is a wide range of RBC materials available, each with different physical properties and handling requirements.

Although some of the RBC materials have the strength and durability to withstand heavy chewing forces and have esthetic properties, they do not release fluoride to adjacent tooth structure and require the use of some form of etching and a bonding agent in order to adhere to the tooth preparation. Because RBCs are extremely sensitive to moisture, isolation and attention to proper technique are critical to the success of these restorations. If proper isolation with rubber dam is not possible, one can expect a higher degree of failure of the restoration. In addition, because extra time is required for the placement of RBC restorations, it is best to reserve these materials for patients with good cooperation.

When using these materials, tooth preparation for limited pit-and-fissure caries does not require extension of the preparation into healthy areas of the tooth (i.e., "extension for prevention"). Also, Class II restorations in primary molars should not extend beyond the proximal line angles. Postoperative sensitivity has been reported when bonding agent is applied to dentin that has not been protected with any form of base or liner. This postoperative sensitivity can be minimized by using a GI base or liner before etching and application of the bonding agent and RBC. To summarize, RBC is indicated for the following:

- Class I restorations—pit-and-fissure caries and caries extending into dentin.
- Class II restorations—where caries does not extend beyond proximal line angles.
- Class V restorations.

RBC is contraindicated for patients with a high risk of developing dental caries, uncooperative patients, and patients for whom ideal tooth isolation is not possible.

Compomers

COs (polyacid-modified RBCs) are another category of dental materials that have been used for the restoration of primary molars. Essentially, these are RBC materials with incorporated chunks of hardened GI cement. Although COs have some of the properties of RBCs, they do not provide the same fluoride release and adaptability of traditional GIs and do not quite have the physical strength of standard RBCs. In addition, because these materials are resin based, a completely dry operating field is critical. There appears to be no significant benefit to the use of COs over RBCs.

Resin-Modified Glass Ionomer Restorative Cements

The GI systems (glass polyalkenoate cements) have a long history of use in pediatric restorative dentistry (Killian & Croll, 1991; Croll *et al.*, 1993; Croll, 1995; Nicholson & Croll, 1997). These materials bond chemically to enamel and dentin, have the ability for uptake and release of fluoride to adjacent tooth structure, have thermal expansion similar to tooth structure, are biocompatible, and are less sensitive to moisture when compared to RBCs and COs. However, GIs do not display the degree of fracture toughness, other physical strengths, and wear resistance that are often required in order to withstand the forces of mastication; this has limited their use as stand-alone restorations in primary molars to Class V and some Class I restorations. GIs may also serve as bases or liners beneath RBC materials, providing chemical adhesion to the dentin and fluoride release to support the overlying RBC restoration.

Since their introduction in the early 1990s, RMGI restorative cements have been used successfully in the primary dentition (Croll *et al.*, 2001). The RMGI cements are recommended for Class I, II, and V restoration of primary molars and have all the benefits of traditional GIs (biocompatibility, fluoride release, chemical adhesion to tooth structure, and thermal expansion coefficient similar to tooth structure). The incorporation of resin into the GI formulation has greatly improved wear resistance, physical strengths such as fracture toughness and fracture resistance, and the esthetics of the RMGIs, when compared to traditional GIs. RMGIs harden both by light-curing and by the acid–base glass ionomer setting reaction. The latest version of this material is called a "nano-ionomer" (Ketac™ Nano, 3M ESPE, St. Paul, MN, USA) (Killian & Croll, 2010). This material combines the fluoroaluminosilicate glass particles with nanofiller and "nanofiller clusters" so that color characteristics and polishability are enhanced, along with some physical properties. We consider the nano-ionomer innovation as another step in the continuum of RMGIs approaching the wear, strength, and esthetics of RBCs. Because RMGIs are hydrophilic materials, there is less concern with exposure to moisture, as is the case with RBCs. Proper isolation is still important, but the placement of these materials is less technique sensitive and less time-consuming than the placement of RBCs. This is especially important when dealing with pediatric patients.

RMGI restorative cements are indicated for treatment of Class I, II, and V lesions in primary molar teeth.

Summary

Regardless of the choice of adhesive material for restoring primary molars, the following basic principles apply to all of the materials discussed.

1. Careful isolation of the teeth being restored will maximize the performance of the chosen material.
2. It is important to be familiar with the specific recommendations of the manufacturer regarding indications, application technique, and use of the restorative material. Each category of material discussed (GI, RBC, CO, RMGI) has technique applications that are unique for that material. In addition, within the specific category, a particular manufacturer will have instructions that are unique to that brand of material. Optimization of performance of the materials is achieved by carefully following the manufacturer's recommendations.
3. Tooth preparation should, in most cases, follow traditional outline form, recognizing that some materials (e.g., RBC) may not require "extension for prevention," and a more conservative preparation may be used.
4. For Class II restorations, the use of a segmented matrix secured by a wooden wedge can facilitate the placement of the restoration while maintaining appropriate proximal contact.
5. Consider using mechanical retention as an adjunct to the overall tooth preparation. Although these materials are "adhesive," some chemically adhering to the tooth directly (GI, RMGI) and others adhering to the tooth via use of a bonding agent (RBC, CO), the use of mechanical retention can support the overall retention of the material.
6. Recognize the need for incremental placement of some materials (RBC, CO, RMGI), particularly in larger, deeper restorations. Light-curing needs to be complete at each level of the restoration, and inappropriate bulk placement and bulk curing may lead to restoration failure. This is especially important with the nano-ionomer, because it does not have a chemical resin curing component as do other RMGIs. Note that it is also important to periodically verify that the light emitted from the light-curing device is of an appropriate wavelength and intensity to cure the desired materials. Manufacturers recommend periodic evaluation of the curing light to verify optimal performance. Inadequate light penetration may also lead to failure of the restoration.
7. After placement and curing of the restoration, use burs and hand instruments as well as finishing strips as needed to insure proper contours, contacts, and occlusal relationships. The authors recommend the use of diamond finishing burs for optimal contouring.
8. Document in patients' office records the form of isolation and the specific material(s) used, including any base or liner, the type

of bonding agent, and whether the material was placed in bulk (smaller, shallower preparations) or in increments, as indicated. This will facilitate future assessment of the material's performance.

Figures 5.2a–h, 5.3a–d, and 5.4a–d illustrate the placement of various categories of adhesive restorations in primary molars (Class I, II, and V). The material used for these illustrations is RMGI, and the technique demonstrated in this case is unique to this material, although the overarching principles of adhesive restoration, as described previously, are common to all materials.

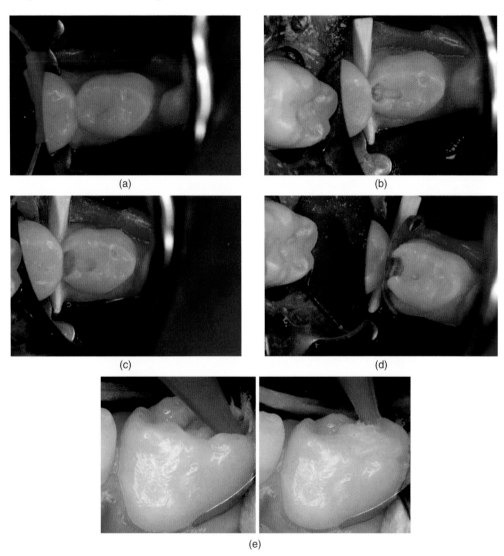

(a)

(b)

(c)

(d)

(e)

Figure 5.2 (a) A 5-year-old child with distal caries lesion of the primary first molar. Tooth isolated using "slit dam" technique. (b) Initial tooth preparation with wooden wedge in place. (c) Carious substance debrided. (d) Contoured matrix strip placed and wooden wedge inserted. (e) First increment of resin-modified glass ionomer (RMGI) material injected and light-polymerized (left). Second increment follows (right). (f) Restoration sculpted with slow-speed round diamond burs. Marginal ridge contoured. (g) RMGI restoration, 2.5 years after placement. (h) Bitewing films, preoperatively (left) and 3 years postoperatively (right).

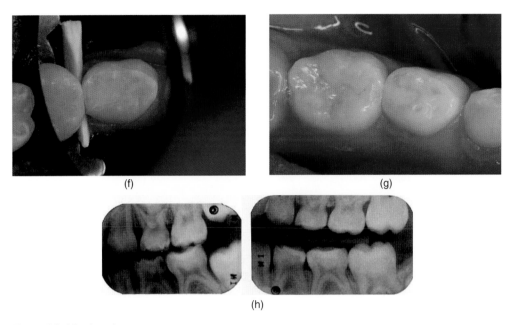

(f)   (g)

(h)

Figure 5.2 (*Continued*)

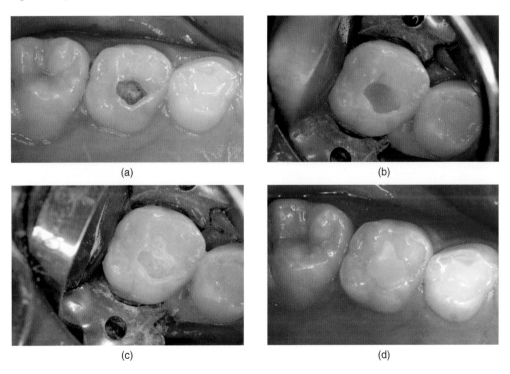

(a)   (b)

(c)   (d)

Figure 5.3 (a) A 6-year-old child with occlusal caries affecting the maxillary second primary molar, tooth isolated for restoration. (b) Carious substance debrided, demonstrating depth of lesion approximating pulp. (c) Hard-setting calcium hydroxide indirect pulp cap placed, followed by the placement of a resin-modified glass ionomer liner. (d) Final restoration, 26 months postoperatively.

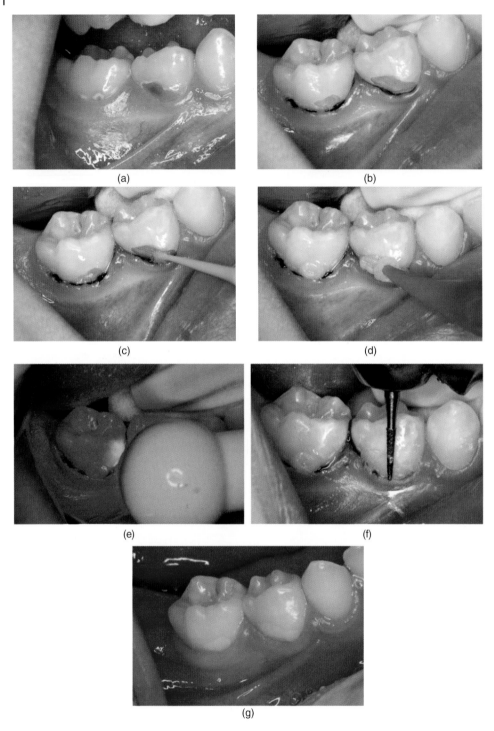

Figure 5.4 (a) A 5-year-old child with Class V caries lesions of the mandibular first and second primary molars. (b) Carious substance debrided and cord in place for hemostasis and gingival retraction. (c) resin-modified glass ionomer (RMGI) primer application; light-polymerization followed. (d) Careful injection of RMGI material into cavity preparation. (e) Light-polymerization. (f) Diamond finishing burs used to contour restoration. (g) Final restoration, 10 months postoperatively.

References

Barbakow, A.Z. (1964) The rubber dam: a 100-year history. *Journal of the Southern California State Dental Association*, 32, 460–464.

Berg, J.H. (1998) The continuum of restorative materials in pediatric dentistry—a review for the clinician. *Pediatric Dentistry*, 20, 93–100.

Christen, A.G. (1977) Sanford C. Barnum, discoverer of the rubber dam. *Bulletin of the History of Dentistry*, 25, 3–9.

Croll, T.P. (1985) Alternative methods for use of the rubber dam. *Quintessence International*, 16 (6), 387–392.

Croll, T.P. (1995) Restorative dentistry for preschool children. *Dental Clinics of North America*, 39 (4), 737–770.

Croll, T.P., Bar Zion, Y., Segura, A., & Donly, K.J. (2001) Clinical performance of resin-modified glass ionomer cement restorations in primary teeth. *Journal of the American Dental Association*, 132, 1110–1116.

Croll, T.P., Killian, C.M., & Helpin, M.L. (1993) A restorative dentistry renaissance for children: light-hardened glass ionomer/resin cement. *Journal of Dentistry for Children*, 60, 89–94.

Francis, C.E. (1865) The rubber dam. *Dental Cosmos*, 7, 185–187.

Hogeboom, F.E. (1953) *Practical Pedodontia or Juvenile Operative Dentistry and Public Health Dentistry*, 6th edn. St. Louis, MO: Mosby; 165–184.

Killian, C.M. & Croll, T.P. (1991) Smooth surface glass ionomer restoration for primary teeth. *Journal of Esthetic Dentistry*, 3, 37–40.

Killian, C.M. & Croll, T.P. (2010) Nano-ionomer tooth repair in pediatric dentistry. *Pediatric Dentistry*, 32 (7), 530–535.

Nicholson, J.W. & Croll, T.P. (1997) Glass-ionomers in restorative dentistry. *Quintessence International*, 28 (11), 705–714.

6

Vital Pulp Therapy for Primary Molars

Jane A. Soxman

Pulpotomy

The goal of vital pulp therapy with pulpotomy is to remove the infected coronal pulp tissue while preserving the healthy radicular pulp. Pulpotomy is recommended in primary molars with extensive caries, complaint of unprovoked spontaneous pain, and with carious or mechanical pulp exposure during caries excavation. Vital pulp therapy is contraindicated with radicular pathology, a sinus tract due to abscess, excessive mobility, presence of purulent material or necrosis in the coronal pulp chamber, or inability to obtain complete hemostasis when performing the pulp therapy (AAPD, 2019–2020a; Winters *et al.*, 2008). The use of a model to describe the pulpotomy procedure to a parent/guardian when obtaining informed consent for the procedure is helpful. Informed consent should include the need for local anesthesia, rubber dam, and a full-coverage crown (Kilgore International, Coldwater, MI, USA) (Figure 6.1).

Radiographic Evaluation

A periapical radiograph should be obtained before performing vital pulp therapy to confirm the health of the radicular pulp, internal or external root resorption, and evaluate caries progression if a period has elapsed since the initial treatment plan (Figure 6.2a). Internal resorption is always associated with extensive inflammation in the primary dentition. The roots of the primary molar are very thin; if internal resorption can be seen on a radiograph, a perforation has usually occurred, and extraction is indicated. The same criteria apply for external resorption (Camp, 2011) (Figure 6.2b).

Local Anesthesia

Local anesthesia with infiltration in the maxilla and inferior alveolar nerve (IAN) block in the mandible should be administered. In younger children, buccal infiltration alone may provide adequate anesthesia in the mandible. A study by Alzahrani *et al.* (2018) found that buccal infiltration with 4% articaine provided equivalent anesthesia to IAN with 2% lidocaine for both pulpotomy and extraction of primary molars in the mandible. If the child appears to be comfortable, with no complaint of pain until the pulp chamber is uncovered, providing immediate additional local anesthesia is indicated. If the discomfort is minimal, a few drops of 2% xylocaine with 1 : 100,000 epinephrine dispensed into the coronal chamber or on a cotton pellet may provide adequate anesthesia to continue the procedure without another injection.

Rubber Dam Isolation

The rubber dam or other equally effective isolation should be routinely used when performing vital pulp therapy (AAPD, 2019–2020a, b).

Handbook of Clinical Techniques in Pediatric Dentistry, Second Edition. Edited by Jane A. Soxman.
© 2022 John Wiley & Sons, Inc. Published 2022 by John Wiley & Sons, Inc.

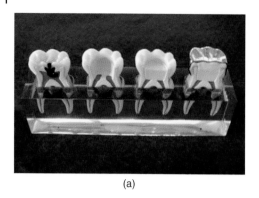

(a)

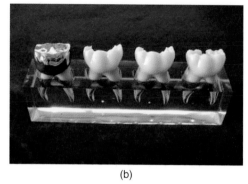

(b)

Figure 6.1 (a, b) Pulpotomy and stainless steel crown model viewed from different sides.

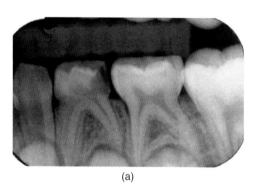

(a)

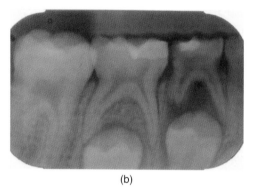

(b)

Figure 6.2 (a) Periapical radiograph of mandibular left first primary molar with carious pulpal involvement. (b) Periapical radiograph with internal and external root resorption.

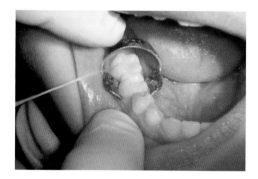

Figure 6.3 W8A rubber dam clamp ligated with floss.

The rubber dam provides a throat partition and protects the oral tissues from exposure to medicaments or injury with the bur or instruments. Multiple colors, nonlatex, and varying thicknesses in $5 \times 5\,\text{in.}^2$ pediatric size are available. The use of a thicker-gauge rubber dam may provide a better seal around the clamp and improved retraction of the surrounding oral tissues. The rubber dam clamp should be ligated with floss to facilitate retrieval should the clamp become dislodged before or during placement of the rubber dam. The W8A rubber dam clamp is typically an ideal fit for a second primary molar (Figure 6.3). If there is difficulty placing the rubber dam over the clamp intraorally, a winged clamp may be used. The rubber dam is placed on the clamp extraorally and then placed on the molar as a single unit with the rubber dam forceps (Figure 6.4a, b). The portion of the rubber dam covering the wings of the clamp is slipped off with an instrument and tucked beneath the wings for good moisture control (Figure 6.4c). Because the tooth is

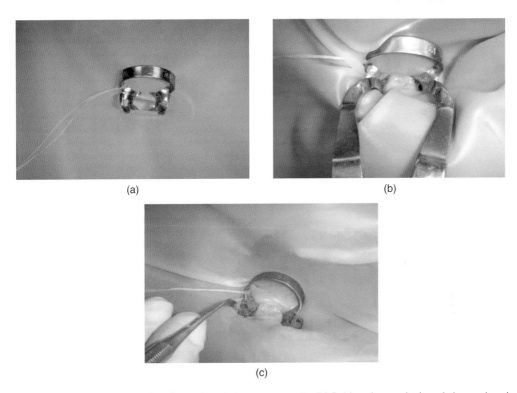

(a)   (b)

(c)

Figure 6.4 (a) Rubber dam placed on winged clamp extraorally. (b) Rubber dam and winged clamp placed intraorally as a unit. (c) Removing rubber dam from wings of clamp.

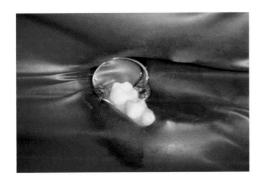

Figure 6.5 Slit technique for rubber dam with floss ligated to clamp under rubber dam.

anesthetized, the rubber dam may be referred to as a blanket to cover the sleeping tooth, when performing "tell–show–do" (discussed in Chapter 23) with a young child. The slit technique may be used to restore a quadrant (Figure 6.5).

Pulpotomy Procedure

Pulpotomy is performed when a pulp exposure occurs during excavation of carious dentin in primary teeth. Direct pulp cap with a biocompatible material is a technique that may be used for a pin-point exposure during caries excavation. This technique has shown limited success and consequently limited acceptance (AAPD, 2019–2020b). Complete caries removal is recommended before entering the coronal pulp. By removing the peripheral caries and prepping from the periphery toward the pulp chamber, the infected tissues will not further contaminate the coronal pulp (Winters *et al.*, 2008).

If a full-coverage crown is the restoration of choice, occlusal reduction for the type of crown selected (stainless steel, zirconia, or preveneered), is performed before unroofing the coronal pulp (Figure 6.6).

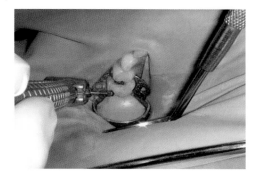

Figure 6.6 Occlusal reduction with large round bur.

After entering the coronal pulp chamber, the pulp tissue is carefully removed to the root canal orifices. Create a large access opening to permit visualization of all canal orifices and remove ledges that could hide tissue tags (Figure 6.7a, b).

A Monoject™ syringe (Kendall Healthcare Products, Seneca, SC, USA) is used for irrigation with sterile saline, sodium hypochlorite, chlorhexidine, or an irrigant of choice. Using water from the dental unit air–water syringe is discouraged unless that water is sterile (Figure 6.8).

Moistened sterile cotton pellets are used to apply pressure and dry the pulp chamber. The tendrils of a dry pellet may pull the clot away from the radicular orifice, inhibiting hemostasis. Size 3 cotton pellets provide more pressure for hemostasis and are more absorbent (Figure 6.9).

A sterile curette may be used to excavate tissue tags causing continued bleeding (Figure 6.10). Follow with irrigation and application of sterile cotton pellets.

Complete hemostasis must be obtained before the medicament of choice is applied. Extensive bleeding indicates degenerative changes; vital pulp therapy is contraindicated. Pulpectomy or extraction should be performed (Winters *et al.*, 2008) (Figure 6.11). Hemostasis should be obtained in 5 minutes. The blood color may provide a diagnostic criterion, with the darkest color indicating more infection and consideration for pulpectomy

(Aaminabadi *et al.*, 2017). Inability to stop hemorrhage indicates a root perforation and extraction is warranted (Figure 6.12).

Medicaments

Primary molar pulpotomy requires a vital radicular pulp, no matter what medicament is used. If the pulp chamber is dry, has an odor, or contains purulent material, extraction is indicated (Seale & Coll, 2010). Various medicaments, along with electrosurgery and laser, have been evaluated by numerous clinical trials. One study reported that if pulpal hemostasis can be obtained within 60 seconds with a cotton pellet, the use of any medicament may not be necessary (Hui-Derksen *et al.*, 2013).

Calcium Hydroxide

A guideline panel convened by the American Academy of Pediatric Dentistry formulated evidence against the use of calcium hydroxide as a pulpotomy medicament (AAPD, 2019–2020b).

Ferric Sulfate

Ferric sulfate (FS) is a hemostatic agent that agglutinates blood proteins. The blood reacts with both ferric and sulfate ions, and the agglutinated protein forms plugs that occlude the capillaries. It provides similar outcomes to formocresol, but offers a nonaldehyde option for those who are concerned about controversy with the use of formocresol. The solution is 15.5% in an aqueous base with a pH of 1 (Fuks, 2012). FS is burnished onto the pulp stumps for 10–15 seconds, rinsed away, and dried with cotton pellets. With decomposition, FS becomes sulfuric acid, which can cause severe burns with contact of oral tissues outside of the coronal pulp chamber (Winters *et al.*, 2008). Internal resorption has been reported with FS (Geneser & Owais, 2018).

Sodium Hypochlorite

Sodium hypochlorite is an effective hemostatic and bactericidal agent that selectively

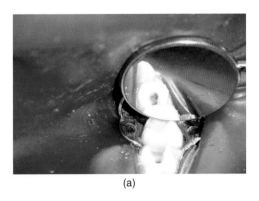
(a)

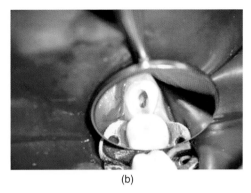
(b)

Figure 6.7 (a) Access opening inadequate to visualize all canal orifices. (b) Enlarged access opening.

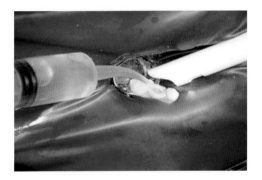

Figure 6.8 Irrigation with Monoject syringe.

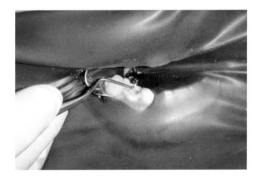

Figure 6.10 Curette to remove tissue tag.

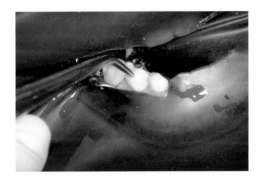

Figure 6.9 Application of sterile cotton pellets.

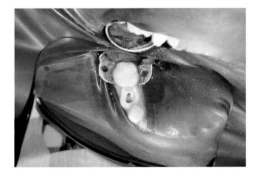

Figure 6.11 Complete hemostasis.

dissolves superficial necrotic tissue without harming deeper tissue. Shabzendedar *et al.* (2013) found that a solution of 3% sodium hypochlorite resulted in the same clinical and radiographic outcomes as diluted formocresol. Other studies show results similar to formocresol and FS. A disadvantage

of sodium hypochlorite is that injection into tissue through a root perforation can result in severe pain, ecchymosis, and swelling. This occurrence is known as a "sodium hypochlorite accident" (Geneser & Owais, 2018).

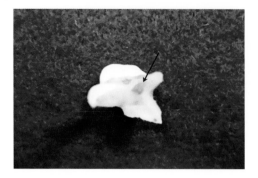

Figure 6.12 Primary molar with root perforation noted following extraction.

Mineral Trioxide Aggregate

Mineral trioxide aggregate (MTA) is a mixture of tricalcium silicate, tricalcium aluminate, tricalcium oxide, bismuth oxide, dicalcium silicate, and calcium sulfate that forms a calcific barrier and is reported to have the highest success rate of all medicaments used in vital pulp therapy (Geneser & Owais, 2018). MTA is highly alkaline, with a pH of 12.5 (Fuks, 2012). It is packaged in a powder form and mixed with sterile water to form a paste. The primary advantage of MTA is an excellent seal provided against bacterial migration, but expense and setting time of about 3 hours are drawbacks. Gray discoloration due to the presence of bismuth oxide has also been cited as a reason for underutilization (AAPD, 2019–2020b; Geneser & Owais, 2018). MTA is covered with a base material such as intermediate restorative material (IRM) before final restoration. MTA dust may cause ocular damage and irritation of respiratory passages. Chemical burns may occur with contact of wet or dry MTA to soft tissues (Winters *et al.*, 2008).

Calcium Silicate

Biodentine® (Septodont, Lancaster, PA, USA) is similar to MTA with its alkaline pH and formation of a calcific barrier. Success rates are comparable to MTA. Advantages are faster setting time and no discoloration of teeth, with the absence of bismuth oxide (Geneser & Owais, 2018). Wong *et al.* (2020) found favorable radiographic and clinical results after 30 months with primary molar pulpotomies using Biodentine.

Formocresol

A guideline panel convened by the American Academy of Pediatric Dentistry formulated evidence-based recommendations for vital pulp therapy in primary molars and found higher evidence supporting the use of MTA and formocresol over other medicaments (AAPD, 2019–2020b). Formocresol has been used for vital pulp therapy for over 80 years, with reported success rates of 62–100%. The formaldehyde component of formocresol provides bactericidal properties and reversible inhibition of numerous enzymes present with the inflammatory process. A superficial layer of fixation, with preservation of the deeper radicular tissues, results with appropriate use of formocresol (Winters *et al.*, 2008; Fuks, 2012). Formocresol was reported to be the most commonly taught medicament for vital pulp therapy taught in training programs (Geneser & Owais, 2018). Rapid metabolism of formocresol to formate and carbon dioxide, with a half-life of 1–2 minutes, occurs with any systemic absorption (Winters *et al.*, 2008).

The liquid formocresol is squeezed from the saturated cotton pellet in a 2 × 2 gauze before snugly being placed over the pulpal stumps in the pulp chamber for 1 minute (Figure 6.13a, b). A 1-minute application of full-strength Buckley's formocresol with a medicated cotton pellet showed comparable success rates to a 5-minute application of the previously recommended one-to-five dilution of full-strength Buckley's formocresol (Kurji *et al.*, 2011; Geneser & Owais, 2018). Only fumes from the pellet are necessary to provide adequate fixation of the superficial pulp tissues. The pulpal floor is very porous in infected primary molars. If the pellet is saturated with formocresol, the agent can penetrate through the accessory canals in the furcation and cause a severe reaction in the furcation tissue. Formocresol cotton pellets are never left in the pulp chamber until a second

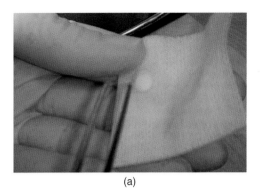

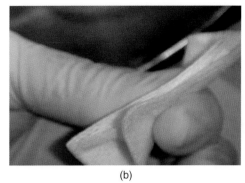

(a)   (b)

Figure 6.13 (a) Saturated formocresol cotton pellet. (b) Compressing formocresol cotton pellet in 2 × 2.

visit, and formocresol is never mixed with IRM because of concern with systemic uptake via the radicular blood supply. Soft tissue burns may occur from contact with formocresol.

The coronal pulp chamber may be filled with IRM, a mixture of reinforced zinc oxide, and eugenol with polymer fibers (Dentsply Caulk, Dentsply Sirona, Charlotte, NC, USA). IRM liquid and powder can be mixed chairside, but triturated capsules save time and clean-up. The mix should be thick enough to form a ball of IRM to be carried to the tooth (Figure 6.14). The IRM is placed in the chamber and compressed with a wet cotton-tipped applicator (Figure 6.15a, b). Although IRM has been traditionally placed in the pulp chamber, the eugenol released has described as cytotoxic (Hilton, 2009). NeoPutty (NuSmile, Houston, TX, USA), glass ionomer, composite, or resin-modified glass ionomer are other filling materials, but cost for multiple layers should be considered and use as a direct pulp cap should be considered. Glass ionomer and resin-modified glass ionomer should not be directly placed over open radicular pulp, as they are not recommended for direct pulp caps. NeoPutty is recommended for direct pulp caps and as such would be a good choice as a base and/or final fill.

MTA may be preferable to IRM for a good seal. Pulpotomized teeth with IRM in the coronal pulp chamber were soaked in methylene blue, sectioned, and evaluated for dye

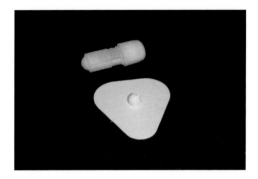

Figure 6.14 Intermediate restorative material (IRM) capsule for trituration with mixed IRM.

penetration. MTA provided a better seal (Farto *et al.*, 2017). However, the cost, set-up time, and discoloration may suggest use of an alternative.

NeoMTA 2

NeoMTA2 (NuSmile) is a bioactive, radiopaque, and nontoxic alternative to formocresol, MTA, and IRM. An inorganic powder of tricalcium and dicalcium silicate is mixed with a water-based gel to a putty-like consistency, with initial setting time of about 15 minutes. One scoop will fill the entire pulp chamber of a first primary molar. A superior seal occurs with the absence of shrinkage during setting and a precipitate of carbonated hydroxyapatite. With no discoloration, the formula is optimized for use under zirconia crowns or composite. A minimum thickness, covering

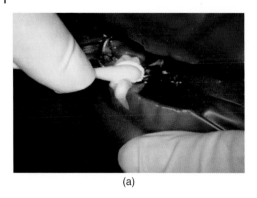

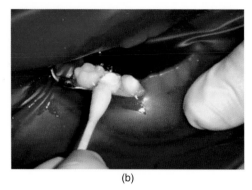

(a)   (b)

Figure 6.15 (a) Intermediate restorative material (IRM) placed with wet cotton-tipped applicator. (b) IRM packed with wet cotton-tipped applicator.

all surrounding dentin, of 1.5 mm is recommended. Restorations can be immediately placed without waiting for setting.

NeoPutty

NeoPutty is a nonstaining premixed MTA-based bioactive, bioceramic material consisting of tricalcium silicate, dicalcium silicate, and a radiopaque agent, titanium oxide. NeoPutty triggers hydroxyapatite and supports healing using the same tri- and dicalcium silicate powders as MTA. With moisture, the silicate cement hardens and calcium hydroxide forms embedded in the cement. An alkaline pH of 12 induces precipitation of calcium phosphate on the surface. This reaction triggers the formation of hydroxyapatite and dentinal bridging. NeoPutty replaces IRM, formocresol, sodium hypochlorite, chlorhexidine, and FS. Different from those materials, NeoPutty is noncytotoxic, hydrophilic, antibacterial, and dimensionally stable. For effectiveness, a 1.5 mm thickness is recommended. If desired by the clinician, NeoPutty may be covered with glass ionomer, composite, resin-modified glass ionomer, or zinc oxide–eugenol (ZOE) to fill the pulp chamber. These materials do not bond to MTA and one cannot etch on top of NeoPutty. If composite is chosen to fill the pulp chamber, a light-cured glass ionomer should first be placed, followed by the composite.

Features include high radiopacity, predictable consistency, no dry-out between uses, immediately washout resistance, and no discoloration of the tooth. Recommended use for direct pulp capping, no mixing with decreased chair time, no discoloration, fast set, and zero waste with a syringe for dispensing are other attractive features.

Restoration

Full-coverage crowns are recommended for the final restoration to insure a good seal, protecting against bacterial infiltration with microleakage. Stainless-steel crowns are typically the restoration of choice, but concerns with esthetics may prompt an alternative restoration. Single-surface (occlusal) restoration with amalgam or composite resin may be performed on a primary molar expected to exfoliate within 2 years (AAPD, 2019–2020b). In a study by Hutcheson *et al.* (2012), primary pulpotomies were treated with white MTA and restored with composite or stainless-steel crowns. More marginal changes were found with composites. After 1 year, 94% of the primary molars restored with composite turned gray (Hutcheson *et al.*, 2012). If esthetics is a priority, preveneered stainless-steel crowns and zirconia crowns offer a more esthetic alternative.

Indirect Pulp Therapy (Indirect Pulp Cap)

Indirect pulp therapy (IPT) is a well-accepted modality to treat deep caries in primary molars without signs or symptoms of pulpal degeneration. The term "indirect pulp cap" may be used synonymously, but IPT is the preferable term. IPT is indicated for asymptomatic primary molars with deep caries approaching the pulp. Percussion elicits no pain, and there is no pathologic mobility. Radiographic examination reveals caries close to the pulp, absence of periapical or furcation radiolucencies, and absence of internal or external root resorption.

The objective of this treatment is to seal and arrest caries, avoid pulp exposure, and maintain pulpal vitality. Peripheral caries and infected dentin are removed and affected dentin, which is remineralizable, is covered with a biocompatible, radiopaque liner to provide the initial seal. The liner may be a dentin bonding agent, resin-modified glass ionomer, ZOE, glass ionomer cement, or calcium hydroxide (CaOH). Although CaOH has a high pH and induces reparative dentin, it has disadvantages of high solubility, inadequate seal, and low compressive strength. Due to these properties, reinforced ZOE or glass ionomer should be placed over CaOH to ensure a seal against microleakage (AAPD, 2019–2020a). A shift from CaOH and ZOE to glass ionomer occurred in 2005. This shift may be the result of using glass ionomer cement as a one-step procedure with liner for IPT and cementing the stainless-steel crown (Dunston & Coll, 2008). Glass ionomer offers additional beneficial properties of an antimicrobial effect on mutans streptococci and a good seal, reducing bacterial microflora due to reduction in nutrients. Vitrebond (3M ESPE, St. Paul, MN, USA), a resin-modified glass ionomer, is commonly used. Bowen *et al.* (2012) reported that IPT studies consistently found success rates of over 90% with CaOH and glass ionomer.

A good seal with the restoration of choice is necessary to insure success. Primary molars with a CaOH base and composite restoration were found to have lower survival compared to total caries removal after 36 months. This was deemed to be due to aprismatic enamel, decreased mineral content of dentin, diminished bond with the CaOH base, and higher water content of the remaining carious dentin in primary molars (Liberman *et al.*, 2020). In general, composite restoration may not be ideal for IPT, because resin's bond to primary teeth is not as strong as to permanent teeth. The combination of poor oral hygiene, high caries history, a multisurface lesion, and soft dentin on the pulpal floor suggest an alternative restoration to insure a good seal.

Re-entry to remove residual caries is not necessary (Dunston & Coll, 2008; Wunsch *et al.*, 2016; Geneser & Owais, 2018; AAPD, 2019–2020a). At 3-year follow-up, Wunsch *et al.* (2016) found that primary molars treated with IPT had significantly greater survival rates compared to pulpotomy with formocresol or FS. Fang *et al.* (2019) had similar findings at 4-year follow-up with IPT showing a significantly higher success rate compared to FS pulpotomy.

IPT is less expensive, has higher success rates with reduced side effects, does not result in the early exfoliation seen with pulpotomy, and is more successful than pulpotomy in treating reversible pulpitis in primary molars (Coll, 2008). However, the decision not to incorporate IPT in practice may be influenced by a low reimbursement rate and the difficulty in accurately diagnosing pulpal status (Bowen *et al.*, 2012). Coll *et al.* (2013) recommends pretreatment with a glass ionomer restoration for 1–3 months. The glass ionomer inhibits progression of caries and may aid in a more accurate diagnosis of pulpal pathology (Coll *et al.*, 2013). Finally, IPT is well accepted, as contemporary caries management and total caries removal may be deemed overtreatment (Liberman *et al.*, 2020).

References

Aaminabadi, N.A., Parto, M., Emamverdizadeh, P., Jamali, Z., & Shirazi, S. (2017) Pulp bleeding color is an indicator of clinical and histohematologic status of primary teeth. *Clinical Oral Investigations*, 21, 1831–1841.

Alzahrani, F., Duggal, M.S., Munyombwe, T., & Tahmassebi, J.F. (2018) Anaesthetic efficacy of 4% articaine and 2% lidocaine for extraction and pulpotomy of mandibular primary molars: an equivalence parallel prospective randomized controlled trial. *International Journal of Paediatric Dentistry*, 28, 335–344.

American Academy of Pediatric Dentistry. (2019–2020a) Pulp therapy for primary and immature permanent teeth. *The Reference Manual of Pediatric Dentistry*. Chicago, IL: American Academy of Pediatric Dentistry; 353–361.

American Academy of Pediatric Dentistry. (2019–2020b) Use of vital pulp therapies in primary teeth with deep caries lesions. *The Reference Manual of Pediatric Dentistry*. Chicago, IL: American Academy of Pediatric Dentistry; 193–206.

Bowen, J.L., Mathu-Muju, K.R., Nash, D.A., Chance, K.B., Bush, H.M., & Li, H.-F. (2012) Pediatric and general dentists' attitudes toward pulp therapy for primary teeth. *Pediatric Dentistry*, 34, 210–215.

Camp, J. (2011) Diagnosis dilemmas in vital pulp therapy. *Pediatric Dentistry*, 30, 197–205.

Coll, J.A. (2008) Indirect pulp capping and primary teeth: is the primary tooth pulpotomy out of date? *Pediatric Dentistry*, 30, 230–236.

Coll, J.A., Campbell, A., & Chalmers, N.I. (2013) Effects of glass ionomer temporary restorations on pulpal diagnosis and treatment outcomes in primary molars. *Pediatric Dentistry*, 35, 416–420.

Dunston, B. & Coll, J.A. (2008) A survey of primary tooth pulp therapy as taught in US dental schools and practiced by diplomates of the American Board of Pediatric Dentistry. *Pediatric Dentistry*, 30, 42–48.

Fang, R.R., Chang, K.Y., Lin, Y.T., & Lin, Y.-T.J. (2019) Comparison of long-term outcomes between ferric sulfate pulpotomy and indirect pulp therapy in primary molars. *Journal of Dental Sciences*, 14, 134–137.

Farto, J., Sahli, C.C., & Boj, J.R. (2017) Microleakage of MTA in primary molar pulpotomies. *European Journal of Paediatric Dentistry*, 18, 183–187.

Fuks, A.B. (2012) Complex pulp therapy. In: Moursi, A.M. (ed.), *Clinical Cases in Pediatric Dentistry*. Oxford: Wiley Blackwell; 89–136.

Geneser, M.K. & Owais A. (2018) Pulp therapy in primary and young permanent teeth. In: Nowak, A.J. & Casamassimo, P.S. (eds.), *The Handbook of Pediatric Dentistry*. Chicago, IL: Academy of Pediatric Dentistry; 137–156.

Hilton, T.J. (2009) Keys to clinical success with pulp capping: a review of the literature. *Operative Dentistry*, 34, 615–625.

Hui-Derksen, E.K., Chen, C.-F., Majewski, R., Tootla, R.G.H., & Boynton, J.R. (2013) Reinforced zinc oxide-eugenol pulpotomy: a retrospective study. *Pediatric Dentistry*, 35, 43–46.

Hutcheson, C., Seale, N.S., McWhorter, A., Kerins, C., & Wright, J. (2012) Multi-surface composite vs stainless steel crown restorations after mineral trioxide aggregate pulpotomy: a randomized controlled trial. *Pediatric Dentistry*, 34, 460–467.

Kurji, Z.A., Sigal, M.J., Andrews, P., & Titley, K. (2011) A retrospective study of a modified 1-minute formocresol pulpotomy technique. Part I: clinical and radiographic findings. *Pediatric Dentistry*, 33, 131–138.

Liberman, J., Franzon. R., Guimaraes, L.F., Casagrande, L., Haas, A.N., & Araujo, F.B. (2020) Survival of composite restorations after selective or total caries removal in primary teeth and predictors of failures: a 36-months randomized controlled trial. *Journal of Dentistry*, 93 (February), 103268.

Seale, N.S. & Coll, J.A. (2010) Vital pulp therapy for the primary dentition. *General Dentistry*, 58, 194–200.

Shabzendedar, M.S., Mazhari, F., Alami, M., & Talebi, M. (2013) Sodium hypochlorite vs formocresol as pulotomy medicaments in primary molars. *Pediatric Dentistry*, 35, 329–332.

Winters, J., Cameron, A., & Widmer, R. (2008) Pulp therapy for primary and immature permanent teeth. In: Cameron, A.C. & Widmer, R.P. (eds.), *Handbook of Pediatric Dentistry*, 3rd edn. St. Louis, MO: Mosby; 95–113.

Wong, B.J., Fu, E., & Mathu-Muju, K.R. (2020) Thirty-month outcomes of biodentine pulpotomies in primary molars: a retrospective review. *Pediatric Dentistry*, 42, 293–299.

Wunsch, P.B., Kuhnen, M.M., Best, A.M., & Brickhouse, T.H. (2016) Retrospective study of the survival rates of indirect pulp therapy versus different pulpotomy medicaments. *Pediatric Dentistry*, 38, 406–411.

7

Pulpectomy for Primary Teeth
James A. Coll

This chapter is intended to give a background on primary tooth pulpectomy and aid the clinician on the step-by-step techniques to successfully perform the procedure.

Clinical Diagnosis

The American Academy of Pediatric Dentistry (AAPD; Coll *et al.*, 2020a) guideline on use of nonvital pulp therapy for primary teeth states that the type of pulpal treatment depends on whether the pulp is vital or nonvital. Pulpal vitality assessment is based on reaching one of three clinical diagnostic assessments: normal pulp (i.e., a tooth with shallow caries, but symptom free and would respond normally to pulp tests); reversible pulpitis (a tooth with an inflamed pulp that is capable of healing); or irreversible pulpitis/necrosis (an inflamed or necrotic pulp incapable of healing). The clinical diagnosis of irreversible pulpitis and/or necrosis is a primary tooth with any one or more of the following:

1. Sinus tract or gingival swelling not associated with periodontal disease.
2. History of spontaneous unprovoked toothache.
3. Excessive tooth mobility not associated with exfoliation.
4. Furcation/apical radiolucency.
5. Internal/external root resorption.

Pain Evaluation

Teeth having no signs or symptoms of irreversible pulpitis or necrosis, but exhibiting provoked pain of short duration relieved by brushing or analgesics or removing the stimulus, are assessed as having reversible pulpitis and are capable of healing. There is evidence in primary molars (Farooq *et al.*, 2000) that pain can last up to 20 minutes and still be reversible pulpitis, because a child may complain while a piece of candy or food is lodged in the cavitated or interproximal lesion. According to Camp (2008), spontaneous pain is a persistent or throbbing pain that occurs without provocation or persists long after the causative factor has been removed. In a histologic study of deep carious lesions in primary teeth (Guthrie *et al.*, 1965), it was demonstrated that a history of spontaneous toothache is associated with extensive histologic pulpal degenerative changes that can extend into the root canals. A child with a history of spontaneous pain in a primary tooth should not receive a vital pulp treatment, because they are candidates for pulpectomy or extraction (Camp, 2008). A normal pulp is a symptom-free tooth with normal response to appropriate pulp tests. For primary teeth, the appropriate clinical tests are palpation, percussion, and mobility, as thermal and electric pulp tests are unreliable (Camp, 2008). Teeth diagnosed as having a "normal

Handbook of Clinical Techniques in Pediatric Dentistry, Second Edition. Edited by Jane A. Soxman.
© 2022 John Wiley & Sons, Inc. Published 2022 by John Wiley & Sons, Inc.

pulp" or "reversible pulpitis" are classified as having vital pulps and treated with vital pulp therapy. Teeth diagnosed as having "irreversible pulpitis or necrosis" are treated with extraction, lesion sterilization tissue repair (LSTR), or pulpectomy for primary teeth (Coll *et al.*, 2020a).

Any planned pulpectomy treatment must include consideration of the restorability of the tooth, the patient's medical history, whether to extract, how long is the likely exfoliation of the tooth in question, and the importance of the tooth to prevent space loss (especially second primary molars before the first permanent molar has erupted).

Interim Therapeutic Restorations for Diagnosis

The diagnosis of the primary tooth's vitality is not always straightforward. A primary molar with deep distal caries near the pulp without gingival swelling, but that has pain of a short duration when the child chews a candy, can be easily misdiagnosed as vital. Performing vital pulp treatment with a pulpotomy on such a tooth can fail because of misdiagnosis (Figure 7.1a, b).

The only way to accurately diagnose the degree of the pulp's inflammation is histologically. There is almost no correlation between the clinical symptoms the child presents with and the histopathologic condition of the tooth, which complicates diagnosis of pulpal health in children (Mass *et al.*, 1995). A patient may present with signs and symptoms that indicate reversible pulpitis, while if the pulp was histologically examined it would demonstrate changes equivalent to chronic total pulpitis and need a pulpectomy or extraction (Seltzer *et al.*, 1963).

A clinical adjunct to help the clinician reliably determine the pulp's vitality has been published. Coll *et al.* (2013) studied 117 primary molars with deep carious lesions that were planned to have vital pulp therapy treatment. It was found that using a glass ionomer interim therapeutic restoration (ITR) before treatment for 1–3 months accurately diagnosed the primary molar's pulp vitality in 94% of the cases, compared to 78% of the teeth when no ITR was used. For teeth with pain, there were 18 patients who presented with pain as the chief complaint, which was not reported by Coll *et al.* (2013). In these 18 patients, the dentist was not sure whether the pain was reversible or irreversible pulpitis. All received ITRs, and 17 of the 18 (94%) were correctly diagnosed with either reversible or irreversible pulpitis. Using a glass ionomer ITR for 1–3 months will reliably diagnose the vitality of those molars with deep caries. If the tooth's

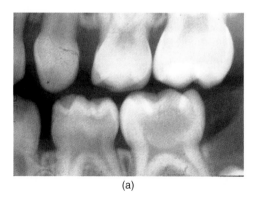
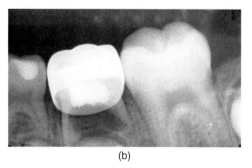

(a)   (b)

Figure 7.1 (a) Diagnosis is not always straightforward, as seen in this second primary molar with deep caries and pain of short duration. A vital pulpotomy was planned because the tooth's pulp was judged as vital. (b) Same tooth 11 months after formocresol pulpotomy showing failure from misdiagnosis.

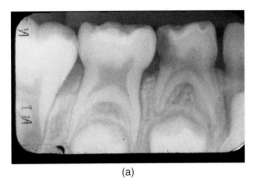 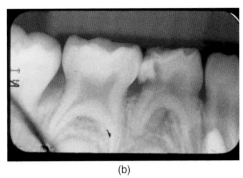

(a)	(b)

Figure 7.2 (a) Pretreatment radiograph of a mandibular first primary molar without soft tissue swelling, but an unclear history of pain that made the dentist unsure of the diagnosis. An interim therapeutic restoration using glass ionomer cement was placed. (b) One week later, the patient had a gingival swelling without pain, finalizing the diagnosis as irreversible pulpitis.

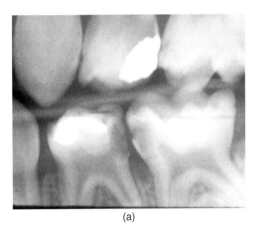 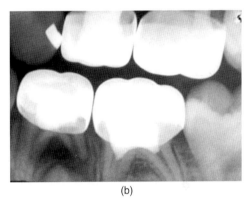

(a)	(b)

Figure 7.3 (a) Pretreatment radiograph of a mandibular first primary molar with distal caries radiographically into the pulp in a patient aged 4.5 years. No interim therapeutic restoration was placed, and a vital formocresol pulpotomy was performed because pulpal bleeding was controlled with a cotton pellet. (b) Same first primary molar showing formocresol pulpotomy failure 24 months later. The tooth's pulp had irreversible pulpitis, which was not clinically apparent and is a contraindication for vital pulp treatment.

pulp is irreversibly inflamed or necrotic after ITR, it will show either a sinus tract, obvious radiographic signs, or pain (Figure 7.2a, b).

One unpublished radiographic finding concerns distal caries in lower primary first molars. If the bitewing shows the caries radiographically into the pulp, it appears from my experience that the pulps of these teeth are irreversibly inflamed, as pulpotomies appear to fail in these situations. From my clinical experience and research I conducted (Coll *et al.*, 2013), distal radiographic decay into the pulp on a bitewing radiograph in mandibular

primary first molars is usually irreversibly inflamed or necrotic (Figure 7.3a, b).

Clinical Evaluation and History

The clinical evaluation involves assessing the child for signs and symptoms of irreversible pulpitis or necrosis clinically or by history. This will include an extraoral examination asking about and looking for facial swelling or tenderness. Question the caregiver as to a history of fever and, if needed, use a thermometer to check for any elevation in temperature. Questioning the child will not always yield reliable information as to the history of pain. Ask the parent or caregiver: "Has your child awakened in the middle of the night, like at 2 a.m., with pain?" Do not simply say: "Has your child awakened with pain at night?" A cavitated lesion in a primary molar may cause pain at bedtime, but not have irreversible pulpitis. The child can have a snack at bedtime and go to bed without brushing the teeth. A reversibly inflamed pulp can then cause the child to complain of "pain at night," which is not spontaneous pain. As stated previously, the duration of pain in a primary tooth is not a critical assessment as to the degree of pulpal inflammation (Farooq *et al.*, 2000). A large cavitated lesion in a primary molar can get a gummy candy or food lodged in it and cause pain for an extended duration in a child, but the pulp may not be irreversibly inflamed. In my opinion, the history of the present toothache is the most important information the dentist can obtain to determine the vitality of the tooth.

Percussion, Mobility, and Pulp Tests

After completing the history, perform an intraoral examination of the area of concern. Be aware that a parent can claim that pain is in the lower right because they see a carious lesion in their child's lower right first primary molar. The child may have held his or her hand on the right side of the face and said his or her tooth hurt. The parent may mistakenly assume that the pain is from the lower right first primary molar. However, the pain is actually from a maxillary right molar the parent never looked at. Look for teeth with caries that show a missing filling, soft tissue redness, fluctuance, or a draining fistula. Percussion can be a valuable aid in diagnosing whether the tooth has irreversible pulpitis due to the infection, causing pressure in the periodontal ligament.

However, the reliability of the child's response has to be assessed due to apprehension and the child's maturity. I recommend using a finger to press on a nonsuspicious tooth first. Then, press on the suspicious tooth and look for any sign of discomfort in the child's expression. Do not use an instrument handle to tap on the tooth, because this can be misunderstood in a child as pain. Tooth mobility in an infected primary incisor may be the only clinical sign of dental infection, especially if diagnostic radiographs are unable to be taken. Maxillary primary incisors in children younger than 4 years that are mobile with large caries are likely infected. The dentist must be aware of physiologic root resorption, but a slightly mobile primary molar in a child aged 6 years or younger would indicate an abscess. However, many infected primary molars do not exhibit mobility. Other pulp tests for primary teeth such as cold, hot, and electric pulp tests are of little use in children due to the unreliable responses (Camp, 2008; Flores *et al.*, 2007).

Tooth Color Change

A temporary tooth color change occurring in primary incisors after trauma in many cases does not indicate necrosis. Holan (2004) studied 97 primary incisors that exhibited dark discoloration after trauma. In 52% of the dark incisors, the color became yellowish, while 48% remained dark. Clinical signs of infection were associated with the incisors that remained dark. The teeth that lightened in color showed pulp canal narrowing or obliteration, but in most cases no infection. Holan (2004) reported on 48 incisors that retained their dark color and found all were clinically and radiographically asymptomatic, but only 2.1% had vital pulps. I did a study on primary incisor trauma that I never published. It was a retrospective analysis of 45 teeth, with concussion blows followed a mean of 47 months. The parents brought most of the children 7–14 days after trauma, because most presented with a gray color within 1 month after trauma. After their final examination or a minimum of 24 months, 86% were a normal or light yellow color and radiographically showed narrowing or obliteration of their root canals. So, in diagnosing traumatized primary incisors for pulp treatment, watchful waiting is a good rule, and if a fistula or other sign of pulp infection is seen, then perform treatment. Be aware that a pulpectomy in a dark primary incisor does not lighten the tooth's color. An avulsed primary tooth should not be reimplanted and have a pulpectomy performed (Flores *et al.*, 2007).

Pulpal Bleeding

When opening into the pulp from a carious exposure, a large exposure likely means the pulpal inflammation is extensive and/or necrotic, so a pulpectomy or extraction is needed (Camp, 2008). It is problematic to assess the color of the pulpal bleeding and correlate the color to the degree of inflammation. In 2018, a study was published by Mutluay *et al.* on primary molars with carious pulp exposures. It showed there was no direct association between the achievement of hemostasis and the inflammatory status of the dental pulp. Coll *et al.* (2020a) state that irreversible pulpitis in a primary tooth should

not be based solely on bleeding that cannot be stopped within 5 minutes, as recommended in the AAPD guidelines, but that controlling bleeding from the exposure site or canal orifices can be misleading for diagnosing vital pulp treatment.

Radiographic Assessment

Radiographic evaluation with good-quality films is essential to help obtain the proper diagnosis of a primary tooth suspected to have irreversible pulpitis or necrosis. In primary molars, the initial irreversible pulpitis radiographic sign is furcation radiolucency (Camp, 2008). Lugliè *et al.* (2012) found that 77% of the primary molars studied had accessory canals in the furcation area, explaining why the radiolucency appears there first. In permanent molars, the radiolucency appears at the apex because it is where most accessory canals are located. The size of the furcation radiolucency in a primary molar is not a contraindication to pulpectomy (Coll & Sadrian, 1996) (Figure 7.4a, b).

As the furcation area in primary molars is critical to evaluate for signs of radiolucency, both a bitewing and a periapical radiograph should be exposed. The bitewing will always be taken with a parallel technique giving the best

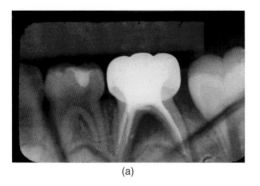
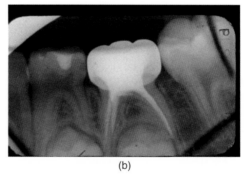

(a)   (b)

Figure 7.4 (a) Immediate post zinc oxide and eugenol pulpectomy radiograph of a mandibular second primary molar showing large radiolucency. Size of radiolucency or gingival swelling is not a contraindication for a pulpectomy. (b) Sixteen months post-treatment radiograph of same second molar that was asymptomatic. It exhibits bone fill and shows that the size of the pretreatment radiolucency is not a contraindication for pulpectomy.

undistorted view of the furcation. Secondly, if there is a proximal or occlusal carious lesion, the bitewing gives a reliable assessment of the depth of decay. The periapical film will help determine any apical root resorption and together with the bitewing allows a proper assessment of the succedaneous tooth's eruption status.

Root Resorption

Owing to the depth of decay and the succedaneous tooth's follicle, radiographic interpretation can be a problem. Proximal lesions in primary molars fail the most often with vital pulp treatments compared to non-proximal lesions (Coll *et al.*, 2013). In maxillary primary molars, the superimposition of the follicle over the primary root makes assessment of root resorption difficult at times. From the study of Coll and Sadrian (1996), the one factor radiographically that predicted primary tooth pulpectomy success was preoperative root resorption. From 81 primary teeth receiving zinc oxide–eugenol (ZOE) pulpectomy and followed over 7 years, it was found that teeth with greater than 1 mm of root resorption had only 23% pulpectomy success ($p = 0.001$) (Coll & Sadrian, 1996). Therefore, examine a primary tooth carefully for any internal or external root resorption. If root resorption is seen, as in the distal root in Figure 7.3b, extraction of the primary tooth is indicated. Pulpectomy is recommended for teeth diagnosed with irreversible/necrotic pulps (Coll *et al.*, 2020b). This recommendation applies to teeth without root resorption, since the 24-month success rates were much higher in teeth without root resorption compared to those with root resorption from a meta-analysis.

LSTR treatment is recommended in teeth with significant internal or external root resorption that one wishes to keep in the arch for up to 12 months (Coll *et al.*, 2020a). The example would be a second primary molar that one wishes to try to maintain until the first permanent molar erupts, and a fixed-space maintainer can be made. If root resorption is found and one wishes to try to maintain a second primary molar for 12 months or so, LSTR using a nontetracycline 3-Mix is the recommended treatment over pulpectomy. LSTR treatment must be monitored closely, with clinical exams and radiographs at least every 12 months. The LSTR technique involves cleaning the pulp chamber after accessing it, then it is dried, 3-Mix paste placed in the floor of the pulp, and then the tooth is restored.

Pulpectomy Filler Research and Resorption

The guideline states that Endoflas® FS (Sanlor, Cali, Colombia) and ZOE may be better choices based on a network analysis compared to the iodoform fillers Vitapex® (Neo Dental International, Federal Way, WA, USA) and Metapex® (Meta-Biomed, Colmar, PA, USA) (Coll *et al.*, 2020b).

ZOE is the most commonly used pulpectomy filler for primary teeth in the United States (Dunston & Coll, 2008). Eugenol is said to have anti-inflammatory and analgesic properties, and ZOE has antibacterial properties, but the disadvantages of ZOE in primary tooth pulpectomy are irritation to the periapical tissues (Praveen *et al.*, 2011), slow and incomplete resorption (Sadrian & Coll, 1993), and alteration to the path of eruption of succedaneous tooth (Coll & Sadrian, 1996) (Figure 7.5a, b).

Vitapex and Metapex are iodoforms, so they easily resorb when extruded out of the apex or into the furcal area (Figure 7.6a, b) (Nurko *et al.*, 2000). Iodoforms will also resorb inside the root canal, so that a Vitapex pulpectomy will always resorb and at times look analogous to a pulpotomy (Howley *et al.*, 2012; Trairatvorakul & Chunlasikaiwan, 2008). Vitapex combines 30% calcium hydroxide with 40.4% iodoform and 22.4% silicone and other oil-type additives in a yellow paste (Praveen *et al.*, 2011). Metapex has in essence the same

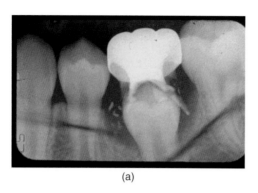
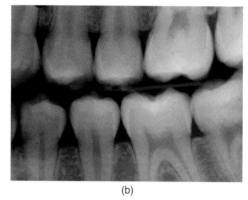

(a)   (b)

Figure 7.5 (a) Same mandibular second primary molar as seen in Figure 7.4 starting to exfoliate 54 months after successful zinc oxide–eugenol (ZOE) pulpectomy. Note small ZOE particles breaking apart around the erupting premolar. (b) Example of ZOE pulpectomy's slow and incomplete resorption 4 years 11 months later. Note one small ZOE particle between the first and second mandibular premolars still present.

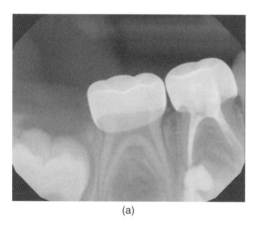
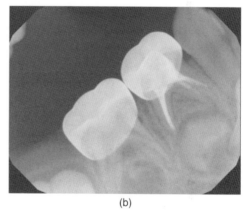

(a)   (b)

Figure 7.6 (a) Example of an immediate post-pulpectomy radiograph showing Vitapex being inadvertently extruded out of the distal canal of this first primary molar. (b) Radiograph of the same first primary molar 6 months later, showing that the Vitapex filler that was extruded has resorbed, and the tooth was asymptomatic without soft tissue pathology from the day of pulpectomy.

composition as Vitapex. Both are supplied in a syringe with disposable plastic tips. Vitapex along with other iodoform pulpectomy pastes has shown bactericidal activity and has no detrimental effect on the succedaneous tooth (Praveen *et al.*, 2011). It never hardens and so it stays as a soluble material. There are no reports of Vitapex filler being over-retained or causing ectopic eruption of the succedaneous tooth.

Endoflas FS is an endodontic paste composed of zinc oxide (56.5%), barium sulfate (1.63%), iodoform (40.6%), calcium hydroxide (1.07%), eugenol, and pentachlorophenol.

Some describe it as Vitapex with zinc oxide (accessed at www.endoflas.com). Endoflas has no published articles indicating that its particles are over-retained after the primary tooth exfoliates, and is not implicated in causing ectopic eruption.

The research on ZOE pulpectomy shows that it is a reliable filler, with success of about 80% with some clinical complications (Casas *et al.*, 2004; Coll & Sadrian, 1996). ZOE is pure ZOE, while intermediate restorative material (IRM) should not be used because the latter resorbs poorly. Coll and Sadrian (1996) retrospectively studied 81 ZOE pulpectomies (51 molars and 30 incisors) followed for a mean of 90.8 months. Overall success was 77.7%, with no difference between molars and incisors. Enamel defects occurred in 18.7% of succedaneous teeth, but they were related to excess pretreatment root resorption of greater than 1 mm. ZOE pulpectomy caused 20% of permanent incisors and premolars to erupt into cross bite or ectopically. One other concern with ZOE filler is its slow resorption. Sadrian and Coll (1993) found that 27% of ZOE pulpectomies had retained filler for a mean time of 40.2 months after pulpectomy tooth loss. Retained filled was related to filler extruded outside the root canal.

In a short-term study of 9 months, Endoflas showed a 95% success rate (Ramar & Mungara, 2010). An 18-month prospective Endoflas study found success of 93%, which was the same as ZOE (Subramaniam & Gilhotra, 2011). Moskovitz *et al.* (2005) has shown long term that Endoflas is a viable alternative to ZOE for use as a pulpectomy filler.

From the aforementioned evidence, the decision of which to use is up to the dentist. However, Endoflas and ZOE seem to have better long-term success than the iodoform fillers.

Pulpectomy Technique

This section describes only primary molar pulpectomy because of space limitations. Primary incisors can also be successfully treated with iodoform pulpectomy fillers in a method similar to that described for molars. The main difference is that the incisor canal is filed with a larger file, such as size #50–60.

After determining that the primary tooth is a candidate for a pulpectomy, recheck that the tooth is restorable. Space loss as a result of large interproximal or excessively deep proximal lesions can make a primary molar difficult to restore. Obtain local anesthesia even if the tooth is necrotic. The soft tissue needs anesthesia, and so the child is not

uncomfortable for the pulpectomy. Plan to perform the final restoration at the same visit as the pulpectomy. I recommend using a rubber dam. The child does not want to taste the hypochlorite that is used, and a rubber dam prevents that from occurring. I have used cotton roll and Isodry® (Zyris, Goleta, CA, USA) isolation techniques for operative dentistry, but would still recommend a rubber dam for the pulpectomy.

After placement of the rubber dam, when doing a steel crown, perform the occlusal reduction first, proximal reduction second, caries removal third, and then enter into the pulp chamber. I use a 330 high-speed bur to enter into the pulp chamber and expose the occlusal part of the pulp chamber. Change to a slow-speed round bur, #4 or #6 depending on the size of the tooth, to remove the overhanging tooth structure. For a first primary molar, I use a #4, but for a second primary molar, I use a #6 slow-speed round bur. One needs to have a good visualization of all the root canal orifices (Figure 7.7).

A mandibular first primary molar will likely have two root canals, but possibly a third canal

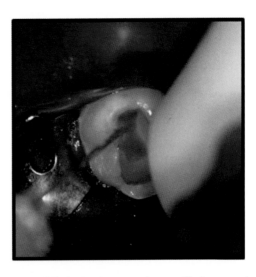

Figure 7.7 Occlusal access of a mandibular second primary molar showing all the root canal orifices without any overhanging tooth structure to hamper visualizing the canals.

in the mesial. A mandibular second primary molar will likely have three canals (mesial buccal, mesial lingual, and one distal canal), but at times there will be two distal canals. A maxillary first primary molar will normally have two canals, but may have a third mesial canal. A maxillary second primary molar will likely have three canals (a mesial lingual, mesial buccal, and a large lingual canal). Identify the canal orifices using a small file, #20 or smaller if needed (Figure 7.8).

Flush the pulp chamber with 5% hypochlorite or dilute the hypochlorite to 2.5% to flush the pulp chamber (Figure 7.9).

I use the #20 file initially to enter each root canal. If the #20 file does not enter the canal very far (<5–8 mm), I will use a #15 or #10 file to negotiate the canal. Usually, a #20 file will negotiate the canal till I can feel an apical resistance point. I use that distance as the working length.

Some dentists advocate using an apex locator, tactile feel, or a digital image for the working length. The AAPD guideline (Coll *et al.*, 2020a) states "that clinicians may choose any of the root length determination methods (tactile, radiographs, apex locators) based on their clinical expertise and individual circumstances." There was no difference in success

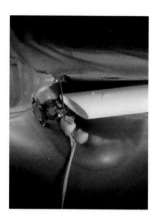

Figure 7.9 Mandibular first primary molar showing liberal use of sodium hypochlorite flushing the canals after each file was used.

using an apex locator versus a radiographic method.

I file each canal by inserting it into the canal till I feel an apical resistance point. Then, I rotate the file 90–180° and withdraw it two or three times. If I feel no resistance point with a size #20, I will go up to a size #25 and then #30. If no resistance point is felt at size #30 (size #40 for large incisors), I assume the tooth has root resorption that was not evident from the preoperative radiograph. At that point, I recommend extraction, rather than a pulpectomy. Assuming there was a resistance point in each canal, I sequentially go through the file sizes up to size #30–35 if I started with a size #20. If I started with a smaller file, I end at size #25–30. Flush the canals with 5 mL or more of hypochlorite after each file. Then, dry the canals with fine-sized paper points. The paper points should come out clean, but may show a slight amount of blood at the tip (Figure 7.10).

The patient's tooth may exhibit excessive bleeding even after filing to size #30–35. If this occurs, either refile the canals, or place into the pulp chamber a slightly moistened full-strength formocresol pellet covered with a temporary filling. After 1–2 weeks, the canals will no longer have excessive bleeding. Or the patient may have a "hot" tooth that will not be adequately anesthetized when one enters the

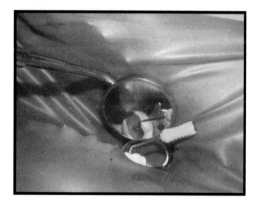

Figure 7.8 A mandibular second primary molar with the initial file inserted using a size #20. It was bent 90° in order to access the mesial buccal canal, which at times is hard to find. The file is rotated 90–180° and withdrawn two to three times in each root canal.

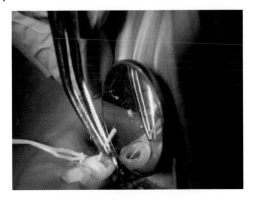

Figure 7.10 Mandibular first primary molar showing the first of multiple fine paper points being used to completely dry the canals. A small amount of blood on the apical tip of the paper point is fine. If there is excessive bleeding, refile the canals.

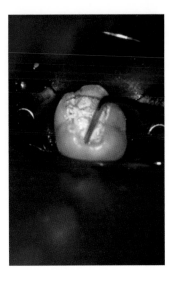

Figure 7.11 Mandibular second primary molar showing zinc oxide–eugenol (ZOE) filler being inserted into the root canals using a root canal plugger. After inserting the ZOE, a slightly moistened cotton pellet is used to compress the ZOE apically.

pulp. If the tooth is too painful when one starts to access the chamber, create a small opening into the pulp chamber. Then, seal in a slightly moistened full-strength formocresol cotton pellet over the small pulpal opening and cover it with IRM or glass ionomer cement. Leave the pellet for 1–2 weeks. The formocresol cotton pellet will denature the vital tissue so that the pulpectomy can be finished without the tooth being painful.

After all the root canal filing is completed and the paper points have been used to dry the canals, it is time to fill the canals. Use pure zinc oxide and eugenol and insert the ZOE with root canal pluggers or with a lentulo (Figure 7.11). Cover the ZOE with IRM or a glass ionomer cement (Ketac™ Molar, 3M ESPE, St. Paul, MN, USA; or Fugi IX GP®, GC Dental, Tokyo, Japan).

Obturating the canals with Endoflas can be done with hand pluggers, lentulo spiral, or a syringe. The Endoflas powder-to-liquid ratio can vary from 1 : 1 if you use a plugger to 1 : 3 for a lentulo and a syringe. Cover the Endoflas with IRM or a glass ionomer cement.

If you are using Vitapex, it is supplied with disposable plastic tips. Place a plastic tip on the Vitapex syringe. Press the syringe plunger till some Vitapex is extruded from the tip. Then,

insert the plastic tip as far as possible into the first canal. Press on the syringe plunger and start withdrawing the tip at the same time out of the root canal. This is a tricky technique. Do the same for each canal. Deposit some of the Vitapex into the floor of the pulp chamber. Use a very slightly moistened cotton pellet to press on the Vitapex that is in the pulp chamber to force it into the root canals (Figure 7.12).

After the Vitapex has been placed, mix a self-setting glass ionomer (Ketac Molar or Fugi IX GP) into the pulp chamber. Use a slightly moistened cotton pellet to apically press the glass ionomer to ensure the glass ionomer is tightly placed over the Vitapex. Then, place the final restoration, which will be a steel crown in most cases. Take a postoperative radiograph for future reference of treatment outcome (Figure 7.13a, b).

Severe postoperative swelling and pain should not occur similarly to what is expected after performing a pulpotomy or indirect pulp cap. One can recommend over-the-counter analgesics for any mild discomfort the child may have. Any preoperative gingival swelling

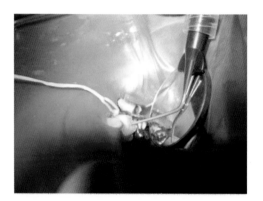

Figure 7.12 Mandibular first primary molar showing the Vitapex syringe with disposable plastic tip being inserted into the distal canal orifice. Press on the syringe plunger with the plastic tip as far into the canal as possible. Begin to slowly remove the plastic tip only when Vitapex filler is seen coming out of the canal opening.

root resorption, or the initial radiolucency is enlarging, or no bone fill after 6–12 months. The whole pulpectomy procedure from rubber dam placement to when the filler is placed, but not including when the final restoration has been placed, takes less than 30 minutes for most teeth.

Lesion Sterilization Tissue Repair Technique

or fistula will resolve on its own without any antibiotic or further surgical treatment within a week or two. If one diagnosed the tooth correctly without any root resorption, one should expect long-term pulpectomy success. Meta-analysis showed significant success rates in obturation with ZOE (92%) and iodoform (71%) at 18 months (Coll *et al.*, 2020a). The Vitapex-filled pulpectomy will likely look analogous to a pulpotomy after a year, but that is not a sign of failure. The signs of pulpectomy failure clinically are pain and/or swelling. Radiographically, failure will show abnormal

LSTR is indicated for primary molars with external and/or internal root resorption that you wish to save for 12 months. Access the pulp chamber and remove any necrotic pulp chamber tissue with a spoon excavator. Then remove any radicular tissue that is easily accessible with broaches or files. Irrigate with 2.5% sodium hypochlorite and rinse with saline and dry chamber. Some dentists enlarge the canal orifices with a round bur to make a "medicated cavity." Use a powdered mixture of the three antibiotics (like clindamycin, ciprofloxacin, and metronidazole) in a 1 : 1 : 1 ratio combined with propylene glycol and/or macrogol to make a paste. Place the antibiotic mixture in the medicated cavity followed by a glass ionomer and a final restoration. The soft tissue pathology should resolve in 7–10 days. The radiologic pathology should resolve or not worsen over the next 12 months.

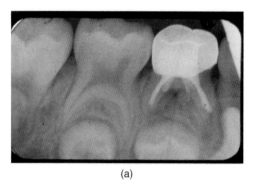

(a)

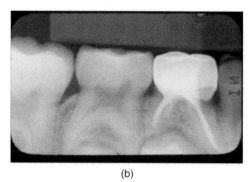

(b)

Figure 7.13 (a) Mandibular first primary molar with a zinc oxide–eugenol pulpectomy showing the day-of-treatment radiograph used as a reference film with a small furcation radiolucency. (b) Same mandibular first primary molar 1 year after treatment, showing bone fill in the furcation compared to the immediate post-treatment film.

References

Camp, J.H. (2008) Diagnosis dilemmas in vital pulp therapy: treatment for the toothache is changing, especially in young, *immature teeth*. *Pediatric Dentistry*, 30 (3), 197–205.

Casas, M.J., Kenny, D.J., Johnston, D.H., & Judd, P.L. (2004) Long-term outcomes of primary molar ferric sulfate pulpotomy and root canal therapy. *Pediatric Dentistry*, 26 (1), 44–48.

Coll, J.A., Campbell, A., & Chalmers, N. (2013) Effects of glass ionomer temporary restorations on pulpal diagnosis and treatment outcomes in primary molars. *Pediatric Dentistry*, 35 (5), 416–421.

Coll, J.A., Dhar, V., Vargas, K., Chen, C.-Y., Crystal, Y.O., *et al.* (2020a) Use of nonvital pulp therapy for primary teeth. *Pediatric Dentistry*, 42 (5), 337–349.

Coll, J.A. & Sadrian, R. (1996) Predicting pulpectomy success and its relationship to exfoliation and succedaneous dentition. *Pediatric Dentistry*, 18 (1), 57–63.

Coll, J.A., Vargas, K., Marghalani, A.A., Chen, C.-Y., AlShamali, S., *et al.* (2020b) A systematic review and meta-analysis of nonvital pulp therapy for primary teeth. *Pediatric Dentistry*, 42 (4), 256–272.

Dunston, B. & Coll, J.A. (2008) A survey of primary tooth pulp therapy as taught in US dental schools and practiced by diplomats of the American Board of Pediatric Dentistry. *Pediatric Dentistry*, 30 (1), 42–48.

Farooq, N.S., Coll, J.A., Kuwabara, A., & Shelton, P. (2000) Success rates of formocresol pulpotomy and indirect pulp therapy in the treatment of deep dentinal caries in primary teeth. *Pediatric Dentistry*, 22 (4), 278–286.

Flores, M.T., Holan, G., Borum, M., & Andreasen, J.O. (2007) Injuries to the primary dentition. In: Andreasen, J.O., Andreasen, F., & Andersson, L. (eds.), *Textbook and Color Atlas of Traumatic Injuries to the Teeth*, 4th edn. Oxford: Blackwell Munksgaard; ch. 22.

Guthrie, T.J., McDonald, R.E., & Mitchell, D.F. (1965) Dental hemogram. *Journal of Dental Research*, 44, 678–682.

Holan, G. (2004) Development of clinical and radiographic signs associated with dark discolored primary incisors following traumatic injuries: a prospective controlled study. *Dental Traumatol*, 20 (5), 276–287.

Howley, B., Seale, N.S., McWhorter, A.G., Kerins, C., Boozer, K.B., & Lindsey, D. (2012) Pulpotomy versus pulpectomy for carious vital primary incisors: randomized controlled trial. *Pediatric Dentistry*, 34 (5), 112–119.

Luglié, P.F., Grabesu, V., Spano, G., & Lumbau, A. (2012) Accessory foramina in the furcation area of primary molars. A SEM investigation. *European Journal of Paediatric Dentistry*, 13 (4), 329–332.

Mass, E., Zilberman, U., & Fuks, A.B. (1995) Partial pulpotomy: another treatment option for cariously exposed permanent molars. *ASDC Journal of Dentistry for Children*, 62 (5), 342–345.

Moskovitz, M., Sammara, E., & Holan, G. (2005) Success rate of root canal treatment in primary molars. *Journal of Dentistry*, 33 (1), 41–47.

Mutluay, M., Arikan, V., Sari, S., & Kisa, O. (2018) Does achievement of hemostasis after pulp exposure provide an accurate assessment of pulp inflammation? *Pediatric Dentistry* 40 (1), 37–42.

Nurko, C., Ranley, D.M., Garcia-Godoy, F., & Lakshmyya, K.N. (2000) Resorption of a calcium hydroxide/iodoform paste (Vitapex) in root canal therapy for primary teeth: a case report. *Pediatric Dentistry*, 22 (6), 517–520.

Praveen, P., Anantharaj, A., Venkataragahavan, K., Rani, P., Sudhir, R., & Jaya, A.R. (2011) A review of obturating materials for primary teeth. *Streamdent*, 20 (20), 1–3.

Ramar, K. & Mungara, J. (2010) Clinical and radiographic evaluation of pulpectomies using three root canal filling materials: an in-vivo study. *Journal of the Indian Society of Pedodontics and Preventive Dentistry*, 28 (1), 25–29.

Sadrian, R. & Coll, J.A. (1993) A long-term follow up on the retention rate of zinc oxide eugenol filler after primary tooth pulpectomy. *Pediatric Dentistry*, 15 (4), 249–253.

Seltzer, S., Bender, I.B., & Ziontz, M. (1963) The dynamics of pulp inflammation: correlations between diagnostic data and actual histologic findings in the pulp. *Oral Surgery, Oral Medicine, Oral Pathology*, 16, 969–977.

Subramaniam, P. & Gilhotra, K. (2011) Endoflas, zinc oxide eugenol and metapex as root canal filling materials in primary molars—a comparative clinical study. *Journal of Clinical Pediatric Dentistry*, 35 (4), 365–369.

Trairatvorakul, C. & Chunlasikaiwan, S. (2008) Success of pulpectomy with zinc oxide-eugenol vs calcium hydroxide/iodoform paste in primary molars: a clinical study. *Pediatric Dentistry*, 30 (4), 303– 308.

8

Full-Coverage Restoration for Primary Molars

Jane A. Soxman, Ehsan N. Azadani, and Paul S. Casamassimo

When Crowns are the Best Restoration

Full-coverage restoration of a primary tooth with a crown is indicated when two or more surfaces are affected by dental caries, or the crown damage from dental caries is too extensive for the remaining tooth structure to support an intracoronal restoration. Primary teeth receiving pulp therapy are best treated with crowns to accommodate physical weakness caused by loss of structure and to prevent leakage of oral fluids into teeth that compromises pulp therapy success. Crowns are also indicated when tooth destruction is extensive from caries or trauma and restoration of occlusion would not be successful with intracoronal restorations. Crowns may also be the best choice for multisurface caries repair in high caries-risk children due to increased susceptibility of remaining enamel to future caries. Although rubber dam isolation is recommended for crown preparation, crowns are also less technique sensitive or compromised by fluid contamination during placement, compared to composite restorations.

Evidence available today supports the choice of a crown as the longest-lasting primary tooth restoration, superior to both amalgam and composite restorations (AAPD, 2019–2020). Maupome *et al.* (2017) recommend a stainless-steel crown (SSC) for proximal caries when the restoration should last longer than 2 years or when the child is under age 6. Mandibular first primary molars initially treated with an SSC compared to amalgam or composite had better longevity (Maupome *et al.*, 2017). SSCs have been shown to be significantly more successful than any other restorative or preventive technique in preventing the need for repeat restorative treatment, especially in very young children who undergo dental general anesthesia (Azadani *et al.*, 2020). A well-done SSC, placed on a primary tooth with good pulpal prognosis, for example, should last the lifetime of that primary tooth. The superiority of an SSC is not only for its physical properties, but also due to the fact that it provides full coverage and prevents future recurrent caries for the tooth. Therefore, SSCs are the best choice for young children with high caries risk. The cost of initial treatment with crowns may exceed that of other restorations, but when retreatment to replace failed complex fillings is considered, as well as the need for repeated pharmacologic behavior management techniques to accomplish replacement, the crown may be most cost-effective restoration in the life span of a primary tooth.

Stainless-Steel Crowns

SSCs are the restoration of choice for primary molars of children with high caries risk, after pulpotomy or pulpectomy, for large, multisurface caries, circumferential caries,

Handbook of Clinical Techniques in Pediatric Dentistry, Second Edition. Edited by Jane A. Soxman.
© 2022 John Wiley & Sons, Inc. Published 2022 by John Wiley & Sons, Inc.

hypoplastic molars, with sedation or general anesthesia, and/or interproximal preparation that extends beyond the line angle (Velan *et al.*, 2018; AAPD, 2019–2020). The use of SSCs may reduce the need for repeated treatment with general anesthesia (Sheller *et al.*, 2003). SSCs provide a good seal and a durable, reliable restoration (Mahoney *et al.*, 2008).

Some parents/guardians find the appearance of the SSC to be unacceptable, so an SSC should be shown when informed consent is being obtained. With uncooperative behavior, an SSC is preferable to an esthetic crown, as an esthetic crown requires extensive tooth reduction that may create the need for vital pulpotomy and, in general, requires longer chair time. After administering local anesthesia and rubber dam placement, primary molar preparation and crown cementation for an SSC can usually be performed in less than 10 minutes.

Precontoured SSCs accurately duplicate the anatomy of the primary molars and require no buccal or lingual reduction during crown preparation. They provide a highly retentive "snap" fit. These SSCs are ready for immediate use and, unlike uncontoured SSCs, which must be customized with trimming and contouring for adaption, they significantly reduce chair time (Figure 8.1).

Procedure for a Stainless-Steel Crown

- Administer local anesthesia.

- Place rubber dam with slit technique and reduce occlusal surface 1mm with coarse diamond or size 6 or 8 carbide round bur or coarse round end taper diamond bur with high speed (Figure 8.2).
- Perform subgingival interproximal reduction with 169 L or 170 L carbide bur with high speed (Figure 8.3).

When prepping the distal of a second primary molar, use caution to avoid disking the mesial of the adjacent first permanent molar. A wooden wedge, placed between the first permanent molar and the second primary molar, will provide protection for the mesial surface of the first permanent molar. Cut just inside the distal marginal ridge and the mesial side of the wooden wedge (Figure 8.4). Remove the wedge and check for a white spot lesion on the mesial of the first permanent molar (Figure 8.5). If

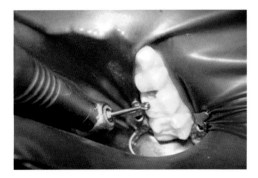

Figure 8.2 Rubber dam with slit technique for 1 mm occlusal reduction with size 8 carbide round bur with high speed.

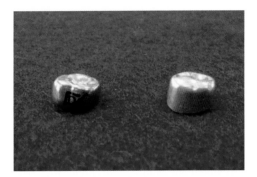

Figure 8.1 Precontoured stainless-steel crown and uncontoured stainless-steel crown.

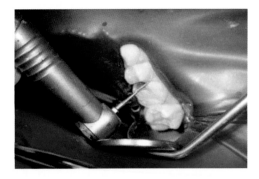

Figure 8.3 Subgingival interproximal reduction with 169 L carbide bur with high speed.

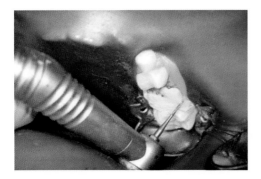

Figure 8.4 Distal reduction of second primary molar with wooden wedge to protect mesial of first permanent molar.

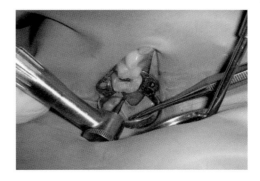

Figure 8.6 Retracting rubber dam with spoon for distal preparation of second primary molar if first permanent molar is unerupted.

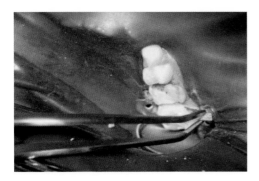

Figure 8.5 Removing wooden wedge and checking mesial of first permanent molar for white spot lesion.

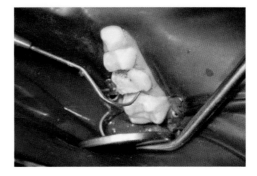

Figure 8.7 Checking for ledge with explorer.

decalcification is noted, fluoride varnish may be applied as a courtesy.

- If the first permanent molar is unerupted and the rubber dam clamp must be placed on the second primary molar, a spoon curette may be used to retract the rubber dam from the distal of the second primary molar during distal interproximal preparation (Figure 8.6). The distal surface, if noncarious, might not need preparation in some instances.
- Check for a ledge on the mesial and distal. Ledges inhibit crown seating (Figure 8.7).
- Select a crown: size 4 is most commonly used.

Measuring the mesial–distal width of the primary molar before preparation with a Boley gauge may be helpful to select the correct size

of SSC. Using this measurement, an SSC is selected (Figure 8.8a, b). After performing the SSC procedure a few times, the clinician will be able to visually estimate the size, and measuring for size selection will no longer be necessary.

- Place the SSC on the tooth, but do not fully seat the crown with the try-in. Check that the SSC covers the entire crown of the primary molar. If fully seated with a "snap" fit, it may be very difficult to remove (Figure 8.9).
- Place the cement of choice inside the crown: carboxylate cement or glass ionomer (GI) is typically used. The wooden end of a cotton-tipped applicator may be used to coat the inside of the crown with the cement (Figure 8.10). Overfilling will cause extrusion of cement and requires more clean-up.

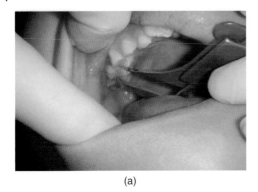

(a)

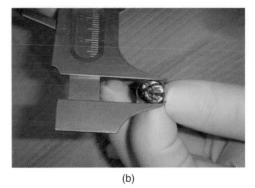

(b)

Figure 8.8 (a) Boley gauge to measure mesial–distal width of primary molar. (b) Boley gauge to measure mesial–distal width of stainless-steel crown.

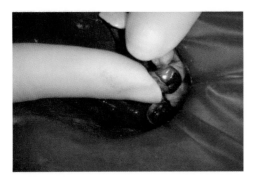

Figure 8.9 Stainless-steel crown checked for size before fully seating.

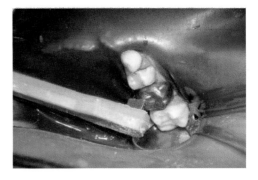

Figure 8.11 Operator seating the stainless-steel crown with a bite stick.

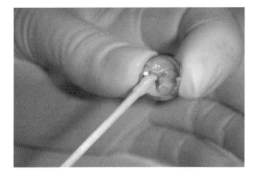

Figure 8.10 Wooden end of cotton-tipped applicator to line inside of stainless-steel crown with cement.

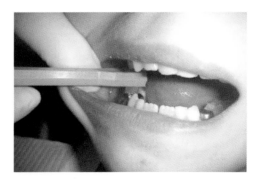

Figure 8.12 Child biting on bite stick to seat stainless-steel crown.

- The crown is first seated by the operator using a bite stick (Figure 8.11). If the crown is not fully seated with a "snap" fit with digital pressure on the bite stick, and the child is capable of cooperating, the rubber dam is removed and the child is instructed to bite on the bite stick as hard as possible (Figure 8.12). The bite stick may initially be placed in the center of the occlusal surface of the crown and then moved to the buccal

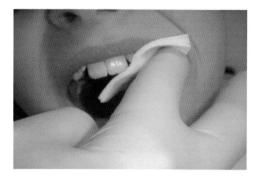

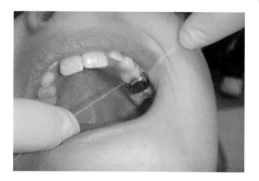

Figure 8.13 Cleaning stainless-steel crown and gingiva with wet 2 × 2 gauze.

Figure 8.14 Floss with knots tied segmentally to remove interproximal cement.

and lingual of the occlusal surface for final seating. Check to be sure that the child's lip is not trapped under the bite stick.

- Gingival tissue may blanch after seating, but this will resolve.
- Cement is cleaned from the crown and gingival tissues with wet 2 × 2 gauze (Figure 8.13).
- Tie five to seven knots segmentally in a strand of floss and pull through the mesial and distal embrasures to remove any excess cement from that area (Figure 8.14).

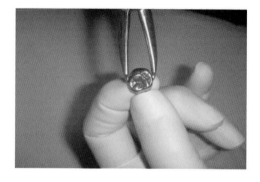

Figure 8.15 Howe plier to reduce mesial–distal size of stainless-steel crown.

Difficulty in Fitting

If space loss has occurred as a result of caries, it may be necessary to reduce the size of an SSC mesial–distally with a Howe plier (Figure 8.15). Because SSCs are not available in half sizes, crimping may be necessary. Crown collars may be crimped with crown and band contouring pliers or band crimping pliers, which perform equally well (Figure 8.16). If unable to find a crown to fit a first primary molar, try a crown from the opposite arch and opposite (contralateral) side. For instance, if unable to

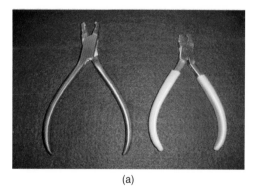

(a)

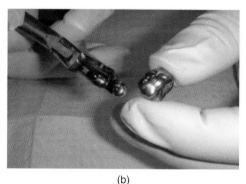

(b)

Figure 8.16 (a) Crown and band contouring and crimping pliers. (b) Crimping a stainless-steel crown with pliers.

find a suitable fit for a maxillary right first primary molar, a crown for a mandibular left first primary molar may be a good fit.

Hall Technique

The Hall technique (HT), developed in the United Kingdom, offers a simplified technique for the SSC procedure without the use of local anesthesia, tooth preparation, or caries excavation. In one study, primary molars with caries radiographically extending greater than halfway into dentin were restored with either HT or standard SSC restoration. The study concluded that the HT, both statistically and clinically, was more successful (Innes *et al.*, 2011). Marginal seal significantly influences crown longevity. In another study, using pre-contoured and pretrimmed SSCs (3M ESPE, St. Paul, MN, USA), microleakage was significantly higher with the HT than with the conventional technique. Regardless of the technique, resin cement showed the lowest microleakage scores, followed by conventional GI and polycarboxylate cements. Buccal margins resulted in higher microleakage scores than lingual margins for both techniques (Erdemci *et al.*, 2014). (HT is also discussed in Chapter 1.)

Esthetic Crowns

When parents/guardians have strong opposition to the appearance of the traditional SSC, preveneered and zirconia crowns offer an esthetic alternative. These crowns are more expensive and require extensive tooth reduction, sometimes creating the need for a vital pulpotomy. Step-by-step clinical instruction may be found on the manufacturer's website, laminated cards with step-by-step instruction, or on a DVD from the manufacturer.

Preveneered Stainless-Steel Crowns

Preveneered crowns (NuSmile Signature, NuSmile, Houston, TX, USA; Kinder Krowns, St.

Louis Park, MN, USA; Cheng Crowns, Exton, PA, USA) are SSCs with composite facings. Light (B1) and extra-light (bleached) shades may be available (Figure 8.17). Preparation of the tooth is more extensive than with SSCs because the veneer is added on to the SSC and crimping may lead to veneer fracture or loss. The inside of the preveneered crown may be sand blasted by the manufacturer to enhance bonding (Figure 8.18). The required interproximal reduction may result in a pulp exposure and need for vital pulpotomy. With inadequate tooth reduction, preveneered crowns can appear bulky. Inability to cooperate for the longer procedure, deep bite, and bruxing may prohibit use of the preveneered crown.

Disadvantages include cost, inability to crimp on buccal or modify the crown

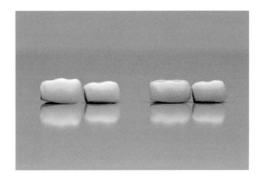

Figure 8.17 Two shades of preveneered stainless-steel crowns. Source: Courtesy of NuSmile.

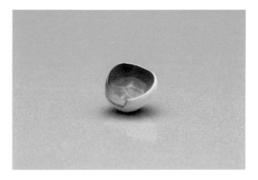

Figure 8.18 Inside view of sand-blasted preveneered stainless-steel crown. Source: Courtesy of NuSmile.

mesio-distally with marked mesio-distal loss of tooth structure due to caries, and fracture or chipping of facings. Adequate occlusal reduction is mandatory to assure light occlusal contact in centric and excursive movement. With bruxing or excessive deep bite, a stainless-steel or zirconia crown may offer a better choice to avoid chipping of the facing.

Heavy occlusal contacts or bruxing can result in fracture of the composite facing. Ram *et al.* (2003) found chipping of facings after 4 years (Figure 8.19). To repair a chipped facing, remove the exposed stainless steel with a high-speed bur, place an opaquer or a resin-modified GI, and follow with light-cured composite resin matching the shade of composite facing.

Informed consent should include possible chipping or loss of facings, longer time required for procedure, and possible addition of a pulpotomy to the treatment plan.

Procedure for Preveneered Stainless-Steel Crowns

Select the crown size before beginning the tooth preparation. Use cotton forceps or a Pic-n-Stic™ (Pulpdent Corporation, Watertown, MA, USA) to hold a preveneered crown next to the primary molar to be restored (Figure 8.20). The preveneered crown will be one to two sizes smaller than a traditional SSC for the same tooth in order to accommodate the addition of the composite facing. Choose a size that looks most similar to the child's tooth.

- Administer local anesthesia and place a rubber dam.
- Reduce occlusal 2 mm with a coarse football diamond or donut diamond bur (Figure 8.21a, b).
- Reduce mesial and distal with fine-tapered diamond or 169 L carbide bur, opening interproximal contacts, and begin circumferential reduction (Figure 8.21c).
- Reduce buccal and lingual with coarse-tapered round-end diamond or carbide bur, creating a circumferential chamfer margin (Figure 8.21d).
- Remove chamfer circumferentially to create a feather-edge margin about 2 mm subgingivally with a fine-tapered round-end diamond bur (Figure 8.21e).

A modified procedure for the preparation may be followed as shown for the zirconia crown in Figures 8.24–8.29. Overall, primary molar reduction is about 30%. Be sure to remove the mesial buccal bulge on the first primary molar. This step will create a smaller preparation and better fit, with a less bulky appearance.

- Check that occlusal reduction is 2 mm before try-in. A 2-mm thick donut diamond bur may be used to check the depth of the reduction or the margin of the adjacent primary molar (Figure 8.21f).

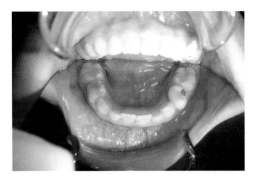

Figure 8.19 Chipped facing on preveneered stainless-steel crown.

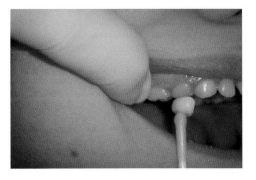

Figure 8.20 Selecting size for preveneered crown.

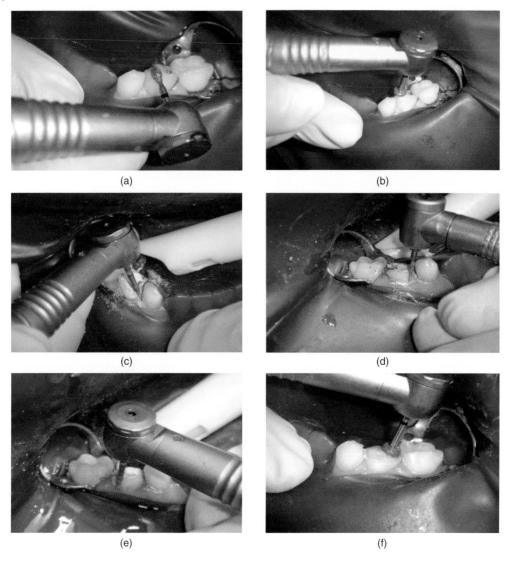

Figure 8.21 (a) Coarse football diamond bur for 2 mm occlusal reduction. (b) Donut diamond bur for 2 mm occlusal reduction. (c) Fine-tapered diamond bur for mesial and distal reduction. (d) Coarse-tapered round-end diamond bur for buccal and lingual reduction, creating a chamfer margin. (e) Fine-tapered round-end diamond bur for circumferential feather-edge 2 mm below gingival margin. (f) Donut diamond bur to check depth of occlusal reduction. (g) Patient biting on cotton roll until cement sets. (h) Checking occlusion with articulating paper. (i) Adjusting occlusion with white stone. (j) Preveneered crown after cementation and checking occlusion with articulating paper.

- Crowns are passively seated with light digital pressure.
- If doing more than one crown, try-in all crowns at the same time, in case additional mesial–distal reduction is required.
- Clean all blood and saliva from the inside of the crown.

- Fill the crown completely with GI cement, or the cement of choice, to prevent voids.
- The crown is seated passively with finger pressure only. There is no "snap" fit as with the traditional SSC, and the collar cannot be crimped. The crown collar should be subgingival.

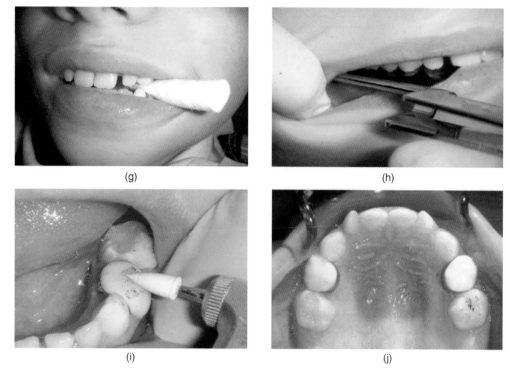

(g)

(h)

(i)

(j)

Figure 8.21 (*Continued*)

- The patient bites on a cotton roll or a cotton-tipped applicator to stabilize the crown until the cement is set, according to the material's setting time (Figure 8.21g).
- Clean with wet 2 × 2 gauze and floss with segmentally tied knots.
- Check the occlusion in centric and excursive movements with articulating paper (Figure 8.21h).
- Adjust the composite facing with a white stone or composite finishing bur (Figure 8.21i). The crown of the opposing primary molar may also be slightly adjusted.
- Check with articulating paper to assure light or no contact on the composite facing (Figure 8.21j).

Common Problems

Inadequate buccal reduction will cause the crown to appear bulky. Inadequate preparation below the gingival margin will impede seating the crown fully and cause occlusion to be high.

Zirconia Crowns

Zirconia crowns (NuSmile; Sprig EZ crowns, Sprig, Loomis, CA, USA; Cheng Crowns, Kinder Krowns) are prefabricated, exceptionally strong ceramic and offer the most esthetic, biocompatible full-coverage primary molar crown. They are anatomically contoured and metal free. The cervical margin is knife-edge to preserve gingival health, and plaque accumulation is reduced with the highly polished finish. Wear is comparable to natural enamel. Depending on the company from which they are purchased, the crowns may be supplied in one universal shade, with additional color added to the cervical and occlusal surfaces, or in shades extra-light and light. The light shade is closer to an A1 or B1

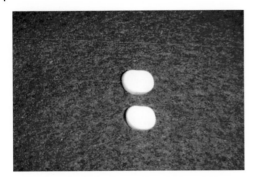

Figure 8.22 NuSmile zirconia crown for mesial–distal space loss compared to regular mesial–distal crown width.

shade and is usually a better match. A narrower crown mesial–distally, with a "squished" design, for first primary molars with space loss due to caries may be purchased from some manufacturers (Figure 8.22). Zirconia crowns cannot be crimped and are not flexible. Passive fit is mandatory. Attempting to seat a zirconia crown with force will result in fracture. Adjustment with a bur will result in microfracture, remove glaze, or create weakened areas. Meticulous attention to proper tooth preparation is necessary.

Procedure for Zirconia Crown

Size selection is done before the preparation. The esthetic advantage may be nullified with a crown that looks too large. Choose the correct size of crown for the space and evaluate the occlusal relationship. Size selection may be accomplished by holding a zirconia crown next to the primary molar to be prepped or with a NuSmile pink try-in crown (Figures 8.23a, b).

The preparation of the tooth for the zirconia crown takes more time than the preparation for an SSC, so this crown would not be recommended for children who are fearful or unable to cooperate for a longer procedure without sedation. Preparation is similar to the preveneered crown. A more recently recommended method for the crown preparation uses depth cuts. Depth cuts provide a visual guide for the necessary amount of reduction and will reduce preparation time.

- *Occlusal reduction*: The tip of a football diamond bur is used to reduce occlusal buccal and lingual cusps to the depth of the central groove, maintaining cuspal inclines and following the natural occlusal contour (Figure 8.24a). The central groove is reduced by about 0.5 mm (Figure 8.24b).
- *Buccal and lingual reduction*: Reduce the buccal and lingual occlusal third of the clinical crown (Figure 8.24c). Adequate occlusal reduction will permit sufficient subgingival margin placement and the correct occlusal plane. The marginal ridge of adjacent teeth can provide a good reference point.

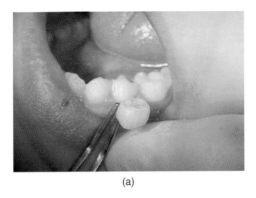

(a)

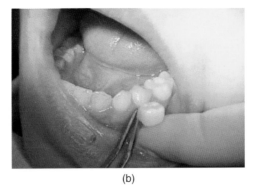

(b)

Figure 8.23 (a) Comparing zirconia crown to primary molar for size selection. (b) Pink try-in zirconia crown for size selection.

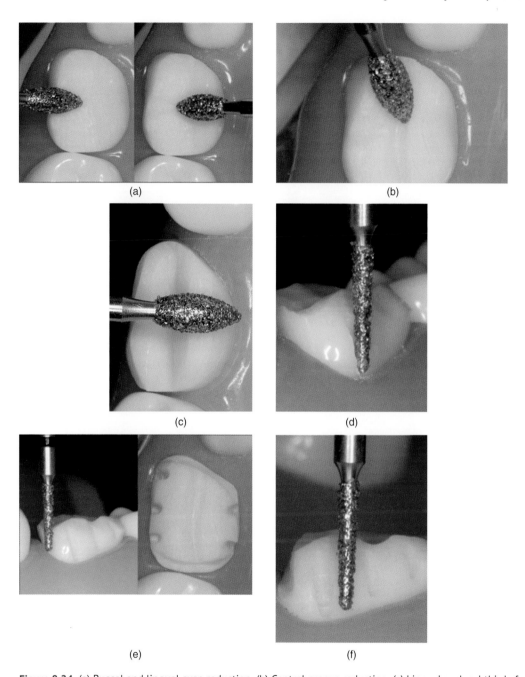

Figure 8.24 (a) Buccal and lingual cusp reduction. (b) Central groove reduction. (c) Lingual occlusal third of crown reduction. (d) Depth cuts. (e) Interproximal slices and depth cuts with shoulder. (f) Level depth cuts. (g) Round facial/lingual interproximal line angles. (h) Shoulder created at gingival margin. (i) Test fit with pink try-in crown. (j) Remove shoulder and extend preparation subgingival to feather-edge. (k) Final test fitting. Courtesy of NuSmile.

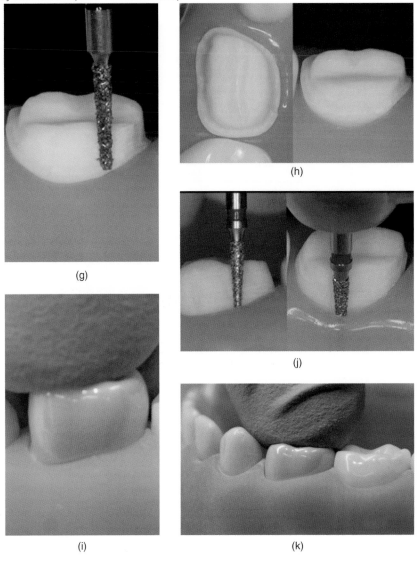

(g)

(h)

(j)

(i)

(k)

Figure 8.24 (*Continued*)

- *Buccal and lingual depth cuts*: A coarse round-end tapered diamond bur is used to create guide cuts for depth of preparation to a depth of about 0.5 mm (Figure 8.24d). The depth cuts insure adequate reduction of the mesial buccal bulge on a first primary molar. Inadequate reduction of this area will compromise fit.
- *Interproximal reduction*: Slices are performed with a coarse round-end diamond bur to a depth of approximately 1 mm, starting at the gingival margin and opening the interproximal contacts (Figure 8.24e). Interproximal reduction is more extensive than preparation for a traditional SSC. Zirconia crowns do not flex and are slightly thicker than the traditional SSC. If adjacent crowns are being placed, the interproximal reduction will be much more extensive. Consent should include first primary molar pulpotomy, as a pulp exposure may occur as a result of deeper mesial and distal reduction.

- *Circumferential reduction*: The buccal and lingual depth cuts are leveled, creating a shoulder (Figure 8.24f). Mesial and distal line angles are rounded (Figure 8.24g). A shoulder is created at the gingival margin (Figure 8.24h). The shoulder permits visualization of the margin during the test fit.
- *Test fit*: The crown fit should be tested at this point in the preparation. If the zirconia crown is too large, a gap between the tooth and the crown will be evident. A second primary molar crown that is too large on the distal may cause impaction of the first permanent molar during its eruption.
- If using a NuSmile zirconia crown, the try-in crown is used for a test fit (Figure 8.24i). Use of a pink try-in crown (NuSmile) will avoid contaminating the zirconia crown with blood and saliva. Pink try-in crowns can be sterilized for repeat use.
- *Subgingival reduction*: A fine, thin round-end tapered diamond bur is used to remove the shoulder and refine the margin to a feather-edge 1–2 mm subgingival to the cementoenamel junction (Figure 8.24j).
- *Final test fitting*: If using a NuSmile zirconia crown, the try-in crown is placed on the preparation. If the fit is good, the matching-size zirconia crown is cemented (Figure 8.24k).

The completed preparation should appear ovoid when viewed from the occlusal. All line angles should be rounded and blended (Figure 8.25). The occlusal plane of proximal teeth is evaluated with a try-in (Figure 8.26).

Common Problems with Preparation

- Inadequate subgingival preparation. Margins should be feather-edge with no undercuts and no ledges. Adequate subgingival extension of 1–2 mm insures that the crown margin will not be exposed, healthy gingival margins, and improved retention. Use of a thin, fine-grit tapered diamond bur avoids tissue maceration.

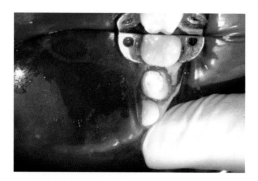

Figure 8.25 Ovoid shape of crown after preparation.

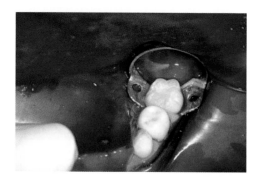

Figure 8.26 Pink try-in zirconia crown on prepared primary molar.

- Inadequate preparation around the cervical collar of the tooth. Proper reduction with this step will not only make the preparation smaller, but also permit the use of a crown closer in size to the original tooth.
- Inadequate removal of mesial buccal bulge.
- Inadequate interproximal reduction. Keep the bur vertical with the long axis of the molar to assure adequate subgingival reduction. Round off line angles and vertical walls as they converge toward the occlusal.
- Slanting bur for preparation. The bur should be vertical at all times during preparation.
- Differing planes of buccal and lingual reduction. Both should converge slightly toward the occlusal.
- Internal binding if vertical walls are not rounded near the occlusal.
- Zirconia crowns, analogous to preveneered crowns, have a passive fit and are placed

with digital pressure only. Forceful seating will fracture a zirconia crown. If a pink try-in was not used during the preparation and occlusion is high, the collar may be reduced with a high-speed fine diamond bur with copious water coolant, as excessive heat may cause microfracture of zirconia. Any adjustment with a bur will remove the crown's glaze and create weakened areas with thin ceramic. Any attempt to adjust the zirconia crown is strongly discouraged. Additional occlusal or interproximal reduction of the primary molar is preferable to attempting to shorten the zirconia crown. If doing multiple crowns, the occlusal table should be maintained to avoid hyperocclusion.

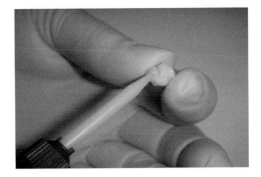

Figure 8.27 Filling the zirconia crown fully with cement to eliminate voids.

Cementation

Rinse the tooth thoroughly, removing all saliva and blood. Saliva will bind to the internal surface of the zirconia crown and impede the cement bond. Depending on the manufacturer, blood may show through zirconia; hemostasis must be achieved before cementation. If a pink try-in crown was not used, clean the inside of the zirconia crown with alcohol, peroxide, Ivoclean (Ivoclar Vivadent, Schaan, Liechtenstein), or sandblast with aluminum oxide before placing cement.

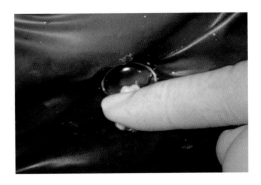

Figure 8.28 Digital pressure holding zirconia crown in place until cement sets.

Completely fill the crown with a resin-modified glass ionomer (RMGI) or GI cement to eliminate voids (Figure 8.27). Seat the crown subgingivally with digital pressure only. Do not permit the patient to bite the crown down into occlusion. The crown should be stabilized with firm finger pressure during the cement's set; movement will interfere with optimal bonding to the tooth, and hydrostatic forces of the cement may lift the zirconia crown away (Figure 8.28).

Pure GI cement is less expensive than RMGI. However, since the marginal seal of the zirconia crown is not seamless, pure GI cement may degrade more rapidly. Carboxylate cement (3M-ESPE) has also been successfully used.

Resin cement resulted in significantly less microleakage than GI in SSCs, preveneered crowns, and zirconia crowns (Al-Haj & Farah, 2018). BioCem (NuSmile), a bioactive cement, chemically bonds with the tooth, creating a strong bond. After the crown is held in place with digital pressure for 15 seconds, a flash cure for 2–5 seconds on the buccal and lingual initially sets the cement. The extruded cement can be easily removed from the margins of the crown with a spoon or explorer. The cement should be peeled toward the gingiva to avoid dislodging the crown. The final light-cure is 60 seconds.

After cementation, check occlusion with articulating paper (Figure 8.29a). If the occlusion is high, it is preferable to reduce the

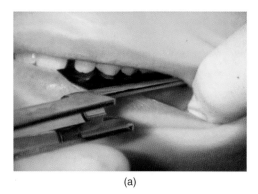

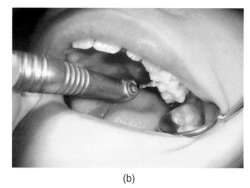

(a)   (b)

Figure 8.29 (a) Checking occlusion with articulating paper. (b) Adjusting occlusion of the opposing primary molar.

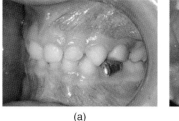
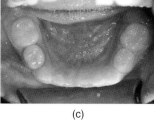
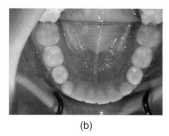

(a)   (c)   (b)

Figure 8.30 (a) Zirconia crown first primary molar in maxilla compared to stainless-steel crown first primary molar in mandible. (b) Occlusal view of zirconia crown mandibular right first primary molar. (c) Occlusal view of zirconia crowns mandibular right and left first primary molars.

Table 8.1 Preveneered versus zirconia crowns

Clinical situation	Zirconia	Preveneered
Bruxing	×	
Deep bite with short crowns	×	
Unable to control gingival bleeding		×
Need a smaller size		×
Minimal tooth structure remaining		×
Larger pulp chambers in younger children		×

occlusal contact on the opposing primary molar (Figure 8.29b).

With proper preparation and cementation, zirconia crowns offer unparalleled esthetics (Figure 8.30).

The crown size, which may be imprinted on the buccal or lingual surface of the crown, may be removed with a spoon or coarse prophylaxis paste. Zirconia crowns may be autoclaved for sterilizing.

While conventional SSCs may be used for various clinical situations, clinicians may have to choose between zirconia and preveneered crowns in different clinical situations, depending on their physical properties or dental characteristics (Table 8.1).

References

Al-Haj, A.S. & Farah, R.I. (2018) In vitro comparison of microleakage between preformed metal crowns and aesthetic crowns of primary molars using different adhesive luting cements. *European Archives of Paediatric Dentistry*, 19, 387–392.

American Academy of Pediatric Dentistry. (2019–2020) Pediatric restorative dentistry. *The Reference Manual of Pediatric Dentistry*. Chicago, IL: American Academy of Pediatric Dentistry; 340–352.

Azadani, E.N., Peng, J., Kumar, A., Casamassimo, P.S., Griffen, A., *et al.* (2020). A survival analysis of primary second molars in children treated under general anesthesia. *Journal of the American Dental Association,* 151 (8), 568–575.

Erdemci, Z.Y., Cehreli, S.B., & Tirali, R.E. (2014) Hall versus conventional stainless steel crown techniques: in vitro investigation of marginal fit and microleakage using three different luting agents. *Pediatric Dentistry*, 36, 286–290.

Innes, N.P., Evans, D.J., & Stirrups, D.R. (2011) Sealing caries in primary molars: randomized control trial, 5-year results. *Journal of Dental Research*, 90, 1405–1410.

Mahoney, E., Kilpatrick, N., & Johnston, T. (2008) Restorative paediatric dentistry. In: Cameron, A.C. & Widmer, R.P. (eds.), *Handbook of Pediatric Dentistry*, 3rd edn. London: Mosby; 341–377.

Maupone, G.,Yepes, J.F., Galloway, M., Tang, Q., Eckert, G.J., *et al.* (2017) Survival analysis of metal crowns versus restorations in primary mandibular molars. *Journal of the American Dental Association*, 148, 760–766.

Ram, D., Fuks, A.B., & Eidelman, E. (2003) Long-term clinical performance of esthetic primary molar crowns. *Pediatric Dentistry*, 25, 582–584.

Sheller, B., Williams, B. J., Hays, K., & Mancl, L. (2003). Reasons for repeat dental treatment under general anesthesia for the healthy child. *Pediatric Dentistry*, 25, 546–552.

Velan, E., Mitchell, S., & O'Connell, A. (2018) Restorative dentistry and dental materials. In: Nowak, A.J. & Casamassimo, P.S. (eds.), *The Handbook of Pediatric Dentistry*, 5th edn. Chicago, IL: American Academy of Pediatric Dentistry; 157–176.

9

Indirect Pulp Therapy for Young Permanent Molars
Patrice B. Wunsch

Young permanent teeth differ from mature permanent teeth in that the roots of young permanent teeth are not fully formed. The length of time for root completion in the permanent molars is approximately three years after full eruption of the tooth (American Academy of Pediatric Dentistry, 2019–2020). This may vary between patients, therefore obtaining a diagnostic radiograph to include the roots of the teeth is recommended before initiating any type of pulp therapy, not only to rule out the possibility of periapical pathology, but also to determine the apical development of the tooth.

There are certain advantages of treating young permanent teeth with immature roots (Figure 9.1). The pulp biology varies, in that permanent teeth with immature roots have a more viable pulp that will respond more favorably to insult and treatment therapies than permanent teeth with fully formed roots (Trope, 2008). This will be discussed in greater detail under the treatment modalities section of this chapter.

Background

As the permanent molars erupt into the oral cavity, there is a likelihood that the pits and fissures of the occlusal surface are composed of uncoalesced enamel, meaning that the enamel surface is not intact and the potential for bacterial invasion of the dentinal subsurface is high. This in itself will predispose the tooth to develop a large carious lesion before the tooth has fully erupted into the oral cavity. Additionally, the position of the partially erupted permanent molars places the tooth at risk for plaque accumulation. Sometimes the molar is not in contact with the opposing teeth, thereby not allowing the self-cleansing action of the occlusal surfaces coming in contact. Also, young patients are not as efficient at brushing the posterior teeth compared to their ability to clean the teeth positioned more anteriorly (Antowson *et al.*, 2012).

Indications for Indirect Pulp Therapy on Young Permanent Molars

In the event of deep caries in a young permanent tooth, the practitioner is faced with numerous factors that will affect the success of treatment:

- Patient behavior and level of cooperation.
- Preoperative symptoms.
- Apical development of the tooth.

In a patient who has minimal coping skills, indirect pulp therapy (IPT) is a viable option, in that it allows one to atraumatically arrest the caries process until trust and cooperation are achieved or some other means of behavior management is successful in order to provide care. There is a two-step (stepwise) method of IPT that would lend itself well to the patient

Handbook of Clinical Techniques in Pediatric Dentistry, Second Edition. Edited by Jane A. Soxman.
© 2022 John Wiley & Sons, Inc. Published 2022 by John Wiley & Sons, Inc.

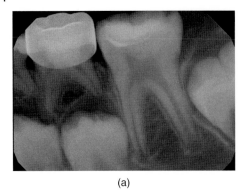 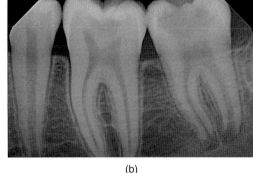

(a)   (b)

Figure 9.1 (a, b) Young immature permanent molar. Courtesy of Dr. Claudia Colorado, VCU Department of Endodontics.

who has poor coping skills. The provider will initially use a spoon excavator to remove gross caries and food debris, followed by placement of a glass ionomer temporary restoration. This has been extremely helpful, since not only does this treatment relieve the symptoms associated with the open lesion, it also affords the dentist time to schedule more definitive care at a later date. The medicament placed on the remaining caries changes the characteristic of the carious tooth structure that is left behind after initial excavation (Maltz *et al.*, 2007; Orhan *et al.*, 2008). The stepwise IPT technique will be described later in this chapter under technique.

Diagnosis

A comprehensive review of the patient's medical and dental history must be initially completed. The clinical exam includes an intraoral and extraoral examination of the hard and soft tissues associated with the area of the patient's chief complaint. Radiographic examination to include a bitewing radiograph and periapical radiograph should be taken. The bitewing is used to evaluate the extent of the caries and its proximity to the pulp. The periapical radiograph is used to look for signs of periapical pathology. The tooth in question should have clinical tests such as percussion and palpation to assess for periapical pathology

or mobility. Electric pulp testing and cold tests can be unreliable in young immature teeth with developing roots (Camp, 2008).

However, cold tests can be useful when the caries as noted on a radiograph approximates the pulp, or when pathosis is noted on the periapical radiograph. To differentiate between reversible and irreversible pulpitis, initial cold tests can be used to provide a baseline upon which the tooth can be monitored for pulpal changes.

Indirect Pulp Therapy is Indicated for Teeth with Signs of Reversible Pulpitis

Symptoms consistent with the diagnosis of reversible pulpitis include pain brought on by a stimulus (usually sweets or cold). The pain will subside after the stimulus is removed. Radiographically, the periapical film shows no signs of periapical pathology and the bitewing film shows caries encroaching upon the pulp, but not into the pulp. Like primary teeth, young immature permanent teeth do not respond reliably to electric pulp testing or cold tests. Therefore, the most reliable indicator for treatment is the history of symptoms and the clinical/radiographic exam.

Signs and symptoms consistent with a diagnosis of irreversible pulpitis are spontaneous pain, sensitivity to cold liquids or cold air, and radiographic signs of a widened periodontal ligament.

Signs and symptoms consistent with a diagnosis of necrotic pulp are spontaneous pain (patient wakes often at night in pain), swelling associated with the tooth, presence of a parulis, and often signs of a radiolucent lesion (periapical pathology). Teeth that have a diagnosis consistent with irreversible pulpitis or a necrotic pulp are not candidates for IPT or other vital pulp therapies.

Due to their highly vascular pulp, young immature permanent teeth have the potential to heal and withstand carious insult better than mature permanent teeth with fully formed roots (Ward, 2002). As early as the 1960s, a comprehensive study was performed by the Eastman Dental Center. Investigators found "after histological evaluation of the teeth selected for indirect pulp therapy, that had all caries been removed, pulpal exposure would have occurred. Additionally, only 3% of 475 teeth treated with indirect pulp therapy resulted in frank clinical failure." This study demonstrated that clinicians should not aggressively remove all carious dentin in an effort to leave none behind and risk exposing the pulp (Ranly & Garcia-Godoy, 2000).

What is Indirect Pulp Therapy?

IPT involves the incomplete removal of carious dentin. Cariously involved dentin is divided into two layers. The layer that is more coronal to the pulp is described as the infected layer or infected dentin. Contained within this layer are viable cariogenic bacteria. This layer is "dead tissue with both organic and inorganic components irreversibly deteriorated, that is deemed infected and non-remineralizable." During the IPT procedure, this is layer is removed. The remaining layer, which is in close proximity to the pulp, is called the affected layer or affected dentin. Within the affected layer are the "organic and inorganic components

present with sound structure and character but are slightly and reversibly degenerated, uninfected, and physiologically remineralizable" (Orhan *et al.*, 2010). It is this layer upon which a biocompatible material is placed to aid in remineralization. In order for the procedure to be successful, the tooth must be sealed from bacterial invasion. It is recommended that the final restoration be one that would not allow for any leakage around the margins. With this in mind, sealing the final restoration has been shown to decrease or prevent marginal leakage, thereby improving treatment success (Mertz-Fairhurst *et al.*, 1998).

Medicaments

Glass Ionomer (Vitrebond) and Calcium Hydroxide (Dycal)

Dycal® (Dentsply Caulk, Milford, DE, USA; Figure 9.2a) is available in hard-setting and light-cured forms. The high pH of the calcium hydroxide in Dycal has a bactericidal effect and calcium hydroxide is able to induce mineralization (Foreman & Barnes, 1990).

Glass ionomer is available as a liner type or restorative type. The most popular glass ionomer liner type is Vitrebond™ (3M ESPE, St. Paul, MN, USA; Figure 9.2a). This lining material can be placed in close proximity to the pulp, where its anticariogenic ability (due to fluoride release) is most effective. Vitrebond is a resin-modified glass ionomer.

Glass Ionomer (Lime-Lite)

Recently, Lime-Lite™ (PulpDent, Watertown, MA, USA; Figure 9.2b) has been introduced to the market as a resin-reinforced glass ionomer cavity-lining material that contains calcium phosphate. Compared to calcium hydroxide (Dycal), the resin-modified glass ionomers such as Vitrebond and Lime-Lite have the ability to create a better seal, since these glass ionomer liners are reinforced with composite resin. Glass ionomer restorative materials

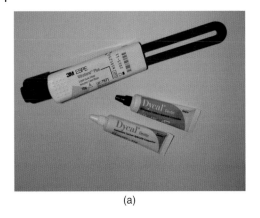

(a)

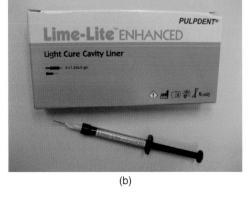

(b)

Figure 9.2 (a) Dycal and Vitrebond (b) Lime-Lite.

include Fugi II/IX GP® (GC America, Alsip, IL, USA), Ketac™ Molar (3M ESPE), and Photac™ Fil (3M ESPE). The glass ionomer restorative materials can be used as temporary restorations (stepwise technique) or as a base over the IPT as added protection for the pulp before the final restoration.

In general, glass ionomers have been shown to inhibit the growth of cariogenic bacteria due to their ability to release fluoride.

How does Fluoride Affect Certain Oral Bacteria *In Vivo*?

Fluoride indirectly affects mutans streptococci (MS) by limiting their ability to produce acid and thereby preventing a decrease in pH (Hamilton, 1990). Chronic exposure to fluoride may decrease the population of MS while increasing the number of more alkaline species (Hamilton, 1990). Glass ionomer releases a high concentration of fluoride after its initial application. Over time, the concentration of fluoride decreases and therefore more importance is placed on the ability of the final restoration to create an adequate seal.

Both calcium hydroxide and glass ionomer are considered good lining materials for IPT in young immature permanent teeth. Marchi *et al.* (2006) have studied IPT in primary teeth. The authors feel that IPT is not a

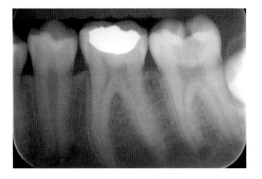

Figure 9.3 Preoperative radiograph of tooth #18.

material-dependent treatment, and that a good marginal seal of the final restoration and controlling the caries-inducing activities of the patient will ensure success.

Indirect Pulp Therapy Technique

After careful assessment of the radiographs (Figure 9.3) and preoperative symptoms, the tooth is anesthetized and a rubber dam is utilized to isolate the tooth.

A number 14A clamp is recommended for the first and second permanent molars. Depending on the age of the child and the presence or absence of the second permanent molar, the clamp is placed on the tooth receiving treatment or on the tooth behind it (Figure 9.4). For example, if deep caries exists

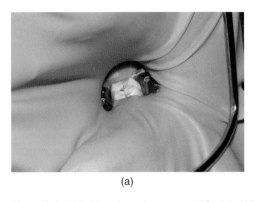
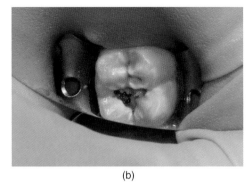

(a)   (b)

Figure 9.4 (a) Rubber dam placement, #18 with #14A clamp. (b) Preoperative photo of tooth #18.

on tooth #19 and the child is 8 years of age, the clamp is placed on tooth #19, since the second permanent molar does not usually erupt until 12 years of age. If the child is 13 years of age and the first permanent molar requires treatment, the clamp can be placed on the second permanent molar and extended into the premolar region.

Once isolation is obtained and the patient is anesthetized, a 557 or 330 bur is used to gain coronal access to the lesion. After initial preparation, the caries is carefully removed with a #6/#8 round bur (Figure 9.5). The larger-diameter round bur decreases the chance of exposure compared to using a #4 round bur. Avoid using a spoon excavator, since using this instrument can result in removing chunks of decay, leading to a pulp exposure. If hand instruments are used, they should be utilized only to remove caries at the dentin–enamel junction, taking care not to produce a pulp exposure (Hargreaves & Cohen 2011).

As the excavation deepens, care must be taken not to place apical pressure on the handpiece in order to avoid pulpal exposure. Rather, the round bur is utilized in a more peripheral manner to remove all of the caries from the preparation walls, and then carefully moved in a circular motion toward the area of deepest caries on the cavity floor (Figure 9.6).

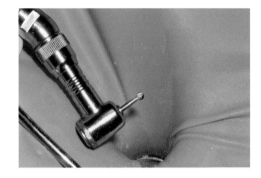

Figure 9.5 Slow-speed handpiece with #8 round bur.

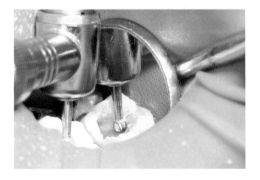

Figure 9.6 Initial excavation with #8 round bur.

At this point caries will be evident on the cavity floor, right above the pulp chamber. Once the operator has reached the point where he or she feels that further apical excavation would result in a pulpal exposure and the cavity walls are clean (Figure 9.7), the handpiece

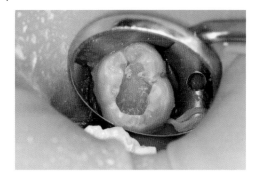

Figure 9.7 Caries excavation nearly completed.

is no longer used and careful examination of the remaining caries is made.

According to the literature, if the remaining caries is hard and dry, either medicament (calcium hydroxide or glass ionomer) is placed (Figure 9.8) followed by the final restoration (Figure 9.9).

If the remaining caries is soft and wet, the operator can make the decision to place calcium hydroxide or glass ionomer and temporize the tooth to allow the medicaments to change the characteristics of the caries, then re-enter the tooth later to complete caries removal. This technique allows for a change in the cultivable flora deep in the carious lesion where, before placement of the medicament, the soft wet caries contains a high bacterial count, whereas afterward the bacterial count is greatly reduced and the caries becomes more dry and hard (Vij *et al.*, 2004; Bjorndal & Larsen, 2000). However, some researchers have found that when the tooth is re-entered, the pulp is exposed in an effort to remove the remaining caries (Leksell *et al.*, 1996). Research has found that there is no difference in the successful outcome between the two-step (stepwise) technique and the one-step technique (Oliveira *et al.*, 2006; Orhan, 2010). In the one-step technique, caries is removed as explained above and whether the remaining caries is wet or dry, the medicaments are placed followed by the final restoration. It is felt that as long as a sealed restoration is placed, the remaining bacteria, whether the count is high or low, cannot survive and the young immature tooth is allowed to heal and continue to develop (Bjorndal & Larsen, 2000).

If the operator is not comfortable leaving wet soft caries and does not feel that patient would tolerate having the tooth temporized and then re-entered (stepwise technique), one can continue to remove the caries until the dryer caries is reached. This poses a risk for exposure and, depending on how deep the caries is, it brings great comfort to know that as long as a sealed final restoration is placed, there is no need to risk exposure, and the operator should stop excavation at the point where the risk of exposing the pulp is evident. IPT is completed after the bulk of carious-involved tooth structure is removed and only a small amount of carious material is left behind to avoid exposing the pulp. Calcium hydroxide or glass ionomer is placed over the remaining caries, followed by a reinforced or nonreinforced glass ionomer base, such as 3M's Ketac Molar, Photac Fil, Fugi II, or Fugi IX.

The two-paste system for calcium hydroxide (Dycal) is also available for the glass ionomer (Vitrebond). These two-paste systems are more favorable than the powder or liquid systems, since there is less chance of incorporating too much liquid or too much powder, thereby altering the intended properties of the material. Lime-Lite is an injectable material that does not require mixing for ease in preparation and application (Table 9.1).

Once the IPT is complete, the liner should be cover with a glass ionomer base for added protection to the pulp. Any of the materials listed in Table 9.2 will serve this purpose well.

Follow-Up

The patient is rescheduled for a follow-up in 6 months, when the results of the treatment are examined both clinically and radiographically. If the treatment is successful, routine recalls are scheduled every 6 months, with radiographs planned at 1-year intervals.

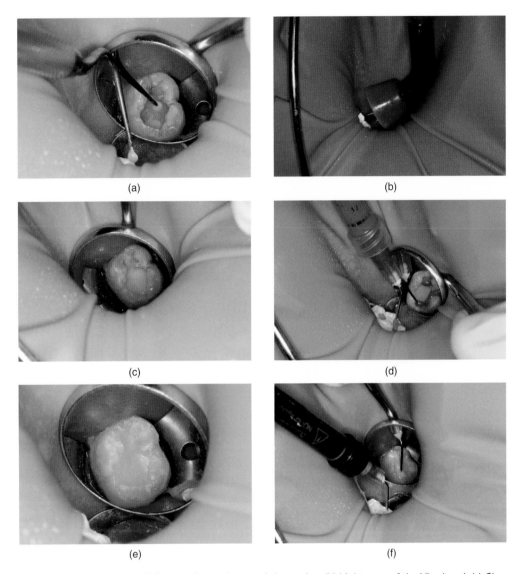

Figure 9.8 (a) Placement of Vitrebond over the remaining caries. (b) Light-cure of the Vitrebond. (c) Glass ionomer liner (Vitrebond) is cured. (d) After placement of glass ionomer base, the tooth is etched in preparation for the final restoration. (e) Final restoration is placed. (f) Sealant is placed over the composite.

Criteria for IPT success include the following:

- Vitality is preserved.
- No pain, sensitivity, or swelling.
- No radiographic evidence of internal or external resorption or other periradicular pathology.
- Continued apexogenesis.

Success Rate

One study has found that there is a high success rate for IPT on permanent teeth with deep carious lesions. In the study, 94 teeth were treated with the stepwise excavation process. Only 5 teeth experienced pulpal exposure on the final excavation; the remaining teeth were

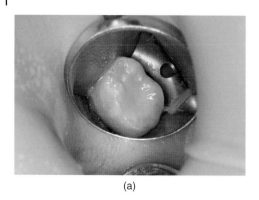
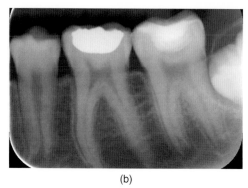

(a)   (b)

Figure 9.9 (a) Tooth #18 with completed restoration. (b) Tooth #18 radiograph of completed treatment.

Table 9.1 Frequently used cavity liner products.

Material	Composition	Radiopaque	Self/Light-Cure	Manufacturer
Vitrebond	Resin-modified glass ionomer	Yes	Light-cure	3M ESPE
Lime-Lite	Resin-modified glass ionomer calcium phosphate	Yes	Light-cure	PulpDent
Dycal	Calcium hydroxide	Yes	Self-cure	Dentsply

Table 9.2 Frequently used glass ionomer–based interim restorative materials.

Material	Composition	Radiopaque	Self/Light-Cure	Manufacturer
Ketac Universal	Conventional glass ionomer	No	Self-cure	3M ESPE
Photac Fil	Resin-modified glass ionomer	Yes	Dual-cure	3M ESPE
Fugi II LC	Resin-modified glass ionomer	Yes	Light-cure	GC America
Fugi IX	Conventional glass ionomer	No	Self-cure	GC America

successful after a 1-year observation period. The authors concluded from this study that it is possible for general dentists to manage deep caries with IPT and thus prolong the vitality of the tooth (Bjornal & Thylstrup, 1998).

In 2010, Gruythuysen *et al.* published a study on the long-term survival of IPT in primary and permanent teeth with diagnosed deep carious lesions. The patients ranged from 4 to 18 years of age. The lesion depth was greater than two-thirds of the dentin thickness. There were 125 primary molars and 45 permanent molars included in the study. One-step IPT was performed (gross caries removed, leaving small amount of affected dentin upon which Vitrebond was placed followed by the final restoration). The survival rate for IPT on the primary molars was 145.6 weeks (2.8 years) and for the permanent teeth 178.1 weeks (3.4 years) (Gruythuysen *et al.*, 2010).

Final Restoration

The type of restoration depends on the size of the preparation and the condition of the remaining tooth structure. If the access preparation is small and the surrounding tooth structure is healthy, either a sealed composite or amalgam is suitable. This can include a conservative Class I or II restoration. If, however, the preparation is large and the supporting tooth structure is weak (demineralized or hypoplastic enamel), the restoration of choice is a stainless-steel crown (SSC) in the young patient, with the understanding that this is a successful interim restoration that is designed to last until the patient has completed their growth, at which time a permanent full cast restoration can be completed.

Composite

After IPT is completed and a therapeutic base material has been placed, the cavity walls should be refreshed by running a bur along them to clean any residual glass ionomer material in preparation for the acid-etch. Next, the cavity walls are etched for 15–20 seconds, then rinsed and dried. The bonding agent is placed and lightly dried with air to create a thin layer; it is then cured for 10 seconds. Packable composite is placed, the occlusion is checked, the surface is re-etched, and bond is placed and thinned with air, followed by a thin application of sealant (they are cured together for 20 seconds). The composite is now sealed to help prevent marginal leakage that can lead to bacterial invasion and possible failure of the IPT procedure (Mertz-Fairhurst *et al.*, 1998).

Amalgam

After IPT and base material placement, the cavity walls are freshened. An amalgam-bonding agent such as Amalgambond® Plus (Parkell, Edgewood, NY, USA) can be used to reduce the chance of marginal leakage. Another way to reduce to chance of marginal leakage is to repeat the steps mentioned above in sealing the composite. Research has shown that a sealed composite or amalgam greatly decreases the chance of marginal leakage resulting in bacterial invasion (Mertz-Fairhurst *et al.*, 1998).

Permanent Stainless-Steel Crown

In the event of a three or more surface restoration, or enamel/dentinal defects, an SSC is the restoration of choice in a growing child. It will provide an adequate seal to ensure therapy success, while giving the strength to resist proximal breakdown that can result in the loss of arch space over time.

Permanent SSCs must be adapted to the tooth with care, since an oversized SSC on a first or second permanent molar can result in creating an ectopic eruption of the permanent molar distal to it, since it can become trapped under a large distal overhang of the SSC upon eruption.

After IPT and base material placement, the tooth is prepped for the SSC. Keep in mind the basic principles of preparation design taught by our prosthodontic colleagues. The concept of parallel walls is just as important while prepping a permanent tooth for an SSC as it is for the full cast crown. First, a football-shaped diamond bur works well for the occlusal reduction. One can utilize either the 169 L or flame-shaped diamond bur for both the occlusal reduction and the interproximal or axial wall reduction. The SSC is an interim restoration that will one day require a full cast crown; therefore, aggressive overpreparation of the tooth should be avoided.

Once ideal preparation has been completed, selection of the SSC is made. There are two types of basic SSC forms available: precontoured and uncontoured. The uncontoured SSC is sometimes referred to as a tin can, since the walls of the crown are straight and lack contour. The advantage of the precontoured

Table 9.3 Glass ionomer cements.

Material	Composition	Self/Light-Cure	Set Time[a]	Manufacturer
FugiCem	Resin-reinforced glass ionomer	Self-cure	4.5 minutes	GC America
Ketac Cement	Glass ionomer	Self-cure	7 minutes	3M ESPE
RelyX Luting Cement	Resin-reinforced glass ionomer	Self-cure	10 minutes	3M ESPE
RelyX Luting Plus Cement	Resin-reinforced glass ionomer	Tack light-cure	5 seconds	3M ESPE
		Self-cure	2 minutes	

[a] Manufacturers set time descriptions vary. Some list the actual hard-set time and others list the amount of time necessary to set before the clinician is able to manipulate the restoration.

SSC is that it is designed to resemble the first permanent molar in its cervical adaptation to the tooth. However, teeth do vary in size and shape, and the cervical constriction of these crowns can make them somewhat difficult to fit.

The advantage of the uncontoured SSC is its disadvantage as well. It requires manipulation to create a good fit, resulting in more chair time, but allowing the crown to have a more customized fit.

Steps for Fitting an Uncontoured Stainless-Steel Crown

1. After tooth preparation is complete, an uncontoured SSC is selected that best fits the tooth.
2. Some brands will be pretrimmed to optimum length to save time, but if that is not the case, after the initial placement of the crown, the crown is marked using an explorer to etch a line along the cervical area where the gingival tissue meets the crown.
3. The crown is then trimmed with a curved crown scissors or a heatless stone to 1 mm below (cervical) to the etched line.
4. The crown is then tried on the tooth to check the fit. If the fit is loose (which should be the case—if not, the crown may be too small), the crown will need to be contoured. This is accomplished by using a contouring pliers or crown crimping pliers, similar to those used by pediatric dentists.
5. Once a tight fit is accomplished, the SSC is ready for cementation.

Stainless-Steel Crown Cements

Glass ionomer cements have gained in popularity and are widely used by pediatric dentists for cementation of primary tooth and permanent tooth SSCs. Some of the more popular cements are listed in Table 9.3.

After the cement has reached its initial set, care must be taken to floss the interproximal areas and clear the sulcus of excess cement. Residual cement left in these areas can make it more difficult to floss and result in gingival inflammation.

References

American Academy of Pediatric Dentistry. (2019–2020) *The Reference Manual of Pediatric Dentistry*. Chicago, IL: American Academy of Pediatric Dentistry; 505.

Antowson, S.A., Antonson, D.E., Brener, S., Crutchfield, J., Larumbe, J., *et al.* (2012) Twenty-four month clinical evaluation of fissure sealants of partially erupted permanent first molars. *Journal of the American Dental Association*, 143, 115–122.

Bjorndal, L. & Larsen, T. (2000) Changes in the cultivable flora in deep carious lesions following a stepwise excavation procedure. *Caries Research*, 34, 502–508.

Bjorndal, L. & Thylstrup, A. (1998) A practice-based study on stepwise excavation of deep carious lesions in permanent teeth: a 1-year follow-up study. *Community Dental Oral Epidemiology*, 26, 112–118.

Camp, J. (2008) Diagnostic dilemmas in vital pulp therapy: treatment for the toothache is changing, especially in young, *immature teeth. Pediatric Dentistry*, 30 (3), 197–205.

Foreman, P.C. & Barnes, I. E. (1990) A review of calcium hydroxide. *International Endodontic Journal*, 23, 283–297.

Gruythuysen, R., van Stijp, G., & Wu, M. (2010) Long-term survival of indirect pulp treatment performed in primary and permanent teeth with clinically diagnosed deep carious lesions. *Journal of Endodontics*, 36 (9), 1490–1493.

Hamilton, I.R. (1990) Biochemical effects of fluoride on oral bacteria. *Journal of Dental Research*, 69 (special issue), 660–667.

Hargreaves, K. & Cohen, S. (2011) Related clinical topics. In: Berman, L. & Hargreaves, K. (eds.), *Pathways to the Pulp*, 10th edn. St. Louis, MO: Mosby; 822.

Leksell, E., Ridell, K., Cvek, M., & Mejare, I. (1996) Pulp exposure after stepwise versus direct complete excavation of deep carious lesions in young posterior permanent teeth. *Endodontics & Dental Traumatology*, 12, 192–196.

Maltz, M., Oliveira, E.F., Fontanella, V., & Carminative, G. (2007) Deep caries lesions after incomplete dentine caries removal: 40-month follow-up study. *Caries Research*, 41, 493–496.

Marchi, J.J., de Araujo, F.B., Froner, A.M., Straffon, L.H., & Nor J.E. (2006) Indirect pulp capping in the primary dentition: a 4 year follow-up study. *Journal of Pediatric Dentistry*, 31 (2), 68–71.

Mertz-Fairhurst, E.J., Curtis, J.W., Jr., Ergle, J.W., Rueggeberg, F.A., & Adair, S.M. (1998) Ultraconservative and cariostatic sealed restorations: results at year 10. *Journal of the American Dental Association*, 129, 55–66.

Oliveira, E.F., Carminatti, G., Fontanella, V., & Maltz, M. (2006) The monitoring of deep caries lesions after incomplete dentine caries removal: results after 14–18 months. *Clinical Oral Investigations*, 10, 134–139.

Orhan, A.I., Oz, F.T., & Orhan, K. (2010) Pulp exposure occurrence and outcomes after 1- or 2-visit indirect pulp therapy vs complete caries removal in primary and permanent molars. *Pediatric Dentistry*, 32 (4), 347–355.

Orhan, A.I., Oz, F.T., Ozcelik, B., & Orhan K. (2008) A clinical and microbiological comparative study of deep carious lesion treatment in deciduous and young permanent molars. *Clinical Oral Investigations*, 12, 369–378.

Ranly, D.M. & Garcia-Godoy, F. (2000) Current and potential pulp therapies for primary and young permanent teeth. *Journal of Dentistry*, 28, 153–161.

Trope, M. (2008) Regenerative potential of dental pulp. *Journal of Endodontics*, 34 (7S), S13–S17.

Vij, R., Coll, J.A., Shelton, P., & Farooq, N.S. (2004) Caries control and other variables associated with success of primary molar vital pulp therapy. *Pediatric Dentistry*, 26, 214–220.

Ward, J. (2002) Vital pulp therapy in cariously exposed permanent teeth and its limitations. *Australian Endodontic Journal*, 28 (1), 29–37.

10

Direct Pulp Therapy for Young Permanent Molars

Patrice B. Wunsch

As discussed in Chapter 9, young immature permanent teeth respond more favorably to insult and treatment therapies. The same principle holds true when considering direct pulp therapy (DPT) in young immature permanent teeth. Young permanent teeth have immature pulps and incomplete root formation. Not only are the root ends not fully closed, but the root canal walls are thin and fragile. In the event of pulp exposure, if the tooth exhibits signs of reversible pulpitis, every effort should be made to maintain pulp vitality and allow the tooth to continue to develop and gain apical root closure naturally (apexogenesis). If DPT is not possible and nonsurgical root canal treatment is indicated before the tooth has fully developed, an apexification procedure would be performed in an effort to obtain root end closure and an adequate apical stop. However, the apexification procedure does not allow for continued development of the root. A tooth that is not able to fully develop will have thin root canal walls and is at risk for fracture (Ward, 2002).

Background

Direct vital pulp therapy in cariously involved teeth is diagnostically and technique dependent. The following are critical for success (Ward, 2002):

- An accurate diagnosis of reversible pulpitis.

- Caries removal to include the infected pulp tissue.
- Use of aseptic technique (rubber dam isolation, irrigation).
- Prevention of bacterial leakage with a permanent restoration.

As early as 1993, Mejare and Cvek wrote a paper reviewing the partial pulpotomy in carious teeth. They surmised that bacteria are able to gain access to the pulp lumen only after some portion of the coronal pulp has become necrotic (Mejare & Cvek, 1993). In order to preserve the remaining pulp, the infected dentin and inflamed pulp must be removed and a biocompatible material that promotes the reparative process is placed over the pulp. In the past, calcium hydroxide $(Ca(OH)_2)$ has been the material of choice for DPT. Long-term follow-up of cariously involved permanent molars that received $Ca(OH)_2$ pulpotomy treatments resulted in a 44.5% failure rate at 5 years and a 79.7% failure rate at 10 years (Witherspoon *et al.*, 2006). Recently, mineral trioxide aggregate (MTA) has proven to be successful in vital pulp therapy. Analogous to $Ca(OH)_2$ (pH of 12), MTA is highly basic (pH of 12.5) and is biocompatible. The goals of a successful pulp capping material are as follows:

- The ability to kill bacteria.
- The ability to promote mineralization.
- The ability to withstand bacterial invasion (bacterial tight seal).

Handbook of Clinical Techniques in Pediatric Dentistry, Second Edition. Edited by Jane A. Soxman.
© 2022 John Wiley & Sons, Inc. Published 2022 by John Wiley & Sons, Inc.

MTA to a great extent fulfills the desired goals of a pulp capping/pulpotomy material. It has the ability to promote mineralization and dentinal bridge formation faster and more effectively than $Ca(OH)_2$. It does, however, have a weak antibacterial effect; in fact, it is less antibacterial than $Ca(OH)_2$. Regardless, MTA does have the advantage of providing an enhanced nonresorbable seal over the vital pulp. Its ability to seal out bacteria is to a great extent why the material has been so successful. According to El Meligy and Avery (2006), $Ca(OH)_2$ does not provide any protection from microleakage.

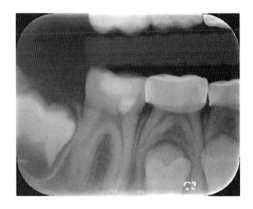

Figure 10.1 Mineral trioxide aggregate direct pulp cap on tooth #30. Courtesy of Dr. Claudia Colorado, VCU Department of Endodontics.

Permanent Tooth Pulp Capping

In the event of a small mechanical or traumatic exposure, the direct application of $Ca(OH)_2$ on the nonbleeding pulp has proven to be very successful in young immature teeth (direct pulp cap or Cvek pulpotomy). Some dentists believe that while using $Ca(OH)_2$ for direct pulp capping is an option, over time it washes out or disintegrates, whereas MTA does not (Farsi *et al.*, 2006). Some now advocate the use of bioactive materials such as MTA for direct pulp capping over the use of $Ca(OH)_2$ (Figure 10.1).

Permanent Tooth Pulpotomy

When the carious exposure is large, as discussed earlier, it is important to remove the infected, necrotic pulp by performing a pulpotomy. $Ca(OH)_2$ has been used to preserve the apical vitality of a carious exposed pulp. But it has been shown that once root end closure has been obtained, the root canals would require obturation in order to prevent dystrophic calcification in the canals, a condition that would later prevent successful root canal therapy (Ranly & Garcia-Godoy, 2000).

It is important to recall the patient every 6 months and obtain a periapical radiograph on a yearly basis. Once root end closure has been obtained and the tooth remains clinically and radiographically within normal limits, it is then determined that nonsurgical root canal treatment is not indicated.

Some studies have shown that the control of pulpal bleeding plays a significant role in the success of the pulpotomy treatment. If a clot is allowed to form, this can result in treatment failure and thus irrigation is an important part of the treatment therapy. Use of either sterile saline or sodium hypochlorite is recommended. However, sodium hypochlorite has the added advantage of being able to provide hemostasis, disinfection, and removal of dentinal chips that remain after excavation (Farsi *et al.*, 2006).

If the pulp is not inflamed, it will not continue to bleed. At this point, MTA is placed onto the pulp. The setting ability of MTA is not affected by blood or water (Figure 10.2) (El Meligy & Avery, 2006).

Indications for Direct Pulp Therapy in Young Permanent Molars

In the event of deep caries in a young permanent tooth that results in a carious exposure, the practitioner must consider the following:

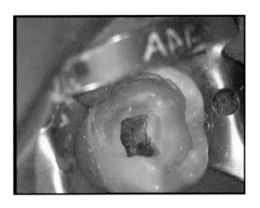

Figure 10.2 Healthy pulp tissue. Courtesy of Dr. Claudia Colorado, VCU Department of Endodontics.

- Patient behavior and level of cooperation:
  - Is the patient able to cooperate for an endodontic procedure such as multiple visit apexification and root canal therapy?
  - If not, DPT *may* be an option.
- Preoperative symptoms:
  - Are the signs and symptoms consistent with a diagnosis of reversible pulpitis?
  - If so, DPT *is* an option.
- Apical development of the tooth:
  - Is the root wall thickness and root end closure complete (has the tooth completed development)?
  - If not, DPT *is recommended* in a tooth with the signs and symptoms consistent with a diagnosis of reversible pulpitis, in order to maintain the vitality of the tooth and allow continued development.

What is Direct Pulp Therapy?

DPT in teeth with deep carious lesions involves the removal of the carious insult as well as the most superficial pulp, which may be characterized by inflammation and bacterial invasion (Horsted-Bindslev & Lovschall, 2002). What is left behind is deemed to be healthy pulp, capable of healing. Placement of $Ca(OH)_2$ (not discussed in the treatment section of this chapter due to its being less successful than MTA) or MTA promotes the formation of a dentinal bridge between the pulp and the material. A sealed restoration will not allow for bacterial invasion and thus allows for the young healthy pulp to heal, and for the young immature tooth to continue to mature and develop.

Diagnosis

As discussed in Chapter 9, a comprehensive review of the patient's medical and dental history must be initially completed. The clinical examination includes an intraoral and extraoral examination of the hard and soft tissues associated with the area of the patient's chief complaint. Radiographic examination to include a bitewing radiograph and periapical radiograph are obtained to adequately assess the extent of caries in the dentin and the periradicular area of the tooth. The periapical radiograph is used to look for signs of periapical pathology. The tooth in question should have clinical tests such as percussion and palpation to assess for periapical pathology or mobility. Electric pulp testing and cold tests are unreliable in teeth with developing root structure (Camp, 2008). However, cold testing performed before the initiation of treatment can be used to provide a baseline from which one can monitor the vitality of the pulp after treatment.

Medicaments

MTA is considered to be a bioactive endodontic cement. A bioactive material promotes healing when it releases $Ca(OH)_2$ as it sets. When the $Ca(OH)_2$ reacts with tissue fluids, a layer of calcium phosphate forms, which is recognized by the body as hydroxyapatite, which in turn induces healing; this is considered a physico-chemical reaction (Sakar *et al.*, 2005). The success rate for DPT with MTA has been studied, and it has been determined that the success rate was significantly higher in those teeth that had open apices than those with closed apices (Parirokh *et al.*, 2018).

Originally MTA had the disadvantage of causing tooth discoloration, which was of great concern, especially with the anterior teeth. MTA White (Figure 10.3) was developed to address this issue, but it did not adequately do so (Hutcheson *et al.*, 2012). There has been controversy over the cause of discoloration, with some studies citing the calcium alumino-ferrite as the cause and others attributing the cause to the bismuth oxide. It has been recommended that after the infected pulp tissue has been removed and before placement of the MTA, sodium hypochlorite is used to prevent clot formation. When the sodium hypochlorite comes in contact with the bismuth oxide in MTA, it can result in tooth discoloration (Camilleri, 2015). Calcium aluminoferrite can cause tooth discoloration and is present in MTA Gray, and also to a much lesser degree in MTA White (Camilleri, 2008; Baroudi & Samir, 2016). Another issue with MTA is the setting time. When first introduced into dentistry, the setting time for MTA was 3–6 hours. It was recommended that a moist cotton pellet be place over the material, then the tooth was temporarily sealed, and the patient was scheduled to complete the treatment at a later time to allow the cement to fully set. This was not desirable for treatment in patients who have dental anxiety and who have difficulty cooperating for appointments. In addition to setting time, MTA had the disadvantage of being expensive and was supplied in unit-dose packets. Mixing and application were technique sensitive and improper technique could affect material performance.

More recently, other bioactive materials have been introduced to overcome the drawbacks of the original MTA (ProRoot MTA, Dentsply Tulsa Dental Specialties, Johnson City, TN, USA); namely, the cost of the material, ease of use, and tooth discoloration. Biodentine® (Septodont, Saint-Maur-des-Fosses, France), NeoMTA/NeoPUTTY™ (NuSmile, Houston,

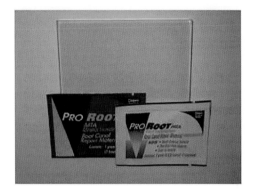

Figure 10.3 Gray and white ProRoot MTA.

TX, USA), and EndoEze™ MTAFlow (Ultradent, South Jordan, UT, USA) are examples of some of the newer bioactive materials used for DPT (Table 10.1). These materials are similar in composition to the original MTA, but are less expensive, easier to use, and have shorter setting times. They also have the added advantage of not turning the tooth dark (Camilleri, 2015; Parirokh *et al.*, 2018).

Biodentine is considered a dentin replacement product that can be placed directly onto the pulp. It is referred to as "dentin in a capsule," since the powder/liquid are triturated for 30 seconds, leaving a putty that can be loaded into an amalgam carrier and directly deposited into the tooth (Figure 10.4). NeoMTA is a gel/powder system. The gel is advantageous in that it resists washout and works to accelerate setting. After the material is mixed, it should be in a putty-like state for ease of handling (Figure 10.5a). More recently, NuSmile developed an injectable MTA called NeoPUTTY, a premixed, bioactive, bioceramic MTA that triggers the formation of hydroxyapatite and supports healing. It contains the same tricalcium and dicalcium silicate powders as do other MTA products, but eliminates the need to measure and mix; one needs to only dispense the material directly into the tooth (Figure 10.5b). EndoEze MTAFlow is a powder/gel system that comes with a syringe for a looser, injectable application of the material, or the material can be applied directly to the tooth

Table 10.1 Comparison of ingredients found in various bioactive materials.

ProRoot MTA	Biodentine	Neo MTA/NeoPUTTY	EndoEze MTA Flow
Tricalcium silicate	Tricalcium silicate	Tricalcium silicate	Tricalcium silicon pentaoxide
Tricalcium aluminate	Dicalcium silicate	Dicalcium silicate	Bismuth trioxide
Dicalcium silicate	Calcium carbonate	Tantalite	Dicalcium silicate
Calcium sulfate dihydrate	Zirconium oxide	Calcium sulfate	Calcium sulfate
Bismuth oxide	Calcium oxide	Tricalcium aluminate	
Tetra calcium aluminoferrite	Iron oxide		
Setting Time			
4 hours	45 minutes[b]	~15 minutes, initial[a]	~15 minutes, initial[a]

[a] Material continues to harden over time.

[b] Short setting time due to the presence of calcium chloride in the mixing liquid.

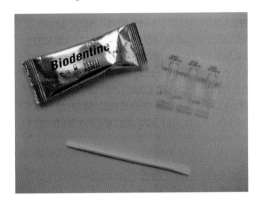

Figure 10.4 Septodont Biodentine.

in putty form. Depending on the consistency, the thinner mix results in a shorter setting time versus the thicker mix having a longer setting time (Figure 10.6).

Mineral Trioxide Aggregate Pulpotomy Procedure (using ProRoot MTA)

The original MTA is a powder consisting of 75% Portland cement, 20% bismuth oxide, and 5% gypsum. The major component (Portland cement) is responsible for the setting and biologic properties. Bismuth oxide provides radiopacity and gypsum is an important determinant of the setting time. The major components of Portland cement are a mixture of dicalcium silicate, tricalcium silicate, tricalcium aluminate, and tetracalcium aluminoferrite. The tetracalcium aluminoferrite contributes to the dark color. Lower amounts of iron are present in white MTA compared to gray MTA (Camilleri, 2008; Steffen & van Waes, 2009). Working time is 5 minutes and setting time is 3–6 hours.

Technique

As stated in an article by Hilton (2009), after a review of the literature on vital pulp therapy, the following are techniques that are recommended for treatment success:

- Teeth are isolated with a rubber dam.
- After isolation, teeth can be cleaned and disinfected.
- A sterile bur is used to initiate cavity preparation and pulp exposure is initiated as atraumatically as possible.
- Hemorrhaging is controlled with sterile materials.

MTA Pulpotomy: Steps to Successful Treatment

1. Local anesthetic is administered and rubber dam placement is completed (Figure 10.7).

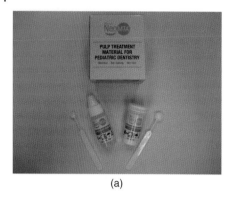

(a)

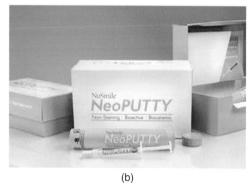

(b)

Figure 10.5 (a) NuSmile NeoMTA. (b) NuSmile NeoPUTTY.

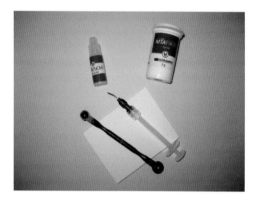

Figure 10.6 Ultradent EndoEze MTAFlow.

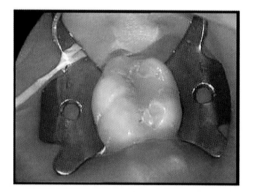

Figure 10.7 Rubber dam placement on tooth with defective restoration resulting in deep recurrent caries. Courtesy of Dr. Claudia Colorado, VCU Department of Endodontics.

2. Removal of caries in the enamel and dentin is initiated with a 330, 245, or 557 in a high-speed handpiece with irrigation (sterile water preferred).
3. A sterile #6 or 8 round bur in a slow-speed handpiece is used to remove the pulp in the pulp chamber. A spoon excavator can be used at this point to decrease the number of dentinal chips that can contaminate the pulp (Figure 10.8).
4. All carious dentin and the infected pulp are removed to the level of the radicular pulp (Figure 10.9).
5. Irrigation can be performed with sterile water or saline. Sodium hypochlorite can be used as well. The exposed pulp is irrigated (Figure 10.10) with 2.5% sodium hypochlorite (Torabinejad & Walton, 2009).

Once hemostasis is achieved, MTA is mixed according to the manufacturer's guidelines.
6. MTA is mixed on a glass slab with a metal spatula. The MTA powder is mixed with sterile saline at a 3 : 1 powder-to-saline ratio (Figure 10.11).
7. The MTA is carried to the pulp stumps with a metal condenser, where a 1–2 mm thickness of MTA is placed directed onto the pulp tissue (Figure 10.12). It is gently condensed with a moistened cotton pellet (Figure 10.13).
8. A moist cotton pellet is left over the MTA to enhance its set (moisture is necessary during the setting process). The MTA

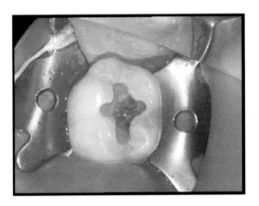

Figure 10.8 Caries excavation. Courtesy of Dr. Claudia Colorado, VCU Department of Endodontics.

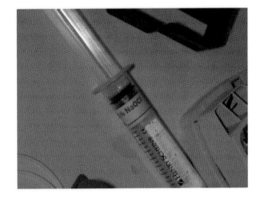

Figure 10.10 Irrigation with 2.5% sodium hypochlorite.

Follow-up

The patient is rescheduled for a follow-up in 3 months, when the result of treatment is examined both clinically and radiographically. If the treatment is successful, routine recalls are scheduled every 6 months, with radiographs planned at 1-year intervals.

Complications

- Root canal obliteration—if the tooth remains vital, this is considered normal, and there is no need for nonsurgical root canal treatment.
- Pulp necrosis—nonsurgical root canal treatment needed.
- Lack of apexogenesis.

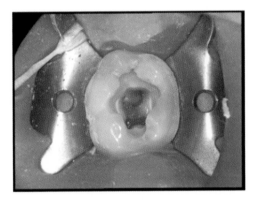

Figure 10.9 Carious dentin and infected pulp removed to level of the radicular pulp. Courtesy of Dr. Claudia Colorado, VCU Department of Endodontics.

and cotton pellet are then covered with a glass ionomer temporary (intermediate restorative material can be used as well).

9. It takes 3–6 hours for the MTA to completely set. Therefore, the patient is rescheduled for the final restoration. The key to pulp survival after vital pulp therapy is a well-sealed restoration. Composites and amalgams can be sealed to prevent microleakage (Mertz-Fairhurst *et al.*, 1998). Full-coverage crowns are recommended if the tooth has enamel or dental defects or the tooth requires a restoration that involves more than two surfaces.

Criteria for Success

- Vitality is preserved.
- No pain, sensitivity, or swelling.
- No radiographic evidence of internal or external resorption or other periradicular disease.
- Continued apexogenesis (Rafter, 2005):
  - Sustain the viability of Hertwig's sheath, thus allowing for continued development of the root length, ensuring a better crown-to-root ratio.

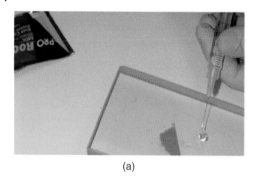
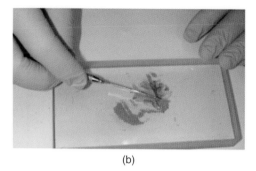

(a)   (b)

Figure 10.11 (a) Mineral trioxide aggregate (MTA)-to-saline ratio is 3 : 1. (b) MTA is mixed on a glass slab.

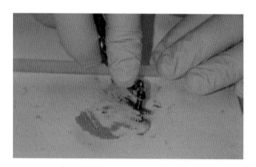

Figure 10.12 Loading amalgam carrier with mineral trioxide aggregate.

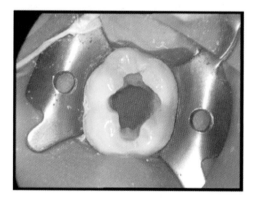

Figure 10.13 Condensing the mineral trioxide aggregate into place. Courtesy of Dr. Claudia Colorado, VCU Department of Endodontics.

○ Maintain pulpal vitality, thus allowing the remaining odontoblasts to lay down dentin, which in turn produces a thicker root wall and less chance of root fracture.
○ Promote root end closure to allow for the natural apical constriction.
○ Generate a dentinal bridge at the site of the pulpotomy. Its presence indicates that the pulp has maintained its vitality.

Success Rate

The success is higher for the MTA pulpotomy than the $Ca(OH)_2$ pulpotomy. This can be due to the fact that MTA produces a thicker dentinal bridge, less inflammation, less hyperemia, and less pulpal necrosis compared with $Ca(OH)_2$ (Witherspoon *et al.*, 2006). MTA also provides a better seal against bacterial invasion.

References

Baroudi, K. & Samir, S. (2016) Sealing ability of MTA used in perforation repair of permanent teeth: literature review. *Open Dentistry Journal*, 10, 278–286.

Camilleri, J. (2008) The chemical composition of mineral trioxide aggregate. *Journal of Conservative Dentistry*, 11 (4), 141–143.

Camilleri, J. (2015) Staining potential of Neo MTA Plus, MTA Plus, and Biodentine used for pulpotomy procedures. *Journal of Endodontics*, 41 (7), 1139–1145.

Camp, J. (2008) Diagnosis dilemmas in vital pulp therapy: treatment for the toothache is changing, especially in young, *immature teeth*. *Pediatric Dentistry*, 30 (3), 197–205.

El Meligy, O.A.S. & Avery, D.R. (2006) Comparison of mineral trioxide aggregate and calcium hydroxide as pulpotomy agents in young permanent teeth (apexogenesis). *Pediatric Dentistry*, 28 (5), 399–404.

Farsi, N., Alamoudi, N., Balto, K., & Al, M.A. (2006) Clinical assessment of mineral trioxide aggregate (MTA) as direct pulp capping in young permanent teeth. *Journal of Pediatric Dentistry*, 31 (2), 72–76.

Hilton, T.J. (2009) Keys to clinical success with pulp capping: a review of the literature. *Operative Dentistry*, 34 (5), 615–625.

Horsted-Bindslev, P. & Lovschall, H. (2002) Treatment outcome of vital pulp treatment. *Endodontic Topics*, 2, 24–34.

Hutcheson, C., Seale, S., McWhorter, A., Kerins, C., & Wright, J. (2012) Multi-surface composite vs stainless steel crown restorations after mineral trioxide aggregate pulpotomy: a randomized controlled trial. *Pediatric Dentistry*, 34 (7), 460–467.

Mejare, I. & Cvek, M. (1993) Partial pulpotomy in young permanent teeth with deep carious lesions. *Endodontics and Dental Traumatology*, 9, 238–242.

Mertz-Fairhurst, E., Curtis, J., Ergle, J., Rueggeberg, F., & Adair, S. (1998) Ultraconservative and cariostatic sealed restorations: results at year 10. *Journal of the American Dental Association*, 129, 55–66.

Parirokh, M., Torabinejad, M., & Dummer, P.M.H. (2018) Mineral trioxide aggregate and other bioactive endodontic cements: an updated overview—part I: vital pulp therapy. *International Endodontic Journal,* 51, 177–205.

Rafter, M. (2005) Apexification: a review. *Dental Traumatology*, 21, 1–8.

Ranly, D.M. & Garcia-Godoy, F. (2000) Current and potential pulp therapies for primary and young permanent teeth. *Journal of Dentistry*, 28, 153–161.

Sakar, N.K., Caicedo, R., Rtiwik, P., Moiseyeva, R., & Kawashima, I. (2005) Physiochemical basis of the biologic properties of mineral trioxide aggregate. *Journal of Endodontics,* 31, 97–99.

Steffen, R. & van Waes, H. (2009) Understanding mineral trioxide aggregate/Portland-cement: a review of literature and background factors. *European Archives of Paediatric Dentistry*, 10 (2), 93–97.

Torabinejad, M. & Walton, R. (2009) Protecting the pulp, preserving the apex. In: *Endodontics*, 4th edn. St. Louis, MO: Saunders Elsevier; 31–32.

Ward, J. (2002) Vital pulp therapy in cariously exposed permanent teeth and its limitations. *Australian Endodontic Journal*, 28 (1), 29–37.

Witherspoon, D.E., Small, J.C., & Harris, G.Z. (2006) Mineral trioxide aggregate pulpotomies. *Journal of the American Dental Association*, 137, 610–618.

11

Diagnosis and Management of Molar–Incisor Hypomineralization

J. Timothy Wright

Molar–incisor hypomineralization (MIH) is a developmental defect of the human dentition that primarily affects the enamel of the first permanent molars and can involve the incisors. Typically, the second permanent molars and premolars are not involved. This condition has been recognized since around 1970 and has been described using a variety of terms (e.g., cheese molars, idiopathic hypomineralization of enamel; Weerheijm *et al.*, 2001a). The term MIH was accepted by leaders in the field who convened at the European Academy of Pediatric Dentistry in 2000, and this continues to be the name most used to describe this condition (Weerheijm *et al.*, 2001b).

The clinical characteristics vary from case to case and between teeth in the same individual. The more severely affected the first permanent molars, the more likely it is that there will be incisor involvement. The defects vary from small, well-demarcated areas of color change to extensive hypomineralization that includes the entire dental crown. Affected teeth form with a normal thickness of enamel and the abnormal areas of enamel have a decreased mineral content and increased protein and water content. Thus, the defects are not hypoplastic, in that the full thickness of enamel develops. Once the tooth begins to erupt and come into function, rapid enamel loss can make the crowns appear hypoplastic, but this is typically the result of enamel fracturing, wear, and dental caries. Discoloration of the involved areas is a result of the decreased

mineral content and increased protein and water content, which change the optical character of the hypomineralized enamel (Fagrell, 2011). The enamel color changes range from white opaque lesions to a creamy yellow or brown. The more severe the level of hypomineralization, the more likely the tooth is to have early loss of enamel. Early enamel loss is often associated with the development and progression of dental caries, which can lead to rapid deterioration of the clinical crown (Figure 11.1) and pulpal involvement if left untreated. The degree of hypersensitivity associated with these defects varies, but can be quite pronounced and appears to be frequently associated with the severity of hypomineralization and enamel loss. Hypersensitivity and difficulty anesthetizing the affected molars can add to the challenge of treating individuals with MIH (William *et al.*, 2006). Numerous studies show that MIH can have a significant impact on a child's quality of life and that treatment of the defective teeth has an immediate and positive effect (Ridell *et al.*, 2015).

Prevalence and Etiology

The prevalence of MIH ranges from about 3% to 40%, with an average worldwide prevalence of 13%, making it quite common and a condition that will regularly challenge clinicians (Jalevik, 2010; Schwendicke *et al.*, 2018). The first permanent molar is the permanent

Handbook of Clinical Techniques in Pediatric Dentistry, Second Edition. Edited by Jane A. Soxman.
© 2022 John Wiley & Sons, Inc. Published 2022 by John Wiley & Sons, Inc.

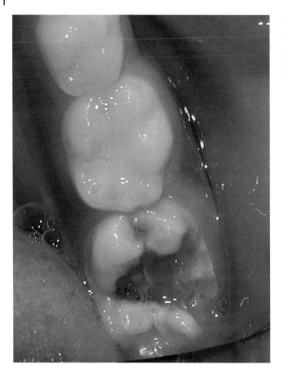

Figure 11.1 This mandibular first permanent molar shows the brown discoloration seen in severe molar–incisor hypomineralization, and the subsequent loss of tooth structure and development of caries is readily evident.

tooth most likely to develop dental caries, and hypomineralized molars are at increased risk for developing dental caries. Caries development can obscure the presence of enamel hypomineralization, which likely contributes to the carious involvement in at least some first permanent molars. The first permanent molars begin to form *in utero* and typically start to mineralize just before or shortly after birth (first permanent molars of girls tend to form earlier than those of boys). The enamel of the permanent first molars and permanent incisors does not fully mineralize until the age of 3–5 years. Having enamel hypomineralization in the primary dentition increases the odds that the individual will have MIH in the permanent dentition (Elfrink *et al.*, 2012).

Attempts to identify the etiology of MIH have largely focused on categorizing environmental insults that might be associated with the condition. Maternal health, premature birth, low birth weight, infant health, use of antibiotics, and a number of other conditions have been associated with MIH (Whatling &

Fearne, 2008; Laisi *et al.*, 2009; Alaluusua, 2010). Most of the environmental stressors associated with MIH appear to occur in the first year of life (Fagrell *et al.*, 2013; Fatturi *et al.*, 2019; Wu *et al.*, 2020). Although there were initially thought to be associations and possible toxins associated with breastfeeding (dioxins), other studies do not support an association of MIH with breastfeeding (Laisi *et al.*, 2008).

Studies evaluating the environmental influences associated with MIH have not ruled out the potential contribution of hereditary factors as participating in the cause of MIH. Indeed genetic loci and even gene interactions have been associated with MIH (Pang *et al.*, 2020), and there are families with a history of MIH in multiple generations and greater concordance in twins with MIH (Kuhnisch *et al.*, 2013; Teixeira *et al.*, 2018). These findings all suggest that there is some genetic component contributing to MIH (Vieira, 2019). This is entirely reasonable, given that we know enamel formation is highly regulated at the molecular level and involves the expression of thousands of genes (Jeremias *et al.*, 2013). Just as genetics contributes significantly to an individual's risk for developing dental caries, it is probable that multiple genetic variations are at play in defining a person's risk for developing MIH and making them more susceptible to environmental insults.

Diagnosis of Molar–Incisor Hypomineralization

Diagnosing MIH can be difficult, and clinicians may confuse MIH with other developmental defects of enamel, such as fluorosis or amelogenesis imperfecta (a group of hereditary conditions that cause a variety of enamel defects). There are hundreds of environmental and genetic conditions that are known to affect enamel formation, and so making a definitive diagnosis can be challenging. The diagnosis of MIH can be further complicated if the tooth begins to decay as it is erupting, thereby destroying the affected crown structure. It is, however, important to accurately diagnosis MIH so that the different approaches for managing the condition can be implemented to achieve optimal treatment outcomes. There often will not be a family history of enamel defects, such as can occur in cases of amelogenesis imperfecta. The hypomineralization defect is primarily limited to the first permanent molars and incisors, whereas most of the teeth of both the primary and permanent dentitions are involved in amelogenesis imperfecta. With fluorosis the primary dentition is typically not affected, but all the permanent teeth tend to be involved, and the enamel defects are more uniformly distributed than appears with MIH (e.g., all four first permanent molars and incisors will be similarly affected).

Clinical evaluation for the presence of MIH ideally involves examining the four first permanent molars and eight permanent incisors, and is often best accomplished in an 8-year-old child (Weerheijm *et al.*, 2003). The examination should be performed when the teeth are clean and moist. They are examined for the presence of demarcated changes in enamel color and translucency (opacities) and areas of enamel loss that most often occur in the affected molars. A severity scale has been developed to classify MIH as mild, moderate, or severe at the tooth level, meaning that one tooth may be mild, and another tooth in the same patient may be severe; seeing this amount of variability is a common occurrence (Table 11.1) (Mathu-Muju & Wright, 2006). Enamel color changes are caused by changes in the enamel composition (amount of mineral and protein) and structure. Enamel that is yellow-brown tends to have less mineral compared to white

Table 11.1 Severity score of teeth affected with molar–incisor hypomineralization.

	Mild	Moderate	Severe
Crown appearance	Demarcated opacities in non-stress-bearing area of molar	Intact atypical restoration present	Posteruptive enamel breakdown present
Enamel loss	Isolated opacities	Occlusal/incisal third of teeth without initial posteruptive enamel breakdown	Posteruptive enamel breakdown on erupting tooth that can be rapid
Caries	No caries associated with affected enamel	Posteruptive enamel breakdown/caries limited to one or two surfaces without cuspal involvement	Often develop widespread caries associated with affected enamel
Sensitivity	Normal dental sensitivity	Usually normal dental sensitivity	Usually history of dental sensitivity
Esthetics	Usually not an issue	Parents often express concern	Parents typically concerned

opacities and is more likely to succumb to enamel loss. These yellow-brown areas tend to lack the shiny, reflective surfaces of normal enamel and have a more ground-glass and slightly rough appearance, indicative of a decreased mineral content. Clinically assessing these characteristics is helpful in determining prognosis for an individual tooth and the likelihood that it will break down over time as a result of enamel loss. These clinical attributes are also helpful in selecting appropriate treatment approaches and optimizing therapeutic success.

Treatment Approaches for Molar–Incisor Hypomineralization

Treatment approaches for MIH will vary substantially, depending on the level of severity of the defect. The treatment goals for molars are to prevent the tooth from developing dental caries, to help prevent or reduce enamel loss, to restore form and function when there is enamel loss, and to address esthetic issues (this is typically more important in the affected incisors and is discussed later in the chapter) (William et al., 2006; Lygidakis et al., 2010). For some moderately and most severely affected molars, another goal is to manage the hypersensitivity associated with the hypomineralized and

lost enamel. Normally, enamel has excellent insulating properties and protects the tooth from chemical and thermal stresses. When the mineral content is reduced and the protein and water content are increased or the enamel is lost, the tooth often becomes easily stimulated, and the level of sensitivity can be quite severe. Treatment approaches thus tend to be predicated on the severity of the MIH and the presence or absence of dental sensitivity (Table 11.2).

Optimizing approaches directed at the prevention of dental caries for individuals with MIH should always be considered, as their caries risk is increased due to having defective enamel. Discussions related to dietary risk factors, fluoride exposure including toothpaste, and other fluoride sources such as topical fluoride applications (fluoride varnish or gel) should be considered. For milder levels of dental sensitivity, the use of toothpaste for sensitive teeth might be of some benefit, although there are no studies to verify their usefulness. Amorphous calcium phosphate–casein phosphopeptide has been suggested, but there is little evidence that it functions with any greater effectiveness than fluoride toothpaste and it is much more costly (Slayton et al., 2018). The use of chlorhexidine rinses at the concentration sold in the United States (0.12%) is not effective for controlling caries and can cause significant staining, so

Table 11.2 Management of molar–incisor hypomineralization.

	Mild	Moderate	Severe
Molars	Desensitizing toothpaste	Fluoride varnish	Glass ionomer coverage
	Silver diamine fluoride	Silver diamine fluoride	Silver diamine fluoride
	Fluoride varnish	Sealants	Interim resins
	Sealants	Resin restorations	Stainless-steel crowns
			Extraction
Incisors	No treatment	Bleach/seal	Bleach/seal
	Resin perfusion	Resin perfusion	Resin perfusion
		Microabrasion	Microabrasion
		Resin restorations	Resin restorations
			Veneers

they are not recommended for caries management (Rethman *et al.*, 2011). Silver diamine fluoride (SDF; 38%) has been shown to help prevent caries in pits and fissures, is highly effective in arresting caries, and can be a useful adjunctive therapy (Liu *et al.*, 2012; Urquhart *et al.*, 2019).

For mild MIH, fissure sealants provide a valuable preventive measure. Sealant retention can be an issue in teeth with MIH, because the enamel is inherently weakened and has increased protein and water content. Studies on sealant retention in MIH-affected teeth have been limited in numbers of teeth studied, but indicate that sealants can be successful; however, retention varies with the material and technique for placement. A number of approaches have been suggested to enhance the bonding to these defective enamel surfaces. Pretreatment of the pits and fissures with 5% sodium hypochlorite (prior to etching) will help reduce the discoloration of the surface and remove proteins and organic material from within the enamel, helping create an intimate resin–enamel interface and increased bond strength (Bayrak *et al.*, 2020). Studies also indicate that the use of a bonding agent before sealant placement will improve retention (Lagarde *et al.*, 2020). The following protocol is recommended for sealant placement in teeth with MIH:

1. Isolate tooth to maintain a dry field.
2. Clean pits and fissures and any discolored tooth surface with pumice and rinse.
3. Apply 5% sodium hypochlorite (NaOCl) for 60 seconds and rinse thoroughly.
4. Apply phosphoric acid etchant for 30 seconds, rinse, and dry.
5. Apply bonding agent and sealant to pits and fissures and treated discolored areas.

Bleaching of the affected enamel and perfusing it with resin can markedly improve the appearance of the enamel (Figure 11.2). Resins that perfuse into enamel are bonding agents, unfilled clear sealants, and the Icon resin systems (DMG America, Ridgefield Park, NJ, USA), designed specifically for treating noncavitated enamel decalcifications or hypomineralized areas. This same technique can be used to manage yellow-brown discolored areas on the anterior and has been called the bleach–etch–seal technique (BEST; Wright, 2002). This can produce excellent esthetic results in some but not all cases. depending on the extent, depth, and type of discoloration. White opacities will tend to remain white, although resin perfusion can markedly diminish this discoloration in some cases as well.

The technique outlined previously uses resin-based sealant systems that have been shown in numerous clinical studies to be highly effective in preventing caries (Gooch *et al.*, 2009). They are relatively technique sensitive to place and require the tooth be isolated. Glass ionomers (GIs) provide another option that can be used as a sealant and, as discussed in the next section, a restorative material. GIs provide an excellent option for partially erupted teeth, teeth with sensitivity to air, or teeth that are difficult to isolate, as they are moisture tolerant and can bond directly to the enamel and be placed without multiple and intermediate steps. MIH-affected molars with caries can be treated with SDF and then restored with a GI restoration. This approach has been referred to as the SDF modified ART technique (SMART) and can help manage MIH lesions where sensitivity is pronounced.

Teeth with moderate degrees of MIH will have more extensive areas of affected enamel, and there is a high likelihood that stress-bearing areas will eventually fracture with function over time. Thus, cuspal and marginal ridge enamel fractures are common in these teeth. If there is no enamel loss, then initial treatment should be placement of a resin or GI sealant that can help protect the enamel surface. If enamel fracturing occurs, then a filled resin or GI-type restoration can be placed to restore the normal tooth contours and help prevent caries from forming

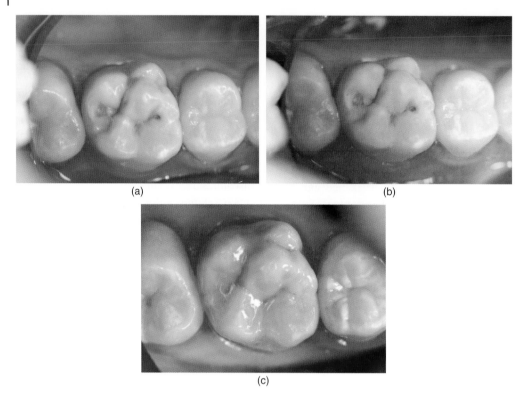

(a)

(b)

(c)

Figure 11.2 (a) This maxillary first permanent molar has moderate molar–incisor hypomineralization, with some enamel loss already occurring in both the mesial and distal occlusal areas. (b) The tooth was cleaned and treated with 5% NaOCl, which shows the improved color change that can occur with this treatment. (c) The tooth was etched, bonding agent placed and polymerized, and then sealed with a white opaque sealant in the lingual area for improved esthetics, and then coated entirely with a highly penetrating clear resin sealant.

in uncleanable and exposed areas. Removal of the severely affected enamel areas to allow for a minimal bulk of material required for fracture resistance, and to allow the restoration to extend to minimally or nonaffected enamel that is adjacent to the fractured area, will improve restoration longevity. The technique for placement of resin restorations is the same as that outlined for resin sealant placement. Amalgam restorations also perform relatively well in the treatment of these teeth (Lygidakis *et al.*, 2010). If this nonadhesive approach is used, the restoration should not end on severely affected areas of enamel that will be stress bearing, as they will likely fracture away from the amalgam.

Teeth with severe MIH are the most challenging to treat. The molars may be losing

enamel and developing caries lesions as they first begin to emerge into the oral cavity. Extreme sensitivity can accompany this clinical presentation. These teeth can often be treated using GI materials that can be placed with no tooth preparation or need for anesthetic. The tooth can be blotted dry with cotton, and either a chemical, light-cured, or resin-modified GI placed (Figure 11.3). If the tooth is early in its course of eruption, then additional material will likely need to be placed at regular intervals until a more definitive restorative approach can be considered. Placement of these materials provides an effective barrier to thermal and chemical stimulation and can provide immediate relief from sensitivity (Figure 11.2). Although these restorations can serve as excellent protective

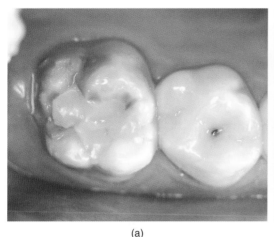
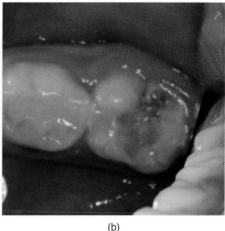

(a)   (b)

Figure 11.3 (a) The maxillary first permanent molar caused extreme sensitivity with temperature changes, and was treated using a protective resin-modified glass ionomer with no tooth preparation other than pumice prophylaxis and blotting the tooth dry. (b) The margins show some deterioration at this 3-year follow-up, but the restoration remains intact, with no development of caries or problems with sensitivity. The mandibular first permanent molar was very sensitive and had a large occlusal caries lesion associated with the molar–incisor hypomineralization defect. This tooth was treated with silver diamine fluoride for 2 minutes, blotted dry, and the lesion filled with a resin-modified glass ionomer material.

treatments, they typically are not definitive, and when the tooth is fully erupted, additional or other treatment can be considered. In some cases, these types of treatments can last for years, allowing additional dentin formation, root apexification, and increased maturity of the patient.

If early treatment is not provided in teeth severely affected with MIH, then extensive destruction and caries development can result in pulp necrosis and teeth requiring more extensive restorations. Many of the severely affected teeth will ultimately need to be restored with crowns. Clinical studies show that stainless-steel crowns (SSCs) and cast crowns provide outstanding results with very few failures (Lygidakis *et al.*, 2010). While Hall technique placement in primary teeth shows good evidence of success, there is no information on this approach in permanent teeth (Boyd *et al.*, 2020). For newly erupted teeth and even in young patients in their early teens, SSCs have many advantages over other types of crowns, as they require a minimal amount of tooth reduction for placement, are

less expensive than cast crowns, and can be completed in one visit.

There are no long-term data on the outcomes of providing root canal therapy and crowns to teeth in young preadult patients. Although excellent results can be achieved using these techniques (Figure 11.4), the long-term prognosis for teeth treated in such a manner should be considered guarded until evidence indicates otherwise. Teeth with a poor or guarded prognosis should be considered as potential candidates for extraction. Individuals having multiple MIH-affected teeth, especially if they are severely affected, may benefit from extracting the first permanent molars. If this is performed when the patient is young and the second permanent molar has less than half of its root formation, then the 12-year molar will often move mesially and close much of the space left from extraction of the first permanent molar (Figure 11.5). Before considering this option, it is optimal to obtain a panoramic radiograph and evaluate whether the second and/or third molars are present and the stage of tooth development, and to have an

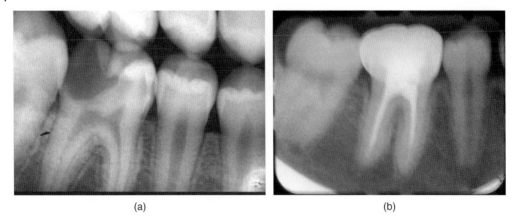

(a)   (b)

Figure 11.4 (a, b) These radiographs show treatment of a mandibular first permanent molar with severe molar–incisor hypomineralization and caries that was treated with root canal therapy and a stainless-steel crown.

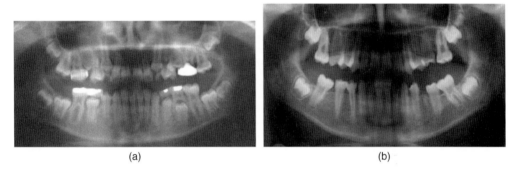

(a)   (b)

Figure 11.5 (a) This child had three first permanent molars with severe molar–incisor hypomineralization that had been restored and had marked crowding in the maxillary arch. (b) All four first permanent molars were extracted, and the position of the 12-year molars and amount of space closure obtained by their eruption are seen before final orthodontic treatment.

orthodontic consultation. Some orthodontic tooth movement may be necessary to achieve optimal space closure, tooth inclination, and alignment.

Pain management can be challenging in patients with severe MIH, as the child associates all stimuli to these teeth with pain. Children with severe MIH are more likely to have restorative or surgical interventions and are more likely than children not affected with MIH to have dental fear and exhibit behavior problems (Jalevik & Klingberg, 2002). Obtaining adequate anesthesia or sedation before using surgical approaches, including restoration where tooth structure is removed, is critical.

Summary

Clinicians are frequently faced with patients who require management of molars and incisors that have hypomineralized defects. Although a specific etiology remains to be established, it appears likely that these defects are the result of a combination of genetic predisposition and environmental insults. Managing patients with MIH requires a variety of patient management approaches, materials, and techniques. The dental hypersensitivity these patients experience and associate with their first permanent molars can make them extremely challenging to manage from a behavioral and anesthetic point of view. Having optimal caries prevention and reducing sensitivity as the teeth erupt using protective restorations and sealants can help reduce the need for more aggressive restorative approaches, assist in maintaining pulp vitality, and thus make patient management from an anesthetic and behavioral aspect potentially less complicated. The materials available to place protective and definitive restorations are excellent and can be applied using a variety of techniques to gain optimal therapeutic results. As we increasingly move to digital restorative approaches, there are opportunities to generate custom-made crowns from polymethyl methacrylate resin or other materials. This can provide esthetic restorations that are modifiable as the tooth erupts and may require less tooth reduction than other approaches such as prefabricated zirconia crowns. The timing of different treatment approaches, including extraction of the first permanent molars, can have a marked impact on the effectiveness of the treatment. By carefully diagnosing MIH and its severity and selectively applying different therapies, clinicians can achieve the goals of having patients with MIH who do not have hypersensitivity and who have a functional and esthetic dentition.

References

Alaluusua, S. (2010) Aetiology of molar-incisor hypomineralisation: a systematic review. *European Archives of Paediatric Dentistry*, 11, 53–58.

Bayrak, G.D., Gurdogan-Guler, E.B., Yildirim, Y., Ozturk, D., & Selvi-Kuvvetli, S. (2020) Assessment of shear bond strength and microleakage of fissure sealant following enamel deproteinization: an in vitro study. *Journal of Clinical Experimental Dentistry*, 12 (3), e220–e226.

Boyd, D.H., Thomson, W.M., Leon de la Barra, S., Fuge, K.N., van den Heever, R., *et al.* (2020) A primary care randomized controlled trial of Hall and conventional restorative techniques. *Journal of Dental Research Clinical and Translational Research*, 2380084420933154.

Elfrink, M.E., Ten Cate, J.M., Jaddoe, V.W., Hofman, A., Moll, H.A., & Veerkamp, J.S. (2012) Deciduous molar hypomineralization and molar incisor hypomineralization. *Journal of Dental Research*, 91, 551–555.

Fagrell, T. (2011) Molar incisor hypomineralization. Morphological and chemical aspects, onset and possible etiological factors. *Swedish Dental Journal.* 5 (Suppl), 11–83.

Fagrell, T.G., Salmon, P., Melin, L., & Noren, J.G. (2013) Onset of molar incisor hypomineralization (MIH). *Swedish Dental Journal*, 37, 61–70.

Fatturi, A.L., Wambier, L.M., Chibinski, A.C., Assuncao, L., Brancher, J.A., *et al.* (2019) A systematic review and meta-analysis of systemic exposure associated with molar incisor hypomineralization. *Community Dental Oral Epidemiology*, 47 (5), 407-415.

Gooch, B.F., Griffin, S.O., Gray, S.K., Kohn, W.G., Rozier, R.G., *et al.* (2009) Preventing dental caries through school-based sealant programs: updated recommendations and reviews of evidence. *Journal of the American Dental Association*, 140, 1356–1365.

Jalevik, B. (2010) Prevalence and diagnosis of molar-incisor hypomineralisation (MIH): a systematic review. *European Archives of Paediatric Dentistry*, 11, 59–64.

Jalevik, B. & Klingberg, G.A. (2002) Dental treatment, dental fear and behaviour management problems in children with severe enamel hypomineralization of their permanent first molars. *International Journal of Paediatric Dentistry*, 12, 24–32.

Jeremias, F., Koruyucu, M., Kuchler, E.C., Bayram, M., Tuna, E.B., *et al.* (2013) Genes expressed in dental enamel development are associated with molar-incisor hypomineralization. *Archives of Oral Biology*, 58, 1434–1442.

Kuhnisch, J., Thiering, E., Heitmuller, D., Tiesler, C.M.T., Grallert, H., *et al.* (2013) Genome-wide association study (GWAS) for molar-incisor hypomineralization (MIH). *Clinical Oral Investigations*, 18, 677–682.

Lagarde, M., Vennat, E., Attal, J.P., & Dursun, E. (2020) Strategies to optimize bonding of adhesive materials to molar-incisor hypomineralization-affected enamel: a systematic review. *International Journal of Paediatric Dentistry*, 30 (4), 405–420.

Laisi, S., Ess, A., Sahlberg, C., Arvio, P., Lukinmaa, P.L., & Alaluusua, S. (2009) Amoxicillin may cause molar incisor hypomineralization. *Journal of Dental Research*, 88, 132–136.

Laisi, S., Kiviranta, H., Lukinmaa, P.L., Vartiainen, T., & Alaluusua, S. (2008) Molar-incisor-hypomineralisation and dioxins: new findings. *European Archives of Paediatric Dentistry*, 9, 224–227.

Liu, B.Y., Lo, E.C., Chu, C.H., & Lin, H.C. (2012) Randomized trial on fluorides and sealants for fissure caries prevention. *Journal of Dental Research*, 91 (8), 753–758.

Lygidakis, N.A., Wong, F., Jalevik, B., Vierrou, A.M., Alaluusua, S., & Espelid, I. (2010) Best clinical practice guidance for clinicians dealing with children presenting with molar-incisor-hypomineralisation (MIH): an EAPD policy document. *European Archives of Paediatric Dentistry*, 11, 75–81.

Mathu-Muju, K. & Wright, J.T. (2006) Diagnosis and treatment of molar incisor hypomineralization. *Compendium of Continuing Education in Dentistry*, 27, 604–610; quiz 611.

Pang, L., Li, X., Wang, K., Tao, Y., Cui, T., *et al.* (2020) Interactions with the aquaporin 5 gene increase the susceptibility to molar-incisor hypomineralization. *Archives of Oral Biology*, 111, 104637.

Rethman, M.P., Beltran-Aguilar, E.D., Billings, R.J., Hujoel, P.P., Katz, B.P., *et al.* (2011) Nonfluoride caries-preventive agents:

executive summary of evidence-based clinical recommendations. *Journal of the American Dental Association*, 142, 1065–1071.

Ridell, K., Borgstrom, M., Lager, E., Magnusson, G., Brogardh-Roth, S., & Matsson, L. (2015) Oral health-related quality-of-life in Swedish children before and after dental treatment under general anesthesia. *Acta Odontologica Scandanavia*, 73 (1), 1–7.

Schwendicke, F., Elhennawy, K., Reda, S., Bekes, K., Manton, D.J., & Krois, J. (2018) Global burden of molar incisor hypomineralization. *Journal of Dentistry*, 68, 10–18.

Slayton, R.L., Urquhart, O., Araujo, M.W.B., Fontana, M., Guzman-Armstrong, S., *et al.* (2018) Evidence-based clinical practice guideline on nonrestorative treatments for carious lesions: a report from the American Dental Association. *Journal of the American Dental Association*, 149 (10), 837–849.e819.

Teixeira, R., Andrade, N.S., Queiroz, L.C.C., Mendes, F.M., Moura, M.S., *et al.* (2018) Exploring the association between genetic and environmental factors and molar incisor hypomineralization: evidence from a twin study. *International Journal of Paediatric Dentistry*, 28 (2), 198–206.

Urquhart. O.,Tampi, M.P., Pilcher, L., Slayton, R.L., Araujo, M.W.B., *et al.* (2019) Nonrestorative treatments for caries: systematic review and network meta-analysis. *Journal of Dental Research,* 98 (1), 14–26.

Vieira, A.R. (2019). On the genetics contribution to molar incisor hypomineralization. *International Journal of Paediatric Dentistry*, 29 (1), 2–3.

Weerheijm, K.L., Duggal, M., Mejare, I., Papagiannoulis, L., Koch, G., *et al.* (2003) Judgement criteria for molar incisor hypomineralisation (MIH) in epidemiologic studies: a summary of the European meeting on MIH held in Athens, 2003. *European Journal of Paediatric Dentistry*, 4, 110–113.

Weerheijm, K.L., Groen, H.J., Beentjes, V.E., & Poorterman, J.H. (2001a) Prevalence of cheese molars in eleven-year-old Dutch children.

ASDC Journal of Dentistry for Children, 68 (259–262), 229.

Weerheijm, K.L., Jalevik, B., & Alaluusua, S. (2001b) Molar-incisor hypomineralisation. *Caries Research*, 35, 390–391.

Whatling, R. & Fearne, J.M. (2008) Molar incisor hypomineralization: a study of aetiological factors in a group of UK children. *International Journal of Paediatric Dentistry*, 18, 155–162.

William, V., Messer, L.B., & Burrow, M.F. (2006) Molar incisor hypomineralization: review and recommendations for clinical management. *Pediatric Dentistry*, 28, 224–232.

Wright, J.T. (2002) The etch-bleach-seal technique for managing stained enamel defects in young permanent incisors. *Pediatric Dentistry*, 24, 249–252.

Wu, X., Wang, J., Li, Y.H., Yang, Z.Y., & Zhou, Z. (2020) Association of molar incisor hypomineralization with premature birth or low birth weight: systematic review and meta-analysis. *Journal of Maternal Fetal Neonatal Medicine*, 33 (10), 1700–1708.

12

Management of Esthetic Concerns
Elizabeth S. Gosnell, Roshan V. Patel, J. Timothy Wright, and S. Thikkurissy

Intrinsic Versus Extrinsic Staining

Tooth discoloration can be one of the most upsetting dental defects a person can encounter in their life. While there is no direct impact on eating and speaking, there are still potential major sequelae associated with discoloration. Tooth discoloration has been shown to impact a person's desire to smile, to freely answer questions from people, and in general their ability to interact with people. Ibiyemi and Taiwo (2011) reported that 87% of respondents noted that their tooth discoloration "made them unhappy." Historically, light, heat, electric current, and chemicals have been used to accelerate "whitening." Noted side effects to the whitening process include gingival irritation and dentinal hypersensitivity. The specific physics of tooth discoloration is related to how light is reflected or absorbed. The most commonly accepted classification system is based on the nature of the stain as intrinsic or extrinsic.

Structural changes within the enamel or dentin (intrinsic discoloration) lead to alterations in light refraction and can lead to what are known as "intrinsic staining" lesions. These may be seen in conditions such as fluorosis, dentinogenesis, and amelogenesis imperfecta. Consumption of antibiotics such as those in the tetracycline class also are associated with

intrinsic discoloration. Table 12.1 lists several etiologies for intrinsic staining. Absorption of various chromogenic compounds (such as polyphenols in food coloring) into the outer enamel surface is known as extrinsic staining.

There are several techniques that can be employed to address esthetic concerns. Techniques addressed in this chapter include whitening agents, microabrasion, resin infiltration, and the bleach–etch–seal technique.

Pharmacology of Whitening Agents

Teeth continue to darken with time due to the process of continued dentin deposition and due to both intrinsic and extrinsic tooth staining, which is created by the buildup of compounds known as chromogens (Carey, 2014). These chromogens can reduce the natural white color and brilliance of the enamel surface. Over the years, teeth whitening products have been marketed to help improve the surface esthetics and overall color appearance of the adult dentition. Commercially and professionally applied tooth whitening agents contain either hydrogen peroxide or carbamide peroxide (American Academy of Pediatric Dentistry, 2020). These whitening agents are made in a variety of forms, including pastes and gels (Carey, 2014).

Handbook of Clinical Techniques in Pediatric Dentistry, Second Edition. Edited by Jane A. Soxman.
© 2022 John Wiley & Sons, Inc. Published 2022 by John Wiley & Sons, Inc.

Table 12.1 Etiologies for intrinsic and extrinsic staining.

Tooth stains		
General classification	**Subgroups**	**Examples**
Intrinsic discolorations	Metabolic disorders	• Congenital hyperbilirubinemia is characterized by yellow-green discolorations caused by the deposition of bile pigments in calcifying dental hard tissues
	Medical treatments	• Tetracyclines chelate to form complexes with calcium ions on the surface of hydroxyapatite crystals primarily within dentin and the affected teeth tend to be yellow or brown-gray in color
	Inherited diseases	• Dentinogenesis imperfecta is an inherited disorder of dentine. The appearance is an amber, gray to purple-blue discoloration or opalescence, thought to be the result of the absorption of chromogens into the porous dentine after exposure of the dentine
	Idiopathic diseases	• Molar–incisor hypomineralization is a condition of unknown etiology that is characterized by severely hypomineralized enamel affecting the incisors and permanent first molars. The appearance of the hypomineralized enamel is asymmetric and yellow or brownish areas could appear
	Traumatic causes	• Enamel hypoplasia, pulpal hemorrhagic products, and root resorption
Extrinsic discolorations	Direct staining	• Tannins found in tea, coffee, and other beverages could promote brown stains on the surface of the teeth • Tobacco smoking is known to cause dark brown and black staining • The oral hygiene is also involved in the direct extrinsic discoloration, accumulations of dental plaque, calculus, and food particles cause brown or black stains
	Indirect staining	• Cetylpyridinium chloride mouthwashes and chlorhexidine mouthwashes are most effective in controlling plaque and gingivitis, but cause the greatest deposition of extrinsic stains

[a] Source: Adapted from Rodriguez-Martinez *et al.* (2019).

There are various formulations available regarding the concentrations of whitening agent. In comparison, a 10% carbamide peroxide is equivalent to a 3.5% hydrogen peroxide solution (American Academy of Pediatric Dentistry, 2020). In-office solutions of hydrogen peroxide are often higher, containing 15–38%, in comparison to home-based products that contain a lower concentration, typically ranging from 3% to 10%.

The whitening effect is a result of either physical removal of extrinsic surface staining or a chemical reaction that causes oxidation (Carey, 2014). Physical or mechanical whitening is the result of the action of detergents and abrasives that help remove surface staining chromogens. In regard to chemical reactions, hydrogen peroxide molecules release hydroxyl ions that easily interact with and break down the molecular bonds in chromogens and other organic compounds (Kugel & Ferreira, 2006). The resulting simpler chromogen molecules reflect less light and thus appear whiter in color (Carey, 2014; Kugel & Ferreira, 2006). Carbamide peroxide reacts with water and chemically breaks down into hydrogen peroxide and urea. The urea compounds are further broken down into ammonia and water.

One of the most common side effects in the use of dental whitening agents is hypersensitivity (American Academy of Pediatric Dentistry, 2020). Hypersensitivity is directly related to the concentration of the peroxide agent and the contact time with the tooth structure. The peroxide ions are able to travel through the dentinal tubules and cause stimulation of the pulp within 5–15 minutes. Use of potassium nitrate dentifrices prior to application and sodium fluoride after application of whitening agents has shown to help patients with sensitivity side effects (Wang *et al.*, 2015). However, excessive bleaching practices over time can lead to enamel crystal breakdown and demineralization of the enamel surface (Lee *et al.*, 2005).

The pharmacologic effects of light activation on whitening agents remain a controversial topic. There are studies that show that the light has a synergistic effect with the active whitening ingredients, while several systematic reviews show no conclusive evidence to support light activation and its efficacy in aiding in the whitening process (Medeiros *et al.*, 2019; SoutoMaior *et al.*, 2019).

Documentation of Staining

As with any procedure, informed consent is a critical aspect of the treatment process. Many offices will have a distinct separate consent process for tooth whitening. This will include adverse effects such as cervical resorption, increased sensitivity, and gingival issues. Documentation of tooth discoloration should be as specific as possible, including shade of sections of the tooth to note any adverse changes. It should be noted that different areas of the stain can respond differently to the whitening agents and this should be discussed as part of the consent process.

Selecting a Vital Bleaching Agent

Selecting a vital bleaching agent is dependent on many factors, such as expected outcome, compliance, and exposure to refractory staining agents. Refractory staining agents include tea, coffee, and tobacco products. The American Dental Association (2010) delineates at-home products into three broad categories:

Whitening Toothpastes

Whitening toothpastes remove stains on the surface of the tooth. It is important to understand that these pastes are not bleaching the tooth or changing its actual color. They are instead focusing on removal of extrinsic discoloration.

Home-Use Bleaching Agents

Home-use bleaching agents come in strips or as gels the patient will paint on their teeth or put in a tray over their teeth. Home-use whiteners can come either from a dentist or over the counter. One benefit of using products from the dentist is that the trays will be fitted to limit the contact that the gel has with gingivae. This is critical, in that one of the most common adverse effects is the discoloration or irritation of gingivae from poorly fitting trays. Most of these agents use hydrogen peroxide.

In-Office Whitening

In-office whitening is performed by a dentist using a peroxide gel—stronger than the one used in at-home whiteners. This treatment may be initiated by a light on the gel to get the whitening reaction started. The whole process takes approximately 1 hour. Because the peroxide is stronger, the results may be more immediately dramatic.

Microabrasion

Enamel microabrasion is an effective method of removing superficial, intrinsic discolored enamel defects (Croll & Cavanaugh, 1986). Lesions that may be effectively removed with microabrasion include mild fluorosis and hypomineralized enamel, which appears as white or brown areas. There are several lesions for which microabrasion is not effective, including deeper lesions or lesions that involve the complete thickness of enamel, amelogenesis imperfecta defects, dentinal discoloration caused by dentinogenesis imperfecta, or tetracycline staining (Opalustre, 2020). Microabrasion is a conservative, nonrestorative method that can be used to improve the appearance of teeth with relatively superficial defects (e.g., the outer quarter of enamel). This procedure involves removal of the superficial enamel, so is permanent. The enamel microabrasion slurry consists of 6.6% hydrochloric acid and silicon carbide microparticles (Opalustre™, Ultradent, South Jordan, UT, USA). It lightly abrades and erodes the enamel surface. There are other products on the market and 37% phosphoric acid with pumice has also been used in studies.

The use of microabrasion produces enamel loss ranging between 25 and 200 μm (Croll & Cavanaugh, 1986), which will depend on the duration and pressure applied. Teeth that have been microabraded show a generalized smoothing effect on the enamel surface, as demonstrated with a scanning electron microscope. The microabrasion results in formation of an amorphous, prismless layer of enamel that appears smooth and lustrous clinically, called the "enamel glaze" (Donly *et al.*, 1992). The highly polished, densely compacted, mineralized structure after microabrasion may be mixed with silica debris. This surface reflects and refracts light, so that mild imperfections in underlying enamel are minimized in appearance. Over time, the smooth appearance is maintained and may improve, potentially by remineralization with saliva

and topical fluorides. Patients with deeper lesions may be managed by a combination of therapies, microabrasion with bleaching. Or if the combination of therapies is not successful in achieving an esthetic result, alternative treatment approaches may be considered.

A systematic review showed enamel microabrasion to be a viable treatment option for mild dental fluorosis lesions, but may be insufficient for moderate or severe fluorosis lesions (Da Cunha Coelho *et al.*, 2019). Esthetic improvement by patients was noted when a higher (10%) hydrochloric acid versus 6.6% hydrochloric acid was used with the microabrasion process, whereas the authors did not note a clinical difference. Caution should be used when considering using higher concentrations of the acid-etch, as it removes more tooth structure (Romero *et al.*, 2018). A prospective clinical trial evaluating the clinical efficacy of enamel microabrasion on mild to severe fluorosis lesions showed that the proportion of patients who required further treatment after microabrasion was significantly higher for the more severe fluorosis lesions. As the severity of fluorosis increases, the degree of hypomineralization and depth of staining increase, making microabrasion less effective (Celik *et al.*, 2013a). A case report showed anterior lesions with mild fluorosis staining. After the application of microabrasion slurry, then a treatment course of at-home bleaching, minor hypocalcified white spots remained (Zuanon *et al.,* 2008). In a clinical study evaluating 10 patients with 118 fluorosed incisors, the combination of at-home bleaching with microabrasion resulted in significantly improved esthetics and patient satisfaction when compared to microabrasion treatment alone.

A study evaluated the enamel loss on exfoliated primary incisors after the use of 37% phosphoric acid and pumice, using manual application with a plastic spatula versus mechanical application with a rubber cup prophy angle. A stereomicroscope was used to evaluate enamel loss and showed that the mechanical technique resulted in significantly higher loss, with 274 μm lost versus the manual technique with 152 μm lost. Due to the thinner enamel layer of primary teeth—0.277 mm thick located 0.125 mm from the cemento-enamel junction (CEJ) and 0.385 mm thick located 0.25 mm from the CEJ, with maximum thickness of 0.5 mm—a conservative approach to removing stains is recommended (DaCunha *et al.,* 2019).

The enamel microabrasion slurry consists of 6.6% hydrochloric acid and silicon carbide microparticles (Opalustre) and is used for superficial (<0.2 mm depth) imperfections, including brown or opaque white congenital enamel defects, fluorosis lesions, or white spot caries lesions. Because some enamel is removed, the facial/lingual thickness of the incisor should be evaluated (Figure 12.1). According to the manufacturer's recommendations, microabrasion should not be used on severe fluorosis or on thin enamel (Celik *et al.,* 2013b). Protective eyewear is recommended. Good isolation is necessary to avoid injury at the gingival margin with the hydrochloric acid and the microabrasion slurry. OpalDam™ (Ultradent), a light-cured resin barrier with syringe delivery, may be purchased along with the Opalustre kit (Figure 12.2). After application to the gingival margin, OpalDam is light-cured, scanning the light across the resin barrier for 20 seconds. If a rubber dam is preferred for isolation, an explorer may be used to pierce a hole in the rubber dam for

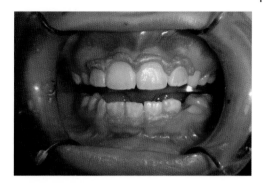

Figure 12.2 OpalDam.

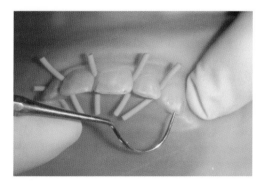

Figure 12.3 Explorer being used to pierce rubber dam for single hole and Wedjets dental dam stabilizing cord for a snug fit at the gingival margin.

each incisor and Wedjets® (Coltene, Altstätten, Switzerland) stabilizing cord used to secure the rubber dam at the gingival margin. Wedjets comes in different thicknesses to accommodate tight contacts or spacing (Figure 12.3).

For lesions that are deeper, it is recommended to complete whitening/bleaching treatments prior to the microabrasion procedure (Opalustre, 2020). Isolate the tooth/teeth with a rubber dam or liquid dam to ensure soft tissue is protected from the acid-etch. Also recommended is to isolate the affected teeth and one tooth on either side. Treatment can be initiated with a fine diamond or carbide finishing bur, abrading the enamel surface prior to application of the slurry. This may hasten the treatment process (Croll, 1993, 1997). In a case report, a bur was first used for 30 seconds. It is noted that bur use leaves markings on

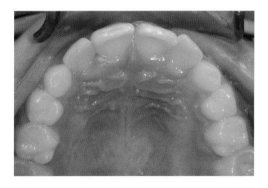

Figure 12.1 Evaluating the facial-lingual thickness of the incisor.

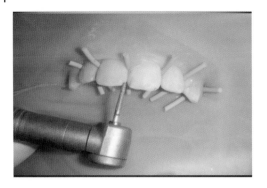

Figure 12.4 Diamond bur for initial microabrasion.

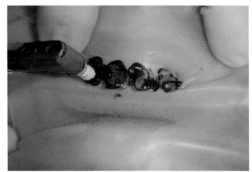

Figure 12.6 Opalustre with medium pressure applied with OpalCup bristle.

the enamel, and the subsequent use of the microabrasion slurry smooths the enamel. The initial use of a bur may reduce treatment time by one-third to one-half, with no discernable differences in results compared to no bur use initially (Figure 12.4) (Croll, 1993).

Procedure

1. Obtain a pretreatment photograph for reference (Figure 12.5).
2. Apply the recommended applicator tip on the Opalustre syringe and ensure flow prior to applying intraorally. Apply a layer of the material over the tooth to be treated. Using an OpalCups™ bristle (Ultradent) at a slow rpm (approximately 500 rpm), apply intermittent medium pressure on each tooth for approximately 60 seconds (Figure 12.6).

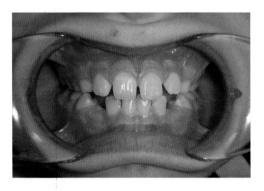

Figure 12.5 Pretreatment photograph for reference.

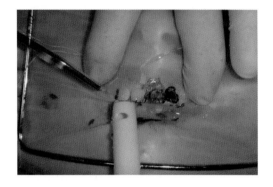

Figure 12.7 Rinsing Opalustre thoroughly.

Using a timer assures the proper time. This can be repeated 4–6 times for each tooth.

3. Remove the paste with suction and rinse thoroughly (Figure 12.7). Evaluate the lesion while the tooth is wet for a more accurate assessment of appearance. If less than 0.2 mm enamel has been removed, repeating application of the Opalustre 4–6 times may be necessary. According to Croll (1997), most superficial enamel defects are removed within 5 minutes of rotary application of the slurry. If during abrasion treatment the tooth appears to be losing its convex form, the lesion is too deep for microabrasion correction and treatment should be halted (Croll, 1997). After the final rinse, remove rubber dam or liquid dam and rinse thoroughly.

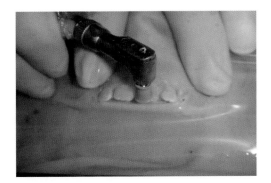

Figure 12.8 OpalCups finishing for surface polishing.

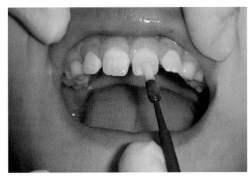

Figure 12.10 Fluoride varnish applied.

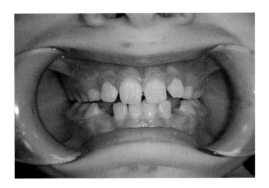

Figure 12.9 Post-treatment photograph.

4. Finishing and polishing are performed with OpalCups and fine prophy paste (Figure 12.8).
5. A post-treatment photograph for reference is obtained (Figure 12.9). Repeat application could have been performed, but the patient was unwilling to permit it to continue.
6. Fluoride application is then recommended (Figure 12.10).

Mild white spot lesions post orthodontic treatment respond well to microabrasion with Opalustre (Figure 12.11a, b).

It is noted in the manufacturer's recommendations that for postoperative sensitivity, potassium nitrate or sodium fluoride varnish products can be used for 30 minutes to 8 hours per day, as recommended.

Areas of deep hypomineralization and some stains may not respond to treatment. A bleaching treatment prior to or after microabrasion may help with improved outcomes. If whitening products are used, and microabrasion is completed and not completely successful in removing superficial stains, additional treatment may be required (Opalustre, 2020). If whitening products are used, wait 7–10 days after bleaching is completed before any esthetic/bonding restorations are placed.

The patient should be re-evaluated 4 weeks after the initial microabrasion attempt. Lesions may improve in appearance once the superficial surface is abraded and the lesion can be remineralized. Take an additional postoperative photograph. At-home bleaching procedures can be done after the 4-week follow-up period if needed. The combination of therapies may improve the esthetic result by first removing the superficial defect, smoothing the enamel surface, then completing a course of bleaching at home (Croll, 1997).

Resin Infiltration

Developmental enamel defects and white spot lesions due to fluorosis, molar–incisor hypomineralization, hypomineralization due to trauma, or initial caries presentation can be esthetically displeasing to a patient, resulting in psychosocial issues and decreased self-esteem (Gencer & Kirzigolu, 2019; Gugnani *et al.*, 2017). There are several approaches to management of these lesions. Noninvasive approaches include vital bleaching,

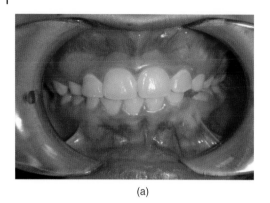

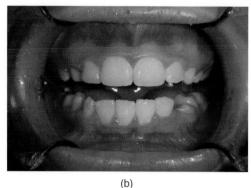

(a)

(b)

Figure 12.11 (a) Pretreatment photograph. (b) Post-treatment photograph.

microabrasion, resin infiltration, or a combination of therapies. More invasive approaches include resin restorations or resin/porcelain veneers. For young patients, minimally invasive approaches are generally recommended as first-line treatment options (MacLean, 2019).

Resin infiltration (Icon, DMG, Hamburg, Germany) was originally used to manage and arrest proximal noncavitated lesions by infiltrating the porous lesion of enamel caries with low-viscosity resin (Kobbe *et al.*, 2019; Gu *et al.*, 2019). The goal is that, once cured, the resin is a barrier and prevents additional caries progression. It is also used to infiltrate anterior porous white spot lesions or enamel defects to improve esthetics. The resin infiltration material has a refractive index similar to enamel, which optically allows it to appear more homogenous.

Orthodontic appliances place a patient at an elevated caries risk due to difficulty with oral hygiene around brackets and prolonged contact with tooth structure. Enamel porosities are caused by an imbalance between demineralization and remineralization. After removal of orthodontics, white spot lesions may remineralize up to 3 months afterward with proper hygiene, saliva contact, and remineralization treatments, such as fluorides (Al-Khateeb *et al.*, 1998). After remineralization efforts, white spot lesions remain 23–97% of the time (Kobbe *et al.*, 2019). There is a wide variation in reported prevalence of white spot lesions post

orthodontics (Senestaro *et al.*, 2013). The characteristic appearance of white spot lesions can be explained by a higher light refraction index within the lesion compared to the surrounding enamel.

In a randomized control trial, resin infiltration significantly improved the clinical appearance of white spot lesions and visually reduced their size (Senestaro *et al.*, 2013). In a systematic review, resin infiltration was shown to be effective in reducing progression or reversing noncavitated carious lesions (Tellez, 2013). Also, in a comparison study with microabrasion in conjunction with fluoride treatments, resin infiltration was found to be the most effective technique in masking fluorosis (Gencer & Kirzioglu, 2019). Gugnani *et al.* (2017) conducted a randomized controlled trial evaluating in-office bleaching versus resin infiltration to improve the esthetics of nonpitted fluorosis stains. They noted that the most significant improvement in esthetics and improvement in stains/opacities occurred with resin infiltration with increased infiltrant time (increased to 3 minutes during second infiltration time; Gugnani *et al.*, 2017). In 2019, Gu *et al.* published a split-mouth randomized clinical trial evaluating esthetic improvements of postorthodontic white spot lesions treated with resin infiltration and microabrasion. The results immediately after application showed that both methods reduced the lesion size and improved color change. Both methods showed stability over 12 months, but resin infiltration showed a better esthetic improvement when compared to microabrasion (Gu *et al.*, 2019). It has been noted in some studies that resin infiltration may be more susceptible to staining (e.g., from coffee) and may lack color stability over time in comparison to enamel microabrasion (Silva *et al.*, 2018).

Procedure

1. The Smooth Surface Treatment Set (Icon, DMG America, Englewood, NJ, USA) is used for enamel defects or white spot lesions on smooth surfaces. The teeth to be treated and adjacent teeth are cleaned and rinsed, removing all residue. The tooth/teeth are isolated with rubber dam with care to keep acid-etch off soft tissues and to ensure a dry field. Varied isolation techniques have been reported, including liquid dam, rubber dam, and lip retractors. Masking the white spot lesion can prove difficult when the resin does not penetrate the surface layer well. Inactive lesions are thought to have a thicker, less permeable surface layer than active lesions, which have larger pores and are less mineralized on the surface. Some studies suggest roughening the surface of the lesion with a disk prior to the initial etching step of resin infiltration (Figure 12.12) (MacLean, 2019; Senestraro

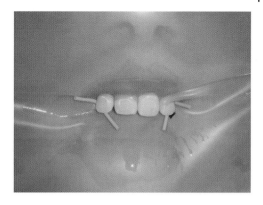

Figure 12.13 Pretreatment photograph.

et al., 2013). Manufacturer's recommendations suggest a medium-grit abrasive disk be utilized if needed prior to the etching process.

2. Take a pretreatment photograph for reference (Figure 12.13).
3. The teeth may be cleaned with pumice after isolation (Figure 12.14).
4. The Icon-Etch (15% hydrochloric acid) is applied with the applicator for 2 minutes and agitated during that time, then rinsed thoroughly for 30 seconds (Figures 12.15 and 12.16).
5. Dry the teeth with oil-free air. The Icon-Dry (ethanol drying agent) is applied (Figure 12.17). The tooth/teeth are evaluated for improvement in opacity or for homogeneity in shade. If this has not improved, the etching process is repeated

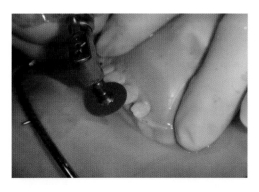

Figure 12.12 Disk to roughen the surface of the lesion.

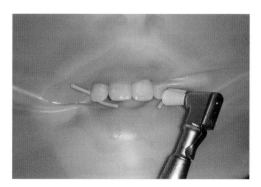

Figure 12.14 Pumice to clean.

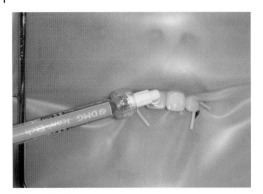

Figure 12.15 Icon-Etch applied with applicator and dispersed over facial surface.

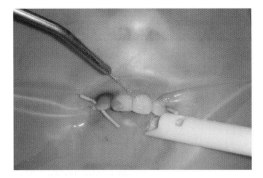

Figure 12.16 Icon-Etch rinsed.

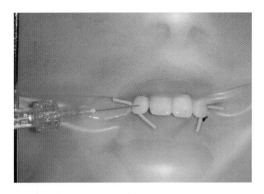

Figure 12.17 Icon-Dry applied.

up to three times to remove the surface layer for deeper penetration of resin. Icon-Dry is reapplied and the tooth is re-evaluated. The Icon-Dry (ethanol) rewetting process serves as a good predictor of the final esthetic result. This process allows evaluation of

the surface layer to determine if it has been sufficiently modified to allow penetration of the resin into the body of the lesion. The refractive index of the Icon-Dry is closer to the surrounding enamel. Once the superficial layer is opened, the fluid enters the lesion and light scattering is reduced (Kobbe *et al.*, 2019). Allow the Icon-Dry to air-dry for 30 seconds. Then dry the lesion thoroughly with oil-free air.

6. Move the operatory light away from the working field when preparing to apply the infiltrant. The low-viscosity resin (Icon-Infiltrant) is applied copiously with the specific applicator tip and left for 3 minutes to allow penetration into the lesion by capillary action (Figure 12.18). If the infiltration soaks into the lesion, it should be continuously added to ensure the lesion remains wet during the 3 minutes. For larger or deeper lesions, the infiltrant can be applied for 6 minutes initially.

7. After 3 minutes (or 6 minutes for larger/ deeper lesions), excess resin is removed with a cotton roll, wiping it away, and dental floss should be passed through interproximally (Figure 12.19).

8. The infiltrant is light-cured for 40 seconds (Figure 12.20). The infiltrant is then applied again for 1 minute, the excess wiped away, floss passed through, then the infiltrant is light-cured again for 40 seconds. The additional application is done to insure that

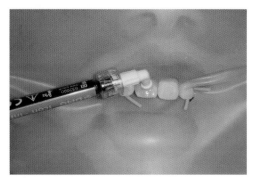

Figure 12.18 Icon-Infiltrant applied.

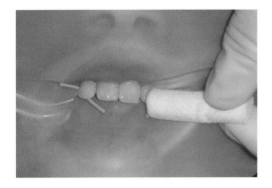

Figure 12.19 Excess resin removed with a cotton roll.

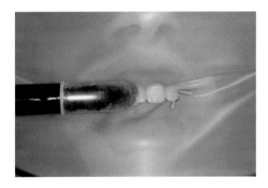

Figure 12.20 Light-cure.

superficial enamel porosities are filled with resin infiltrant.

9. Remove the rubber dam/OpalDam™ (Ultra-dent) and finish the surface with polishing disks or points. Obtain a post-treatment photograph (Figure 12.21).

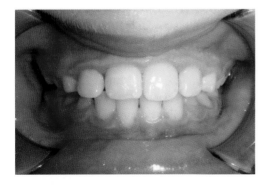

Figure 12.21 Post-treatment photograph.

Bleach–Etch–Seal Technique

The bleach–etch–seal technique (BEST) is an approach for managing intrinsic discoloration of anterior teeth and can be used to enhance bonding of hypomineralized enamel on any tooth (Wright *et al.*, 1995). The genesis of the technique was based on the finding that discolorations of enamel are typically caused by hypomineralization and retention or incorporation of proteins into the enamel porosities (Wright, 2002) Enamel is typically about 85% mineral per volume (about 96% by weight) and contains very little protein. Hypomineralized enamel, on the other hand, has a diminished mineral content and elevated protein content. The proteins are what appear to cause the yellow-brown discolorations commonly seen in hypomineralized enamel defects. Investigation on removing proteins from enamel showed that several agents could accomplish this, with one commonly used in dentistry being especially effective, sodium hypochlorite (NaOCl). Subsequent studies have gone on to show that treating hypomineralized enamel with NaOCl not only helps remove proteins and the associated yellow-brown discoloration, but also can improve the penetration into and bond strength of resins to the affected enamel (Lagarde *et al.*, 2020; Venezie *et al.*,1994). Thus, the introduction of BEST was an approach to managing what are typically isolated yellow-brown discolored areas of hypomineralized enamel lesions that occur in a variety of conditions such as fluorosis or molar–incisor hypomineralization, or may be idiopathic.

Case selection helps achieve optimal results using BEST and with outcomes typically being most successful for isolated yellow-brown discolored areas of hypomineralized enamel (Figure 12.22). Bleaching can be used in combination techniques including microabrasion, resin infiltration, and restoration, with the latter being indicated for most hypoplastic enamel situations (Hasmun *et al.*, 2018). If there is concern over the white opaque

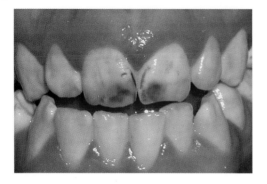

Figure 12.22 Yellow-brown discolorations may respond well to the bleach–etch–seal technique.

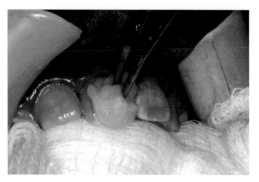

Figure 12.23 Keep the enamel moistened with sodium hypochlorite (NaOCl) using a cotton pellet or swab until the discoloration is removed.

appearance of the adjacent enamel surrounding a discolored lesion, then using BEST will likely increase the white opaque appearance and adjunctive therapy using a more penetrating resin perfusion technique may be helpful. Bleaching is the least invasive approach for managing discolorations; however, the extent, color, depth of the lesion, and other factors will be determinants in color change and esthetic results.

Technique

The agents used for this procedure have a low soft tissue causticity, therefore isolation can be achieved without a rubber dam. If you combine it with other techniques where more caustic agents are used (e.g., hydrochloric acid, microabrasion, Icon), then rubber dam isolation is indicated. Be sure to use patient eye protection and protect clothing from possible bleach exposure. Clean the teeth to remove surface biofilm using a plain flower of pumice. Etch the tooth for 60 seconds with phosphoric acid, which is supplied with most resin bonding systems (typically 35–37% phosphoric acid). This will provide initial proteolysis of proteins and increase the enamel porosity, thus aiding in the penetration and wetting of the NaOCl.

The NaOCl can be used at full strength (~5.25%) and is applied with a cotton pellet or cotton swab (Figure 12.23). Keep the enamel moistened with NaOCl using a cotton pellet or swab until the discoloration is removed, or for enhanced bonding of hypomineralized enamel for 90 seconds.

The goal is to keep the affected area moist and let the chemical penetrate and hydrolyze the underlying proteins. The tooth can be covered with a thin cotton veneer to help retain the NaOCl and keep the surface moist, or you can continue to periodically replenish the bleach to keep the surface moist. The duration of application will depend on the depth and size of the lesion and how accessible the proteins are to the bleach. Typically changes will become observable in 5–10 minutes. Complete protein hydrolysis and removal of yellow-brown discoloration can require 30 or more minutes, and in some instances need a second visit and bleaching. Once you feel you have achieved a definitive result from bleaching, hydrate the tooth and evaluate for color and esthetic result. The bleached area will often take on the mottled appearance of the adjacent enamel and may appear opaque. If the result is not adequate, then additional treatment using microabrasion, resin perfusion, and/or restoration may be necessary.

Once the yellow-brown discoloration has been removed and an adequate esthetic appearance achieved, the enamel surface is thoroughly rinsed to remove all bleach and then etched for 20–30 seconds with phosphoric

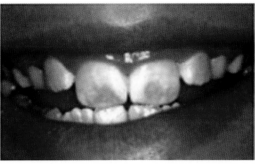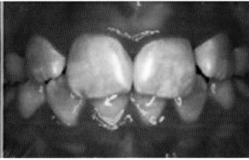

Figure 12.24 Before and after results of bleach–etch–seal technique on yellow-brown staining.

acid. The tooth is then perfused with a clear bonding agent, allowing it to penetrate the treated enamel and then light-cure the material. A clear sealant or second coat of bonding agent is then placed and cured to help insure complete coverage and good resin penetration (Figure 12.24). The goal of this step is to improve the optics of the enamel by filling porosities with resin that will change light refraction and reflection, and to occlude the porosities to prevent restaining of the area due to protein infiltration from saliva and oral exposure to chromogens.

References

Al-Khateeb, S., Forsberg, C.M., de Josselin de Jong, E., & Angmar-Månsson, B. (1998) *A longitudinal laser fluorescence study of white-spot lesions in orthodontic patients. American Journal of Orthodontics and Dentofacial Orthopedics*, 113, 595–602.

American Academy of Pediatric Dentistry. (2020) *Policy on the use of dental bleaching for child and adolescent patients. The Reference Manual of Pediatric Dentistry.* Chicago, IL: American Academy of Pediatric Dentistry; 112–115.

Carey, C. (2014) Tooth whitening: what we now know. *Journal of Evidence Based Dental Practice*, 14 (Suppl), 70–76.

Celik, E.U., Yildiz, G., & Yazkan, B. (2013a) Clinical evaluation of enamel microabrasion for the aesthetic management of mild-to-severe dental fluorosis. *Journal of Esthetic and Restorative Dentistry*, 25, 422–430.

Celik, E.U., Yildiz, G., & Yazkan, B. (2013b) Comparison of enamel microabrasion with a combined approach to the esthetic management of fluorosed teeth. *Operative Dentistry*, 38, E134–E143.

Croll, T. (1993) Hastening the enamel microabrasion procedure: eliminating defects, cutting treatment time. *Journal of the American Dental Association*, 124, 87–89.

Croll, T. (1997) Enamel microabrasion: observations after 10 years. *Journal of the American Dental Association*, 128, 45S–50S.

Croll, T. & Cavanaugh, R.R. (1986) Enamel color modification by controlled hydrochloric acid-pumice abrasion. *I. Technique and examples. Quintessence International*, 17, 81–87.

Da Cunha Coelho, A.S.E., Mata, P.C.M., Lino, C.A., Pereira Macho, V.M., Pereira Areias, C.M.F.G., *et al.* (2019) Dental hypomineralization treatment: a systematic review. *Journal of Esthetic Restorative Dentistry*, 31 (1), 26–39.

Donly, K.J., O'Neill, M., & Cross, T.P. (1992) Enamel microabrasion: a microscopic evaluation of the "abrosion effect." *Quintessence International*, 23, 175–178.

Gencer, M.D.G. & Kirzioglu, Z. (2019) A comparison of the effectiveness of resin infiltration and microabrasion treatments applied to developmental enamel defects in color masking. *Dental Materials Journal*, 38, 295–302.

Gugnani, N., Pandit, I.K., Gupta, M., Gugnani, S., Soni, S., & Goyal, V. (2017) Comparative evaluation of esthetic changes in nonpitted fluorosis stains when treated with resin infiltration, in-office bleaching, and combination therapies. *Journal of Esthetic Restorative Dentistry*, 29, 317–324.

Gu, X., Yang, L., Yang, D., Gao, Y., Duan, X., *et al.* (2019) Esthetic improvements of postorthodontic white-spot lesions treated with resin infiltration and microabrasion: a split-mouth, randomized clinical trial. *Angle Orthodontist*, 89, 372–377.

Hasmun, N., Lawson, J., Vettore, M.V., Elcock, C., Zaitoun, H., & Rodd, H. (2018) Change in oral health-related quality of life following minimally invasive aesthetic treatment for children with molar incisor hypomineralisation: a prospective study. *Dental Journal*, 6 (4), 61.

Ibiyemi, O. & Taiwo, J.O. (2011) Psychosocial aspect of anterior tooth discoloration among adolescents in Igbo-Ora, *southwestern Nigeria. Annals of Ibadan Postgraduate Medicine*, 9 (2), 94–99.

Kobbe, C., Fritz, U., Wierichs, R.J., Meyer-Lueckel, H. (2019) Evaluation of the value of re-wetting prior to resin infiltration of post-orthodontic caries lesions. *Journal of Dentistry*, 91,103243.

Kugel, G. & Ferreira, S. (2006) The art and science of tooth whitening, *Inside Dentistry*, 2 (7), 84–89.

Lagarde, M., Vennat, E., Attal, J.P., & Dursun, E. (2020) Strategies to optimize bonding of adhesive materials to molar-incisor hypomineralization-affected enamel: a systematic review. *International Journal of Paediatric Dentistry*, 30, 405–420.

Lee, S.S., Zhang, W., Lee, D.H., & Li, Y. (2005) Tooth whitening in children and adolescents: a literature review. *Pediatric Dentistry*, 27, 362–368.

MacLean, J.A. (2019). Minimally invasive treatment option for post-orthodontic white spot lesions. DMG America. Retrieved from https://dmg-connect.com/articles/a-minimally-invasive-treatment-option-for-post-orthodontic-white-spot-lesions. Accessed November 28, 2020.

Medeiros, M.B., Ziegelmann, P.K., Burey, A., de Paris Matos, T., Loguercio, A.D., & Reis, A. (2019) Different light-activation systems associated with dental bleaching: a systematic review and a network meta-analysis. *Clinical Oral Investigations*, 23, 1499–1512.

Opalustre. (2020) Opalustre enamel microabrasion slurry IFU instructions for use. Retrieved from https://assets.ctfassets.net/wfptrcrbtkd0/77KvbclixWh3aRJxFgS2mu/08af48161fd164eaffbd11888a193dbb/Opalustre-IFU-55424-UAR12.pdf.

Rodríguez-Martínez, M., Valiente, M., & Sánchez-Martí, M.J. (2019) Tooth whitening: from the established treatments to novel approaches to prevent side effects. *Journal of Esthetic Restorative Dentistry*, 31, 431–440.

Romero, M.F., Babb, C.S., Delash, J., & Brackett, W.W. (2018) Minimally invasive esthetic improvement in a patient with dental fluorosis by using microabrasion and bleaching: a clinical report. *Journal of Prosthetic Dentistry*, 120, 323–326.

Senestraro, S.V., Crowe, J.J., Wang, M., Vo, A., Huang, G., *et al.* (2013) Minimally invasive resin infiltration of arrested white-spot lesions: a randomized clinical trial. *Journal of the American Dental Association*, 144, 997–1005.

Silva, L.O., Signori, C., Peixoto, A., Cenci, M.S., & Farie-e-Silva, A.L. (2018) Color restoration and stability in two treatments for white spot lesions. *International Journal of Esthetic Dentistry*, 13, 394–403.

SoutoMaior, J.R., de Moraes, S., Lemos, C., Vasconcelos, B. do E., Montes, M., & Pellizzer, E.P. (2019) Effectiveness of light sources on in-office dental bleaching: a systematic review and meta-analysis. *Operative Dentistry*, 44, E105–E117.

Tellez, M., Gomez, J., Kaur, S., Pretty, I.A., Ellwood, R., & Ismail, A.I. (2013) Non-surgical management methods of noncavitated carious lesions. *Community Dentistry and Oral Epidemiology*, 41, 79–96.

Venezie, R.D., Vadiakis, G., Christensen, J.R., & Wright, J.T. (1994) Enamel pretreatment to enhance bonding in hypocalcified amelogenesis imperfecta: case report and SEM analysis. *Pediatric Dentistry*, 16, 433–436.

Wang, Y., Gao, J., Jiang, T., Liang, S., Zhou, Y., & Matis, B.A. (2015) Evaluation of the efficacy of potassium nitrate and sodium fluoride as desensitizing agents during tooth bleaching treatment—a systematic review and meta-analysis. *Journal of Dentistry*, 43, 913–923.

Wright, J.T. (2002) The etch-bleach-seal technique for managing stained enamel defects in young permanent incisors. *Pediatric Dentistry*, 24, 249–252.

Wright, J.T., Deaton, T.C., Hall, K.I., & Yamauchi, M. (1995) The mineral and protein content of enamel in amelogenesis imperfecta. *Connective Tissue Research*, 31, 247–252.

Zuanon, A.C.C., Santos-Pinto, L., Azevadeo, E.R., & Lima, L.M. (2008) Primary tooth enamel loss after manual and mechanical microabrasion. *Pediatric Dentistry*, 30, 420–423.

13

Extraction of Primary Dentition

Jane A. Soxman

Before extraction of any of the primary dentition, a periapical radiograph to evaluate the location, presence, or absence of the permanent successor and informed consent should be obtained. The length of unresorbed roots after a primary tooth's extraction may surprise the parent/guardian. The use of the pre-extraction radiograph and/or the use of a mixed-dentition typodont (Kilgore International, Coldwater, WI, USA) are good methods to show root length before an extraction (Figure 13.1).

Curette

After administration of local anesthesia, a sterile curette may be used to sever the gingival attachment (Figure 13.2). This first step of the procedure may predict the behavior for the remainder of the procedure, as a very anxious child will respond negatively to even slight pressure with the curette. Anxiety is the biggest predictor of poor pain control (Nakai *et al.*, 2000).

Elevation

Elevation is the most important technique to facilitate extraction and avoid root fracture of a primary molar. Elevator instruments luxate the tooth, sever the periodontal ligament around the roots, and expand the alveolar bone. The interproximal contacts of primary molars are broad, flat, and without cervical constriction. The tip of the instrument for elevation should be narrow enough to be placed through the embrasures of the primary molars (Figure 13.3a, b). This step may not be necessary for primary incisors and canines with conical, single roots, but may be helpful in some cases. During elevation, use caution not to include adjacent teeth, causing mobility. If an adjacent tooth is mobile, nearing normal exfoliation before the extraction, the parent/guardian should be informed of the possibility of unintentional inclusion.

The feeling of pressure during the elevation and extraction should be explained. Pushing on the child's shoulder may demonstrate this sensation. If a previously cooperative child begins to cry, exhibiting pain during elevation, administration of additional local anesthesia is indicated. Injections through the mesial and distal papilla from buccal to lingual, along with injection into the gingival sulcus, are very effective (Figure 13.4a–c). Palatal injection using the DentalVibe® (DentalVibe, Boca Raton, FL, USA) significantly reduces injection discomfort (Figure 13.5).

Extraction

Primary incisors' roots are conical in shape. Place a straight-beak pediatric forceps, designed for primary incisor and canine extractions, vertically on the long axis of the

Handbook of Clinical Techniques in Pediatric Dentistry, Second Edition. Edited by Jane A. Soxman.
© 2022 John Wiley & Sons, Inc. Published 2022 by John Wiley & Sons, Inc.

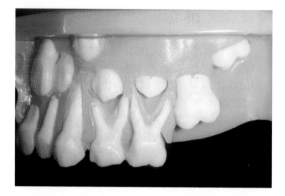

Figure 13.1 Mixed-dentition typodont to show root length of primary dentition.

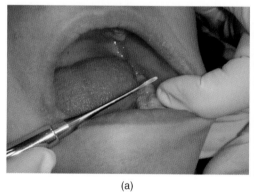

Figure 13.2 Curette severing the gingival attachment.

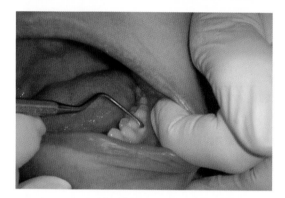

| (a) | (b) |

Figure 13.3 (a) Elevation instrument with narrow tip. (b) Elevation of primary molar.

tooth (Figure 13.6a, b). In this case, elevation may not be necessary. A rotational movement is used for extraction. Primary molars present more of a challenge because their roots are thin and diverge beyond the crown. Root fracture may occur during extraction of a primary molar if too much pressure is placed during luxation with the forceps. Elevation, achieving

Class III mobility of the primary molar before use of the forceps, will significantly reduce the incidence of root fracture. After adequate elevation, minimal buccal/lingual (palatal) force is applied with the forceps to expand the alveolar bone and lift the tooth out of the socket. Serrated-beak pediatric forceps provide a firmer grasp than the traditional

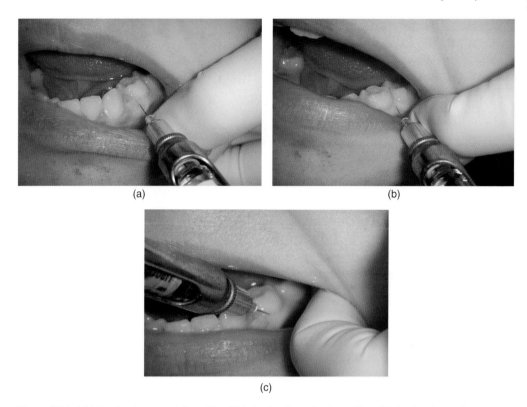

(a)   (b)

(c)

Figure 13.4 (a) Injection into mesial papilla. (b) Injection into distal papilla. (c) Injection into sulcus.

Figure 13.5 Palatal injection with DentalVibe.

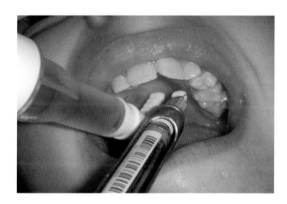

smooth-beak forceps to retain the short crown of a primary molar (Figure 13.7a). The capture forceps is designed to retain the extracted primary molar within the forceps, avoiding aspiration (Figure 13.7b).

The premolars develop in the furcation between the roots of the primary molars. If the roots of the primary molar encircle the crown of the permanent successor, the primary molar should be sectioned before extraction to avoid inadvertent extraction of the permanent successor (AAPD, 2019–2020b). A subgingival slice through the center of the primary molar with a 557 or 558 cross-cut fissure carbide bur from buccal to lingual (or lingual to buccal) is performed (Figure 13.8a, b). The subgingival slice should be deep enough to cut through the furcation. An elevator may be used to place

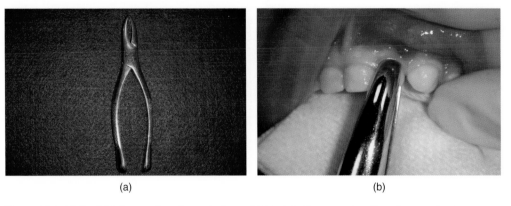

(a)   (b)

Figure 13.6 (a) Straight forceps for primary incisors. (b) Straight forceps extracting abscessed primary lateral incisor.

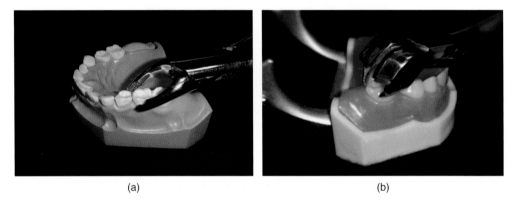

(a)   (b)

Figure 13.7 (a) Serrated split-beak forceps for primary molar extraction. (b) Capture forceps.

pressure on the segments, separating the coronal portion into two halves. The two halves are lifted out of the socket (Figure 13.8c–g).

Damage to the developing succedaneous tooth is the primary concern regarding retrieval of a fractured root. A periapical radiograph may be obtained to determine the presence or location of the root or root tip. Removal may be performed with a root tip pick or a surgical suction tip. If retrieval cannot be achieved after a few attempts, the root or root tip should be left for resorption. Active surveillance is recommended to monitor postoperative infection or delayed eruption of the permanent successor. The parent/guardian should be informed along with documentation in the patient's chart (AAPD, 2019–2020b).

Considerations with Abscesses

With localized infection, antibiotic coverage, before or after extraction, is not necessary for an asymptomatic, healthy child. Most localized odontogenic infections can be treated with extraction, pulp therapy, or incision and drainage. (AAPD, 2019–2020b,c). Any purulent material is gently curetted from the socket after the extraction. The source of infection has been removed, and so antibiotic coverage would not be prescribed after the extraction.

With a concomitant temperature of 102–104 °F, mild facial swelling, or induration of the surrounding mucosa, an antibiotic should be prescribed (AAPD, 2019–2020b). This coverage should begin several days prior

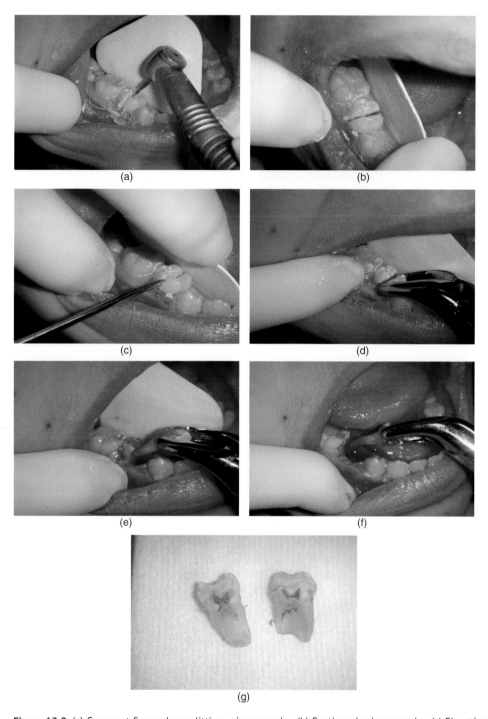

Figure 13.8 (a) Cross-cut fissure bur splitting primary molar. (b) Sectioned primary molar. (c) Elevation instrument to separate primary molar at furcation. (d) Extraction of mesial root of primary molar. (e) Extracting mesial root of primary molar from socket. (f) Extracting distal root of primary molar from socket. (g) Extracted, sectioned primary molar.

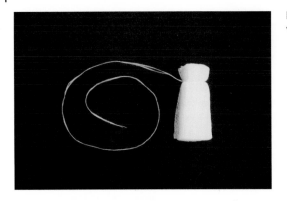

Figure 13.9 Ghost made with 2 × 2 gauze tied with long strand of floss for young child.

to the extraction to provide immediate control and stop spread of the infection. Antibiotic therapy should continue for a minimum of 5 days after significant improvement or resolution. The course of treatment is typically 5–7 days (AAPD, 2019–2020c). Follow-up in 48 hours to insure improvement is recommended. If there is no improvement at that time, the child should be seen and a different antibiotic prescribed. Adequate local anesthesia may be delayed or unobtainable due to the lower pH of the tissues with an acute infection. Physiologic pH is 7.4, but pH may be 6 or lower with infection and the inflammatory process, inhibiting uptake of the local anesthetic across the nerve sheath. (AAPD, 2019–2020a). Emergency care with intravenous antibiotics is indicated for signs of systemic involvement or septicemia, such as facial swelling or cellulitis, fever, malaise, dysphagia, respiratory distress, tachycardia, or lymphadenopathy (AAPD, 2019–2020b,c). Children are at greater risk than adults with cellulitis due to airway involvement and spread of infection through facial planes. Rapid emergency treatment is not only indicated, but reduces length of stay and costs of hospitalization (Thikkurissy *et al.*, 2010).

After Extraction

Prepare the parent/guardian for more bleeding with an abscess. One drop of blood mixed with copious saliva appears to be much more blood than in actuality. This is important for both the parent/guardian and the child to understand. Sterile 2 × 2 folded gauze should remain in place, with teeth firmly held together for 10–15 minutes. Remind the parent/guardian and child that the gauze should not be repeatedly taken in and out of the mouth, interrupting blood clotting, during that period. Extra sterile gauze may be provided for use as needed, along with a plastic sandwich bag to discard saturated gauze after leaving the office.

For a very young child, a "ghost" can be made using 2 × 2 sterile gauze (Figure 13.9). A long strand of floss, tied to the gauze, will facilitate retrieval if necessary. The gauze should always be visible in the child's mouth. The extracted tooth is placed in a plastic treasure chest selected by the child before the extraction. Without the child present, sparkles in a small envelope may be given to the parent/guardian. These sparkles are said to be from the tooth fairy's wings and are sprinkled on the floor by the child's bed that night.

If bleeding continues beyond 20 minutes, advise rinsing vigorously with room temperature water and biting on a wet tea bag. The tannic acid in tea aids in hemostasis. Plain tea is preferable to herbal tea. Tylenol may be recommended after extractions requiring more forceful elevation or luxation. Nonsteroidal anti-inflammatory drugs may also be suggested, but use caution with asthmatics (Debley *et al.*, 2005).

A follow-up phone call from the dentist or a staff member the following day to check

on the child is always appreciated by the parent/guardian.

References

American Academy of Pediatric Dentistry. (2019–2020a) *Use of local anesthesia for pediatric dental patients. The Reference Manual of Pediatric Dentistry.* Chicago, IL: American Academy of Pediatric Dentistry; 286–292.

American Academy of Pediatric Dentistry. (2019–2020b) *Management considerations for pediatric oral surgery and oral pathology. The Reference Manual of Pediatric Dentistry.* Chicago, IL: American Academy of Pediatric Dentistry; 402–411.

American Academy of Pediatric Dentistry. (2019–2020c) *Use of antibiotic therapy for pediatric dental patients. The Reference Manual of Pediatric Dentistry.* Chicago, IL: American Academy of Pediatric Dentistry; 412–415.

Debley, J.S., Carter, E.R., Gibson, R.L., Rosenfeld, M., & Redding, G.J. (2005) The prevalence of ibuprofen-sensitive asthma in children: a randomized controlled bronchoprovocation challenge study. *Journal of Pediatrics*, 147 (2), 233–238.

Nakai, Y., Milgrom, P., Mancl, L., Coldwell, S.E., Domoto, P.K., & Ramsay, D.S. (2000) Effectiveness of local anesthesia in pediatric dental practice. *Journal of the American Dental Association*, 131 (12), 1699–1705.

Thikkurissy, S., Rawlins, J.T., Kumar, A., Evans, E., & Casamassimo, P.S. (2010) Rapid treatment reduces hospitalization for pediatric patients with odontogenic-based cellulitis. *American Journal of Emergency Medicine*, 28, 668–672.

14

Traumatic Injury to the Primary Incisors
Patrice B. Wunsch

Incidence of Injuries

The peak incidence of injury occurs during the toddler stage of development (2–3 years of age), at the time the child is learning to walk and experiences injury due to falls. A recent study of 628 traumatically injured primary anterior teeth discovered that the highest frequency of traumatic dental injuries occurred between 2 and 4 years of age (Goettems *et al.*, 2020). The maxillary central incisors are the most commonly injured teeth, followed by the maxillary lateral incisors and the mandibular incisors (McTigue, 2013). Therapy for the primary dentition most frequently includes follow-up of the traumatized tooth, followed by extraction of the traumatized tooth (Atabek *et al.*, 2014).

Primary Cause of Injuries

- *Falls*—toddler years (primary dentition).
- *Sports*—school-age years (mixed or early permanent dentition).
- *Automobile*—adolescent to young adult years (permanent dentition).

Dental trauma may possibly be related to child abuse. The provider can differentiate an accidental trauma from an intentional one by looking for the following potential signs of child abuse (McTigue, 2013):

- Bruises in various stages of healing, indicating multiple traumatic incidents.

- Torn upper labial frenum.
- Bruising of the labial sulcus in young, preambulatory patients.
- Bruising on the soft tissue of the cheek.

Background

Primary Tooth Fractures Versus Tooth Movement

Since the bone is less dense and the primary teeth have shorter roots, fractures are less common in the primary dentition than tooth movement (luxation, intrusion, avulsion) (Camp, 2008). One of the most common tooth injuries during early childhood is intrusion of the primary anterior teeth (Colak *et al.*, 2009). Furthermore, luxation injuries involve damage to the periodontal ligament and are the most common injury in the primary dentition (McTigue, 2013). With luxation type of injuries, the proximity of the developing permanent successor to the injured primary tooth will determine the type of treatment (Figure 14.1). Depending on the direction of the impact, the apex of the intruded tooth is most often displaced labially, thereby leaving the permanent successor tooth bud unaffected (Colak *et al.*, 2009).

Post-Traumatic Injury Color Change

Coronal color change is a common complication following luxation injuries (Andersson

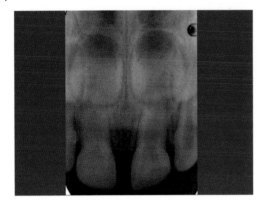

Figure 14.1 Radiograph showing the proximity of the primary tooth root to the developing permanent successor.

et al., 2012). Nearly half of traumatized primary anterior teeth develop transient or permanent discoloration within 1–3 weeks post trauma (Camp, 2008). Tooth color can range from yellow to dark gray (Figure 14.2a,b). Neither pink nor yellow discoloration reflects devitalization of the pulp (Holan & Fuks, 1996). Primary teeth that are yellow in color usually present with pulp canal calcification/obliteration and do not require further treatment. Primary teeth that are dark gray in color require follow-up, since this can either be a transient situation where the tooth will become light in color again, or the tooth will remain dark. In both instances, the traumatized tooth must be monitored for signs of pulpal necrosis. Factors that can determine the likelihood of pulpal necrosis are the age of the patient, the degree of tooth

displacement, and concurrent crown fracture (Camp, 2008). According to Goettems *et al.* (2020), the frequency of crown discoloration was higher in teeth that suffered subluxation, followed by teeth that exhibited enamel–dentin fractures. Some providers will prophylactically perform pulp therapy on primary teeth that have experienced trauma and are dark in color; however, this practice is controversial, since it is difficult to predict whether the tooth will become necrotic after a traumatic dental injury.

In a study performed by Soxman *et al.* (1984), the investigators extracted pulp tissue from 23 traumatically injured primary incisors that experienced color change. Histologic examination of the extracted pulps revealed that the pulps of 11 teeth experienced total necrosis as early as 10 days after injury, 7 had experienced total autolysis (absence of pulp tissue) between 3 and 24 months after injury, and 1 experienced complete calcification, while the remaining 4 teeth exhibited minimal to moderate degrees of necrosis. The authors concluded, "While this study failed to demonstrate a positive correlation between the shade of discoloration and histological status of the dental pulp, there was a high degree of correlation between discoloration and pulpal necrosis" (Soxman *et al.*, 1984).

In another study (Holan, 2006), the author compared traumatized primary anterior teeth where dark discoloration was the only sign

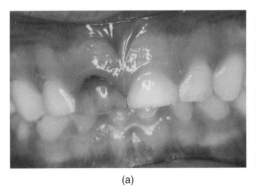
(a)

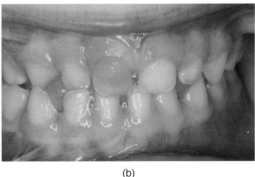
(b)

Figure 14.2 (a, b) Dark color due to intracoronal hemorrhage.

Table 14.1 Study results show that root canal treatment (RCT) for traumatized discolored incisors does not improve outcomes.

	RCT n=25, %	Monitor n=28, %
Primary tooth, early extraction	28	32
Permanent tooth, early/delayed eruption	20	21
Permanent tooth, ectopic eruption	64	78
Permanent tooth, hypocalcification/hypoplasia	36	36

Source: Data from Holan (2006).

of injury. Half received root canal treatment (RCT) and half were monitored. The study revealed that traumatized anterior teeth with dark discoloration as the only sign of injury resulted in early extraction of the injured primary tooth at 28% for those that received RCT and 32% for those that were monitored. Early or delayed eruption of the succedaneous tooth occurred at 20% for the primary predecessors that received RCT, versus 21% for those that were monitored. Permanent successors that erupted ectopically occurred in 64% and 78% for those that received RCT or were monitored, respectively. Lastly, permanent successors that experienced hypocalcification/hypoplasia occurred at 36% for both the RCT and monitored groups (Table 14.1). The author concluded that primary incisors that experienced dark gray color change post trauma and that had no other clinical or radiographic symptoms did not require RCT, as it did not result in better outcomes for the primary teeth and their permanent successors (Holan, 2006).

Evaluation

History of The Traumatic Event

Asking when, where and how the injury took place will aid the provider in assessing the severity of the injury and the best treatment options (McTigue, 2013).

- *When*—the period of time between when the injury occurred and when patient receives treatment is important, since immediate treatment after dental trauma can positively affect the prognosis of traumatized teeth. According to Atabek *et al.* (2014), the percentage of patients who present for treatment within an hour of an injury is low, leaving one to believe that parents in our society do not feel the immediacy for care after traumatic injury and will often allow a significant amount of time to elapse, until the appearance of acute signs or symptoms, before seeking care (Atabek *et al.*, 2014).
- *Where*—to determine the contamination level of the injury (outside versus inside).
- *How*—to determine the force of impact. For example, if the patient fell and hit their front teeth on the floor, the force of impact on the primary tooth crown would be lingual with the root apex moving labial, away from the permanent successor tooth bud. If, however, an object was forcibly pulled from the patient's mouth, the force of impact on the primary tooth crown would be facial, with the root apex moving in a less favorable lingual direction toward the permanent successor tooth bud.

Neurologic History

Since dental injuries are a subset of head trauma, the patient should be referred for medical evaluation if any of the following are present (McTigue, 2013):

- Dizziness.
- Headache.
- Nausea/vomiting.
- Loss of memory.
- Loss of consciousness.
- Lethargy or irritability.

If the patient's neurologic condition is not obvious to assess, the simple acronym

PERRLA provides an easy way to remember how to check for a concussion:

P = **Pupils** are in the center of the iris

E = Pupils are **Equal** in size

R = Pupils are perfectly **Round** in shape

R = Pupils are **Reactive** to...

L = **Light**

A = Eyes **Accommodate** to see things up close and far away

Clinical Examination

A thorough clinical exam should be completed to include the facial skeleton and temporomandibular joint, intraoral and extraoral soft tissues. All the teeth should be examined for mobility, tenderness, and sensitivity, fractures, and pulp exposures. The occlusion should be checked to determine if tooth luxation or an alveolar fracture is preventing the child from occluding properly (McTigue, 2013).

Radiographic Examination

A radiographic examination is important in gathering the necessary information to make an accurate diagnosis and plan of treatment. It is important to obtain a baseline radiograph to compare with future radiographs obtained at follow-up appointments.

Things to look for (McTigue, 2013):

- Extent of root development.
- Position of unerupted teeth.
- Size of pulp chambers.
- Relation between traumatized primary tooth and permanent successor.
- Periapical radiolucency.
- Root fractures.
- Extent and type of root resorption.
- Degree of tooth displacement.
- Jaw fractures.
- Presence of tooth fragments or other foreign bodies in the soft tissues (Figure 14.3).

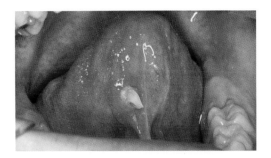

Figure 14.3 Fragment of tooth structure lodged in the ventral surface of the tongue. Courtesy of American Academy of Pediatric Dentistry members' library.

Fractures

A force that causes a tooth or root to fracture will most likely result in some form of movement as well. It is important when evaluating fractured teeth to evaluate the possibility of some type of luxation injury.

Enamel Fracture

- *Diagnosis*—clinically, the fracture will involve the enamel only (Figure 14.4); radiographically the tooth is normal.
- *Treatment*—smooth sharp edges with finishing bur or sandpaper disc.
- *Follow-up*—not required.
- *Complications*—unlikely to have any complications.
- *Criteria for success*—tooth remains healthy and exfoliates normally.

Enamel–Dentin Fracture

- *Diagnosis*—an enamel–dentin fracture is clinically evident (Figure 14.5); the radiograph confirms pulp is not involved.
- *Treatment*—type of treatment depends on patient behavior and size of the fracture. If small and/or patient lacks the cooperation necessary for restorative care, complete coverage can be achieved by placing resin-reinforced glass ionomer such

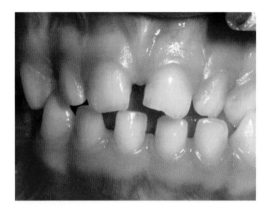

Figure 14.4 Enamel fracture of maxillary left primary central incisor. Courtesy of Dr. Paul Cassamassimo, Nationwide Children's Hospital, Columbus, OH.

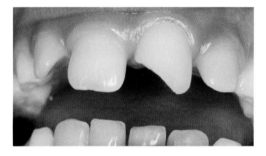

Figure 14.5 Enamel–dentin fracture of maxillary left primary central incisor. Courtesy of American Academy of Pediatric Dentistry members' library.

as Vitrebond™ (3M ESPE, St. Paul, MN, USA) or Fugi II LC (GC America, Alsip, IL, USA). If the fracture is large and the patient is cooperative, a composite restoration is the treatment of choice. However, if the patient is uncooperative, glass ionomer will suffice until a final restoration can be completed with proper behavior management techniques.
- *Follow-up*—the patient can be followed up in 3–4 weeks to ensure the restoration is intact.
- *Complications*—none.
- *Criteria for success*—the restoration provides structural form and adequate seal to prevent leakage.

Enamel–Dentin–Pulp Fracture

- *Diagnosis*—whereas enamel and enamel–dentin fractures are considered uncomplicated crown fractures, the enamel–dentin–pulp fracture is considered to be a complicated fracture. This fracture involves the enamel and the dentin, and the pulp is exposed (Figure 14.6 and see later Figure 14.10). A radiograph is obtained to determine the stage of root development. If the primary tooth root is significantly resorbed, extraction may be the treatment of choice. If the primary tooth root is not resorbed, pulp therapy will be necessary:
- *Treatment*—ideal treatment (preservation of the pulp) options are as follows, but if the patient is unable to cooperate the tooth may need to be extracted.
  - Small exposure:
    a. Rubber dam isolation.
    b. Clean area and remove 2 mm of pulp.
    c. Place calcium hydroxide or a bioactive material (mineral trioxide aggregate/Biodentine®, see Chapter 10) is preferred, since they will prevent microleakage better than calcium hydroxide.
    d. Provide restoration that will prevent microleakage.
  - Large exposure:
    a. Rubber dam isolation.
    b. Pulpotomy with bioactive material.
    c. Provide restoration that will prevent microleakage.
- *Follow-up*—6–8 weeks and 1 year.
- *Complications*—irreversible pulpitis or nonvital pulp requiring one of the following:
  - Pulpectomy with an iodoform–calcium hydroxide product such as Vitapex® (Neo Dental International, Federal Way, WA, USA).
  - Extraction.
- *Criteria for success*—a traumatized primary incisor that has received vital pulp therapy remains vital and exfoliates normally,

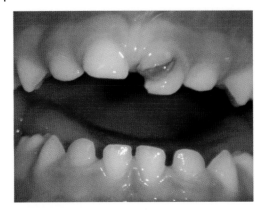

Figure 14.6 Maxillary left primary central incisor with an enamel–dentin–pulp fracture.

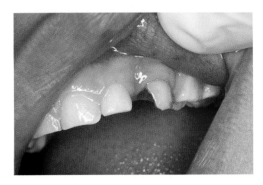

Figure 14.7 Maxillary left primary canine with crown–root fracture. Fractured crown segment removed. Courtesy of American Academy of Pediatric Dentistry members' library.

without complications for the permanent successor.

Crown–Root Fracture

- *Diagnosis*—clinically the crown is intact. Radiographic image to determine presence and extent of fracture.
- *Treatment*—once the coronal portion is removed (Figure 14.7), it is determined whether the fracture involves a small or large portion of the root. If a large portion of the root is involved, extraction will be necessary. If only a small portion of the root is involved without pulpal involvement and coronal restoration is possible, the final restoration will preferably be a full-coverage restoration such as a stainless-steel crown with esthetic facing (Signature Series, NuSmile, Houston, TX, USA) or zirconia crown (EZPedo, NuSmile).
- *Follow-up*—1 week, 8 weeks, and 1 year.
- *Complications*—restoration failure and leakage, resulting in reversible/irreversible pulpitis, necessitating extraction of the involved tooth.
- *Criteria for success*—restoration performs adequate form and function until tooth is ready to exfoliate as permanent successor erupts.

Root Fracture

- *Diagnosis*—clinically the coronal fragment may be mobile or displaced. Radiographically, the fracture will be visualized in the middle or apical third of the root (Figure 14.8).
- *Treatment*
  o If the coronal fragment is not mobile/displaced, no treatment is necessary.
  o If the coronal fragment is mobile/displaced:
    a. Fragment can be repositioned and possibly splinted (requires cooperative patient).
    b. Fragment can be extracted and root portion can be left to resorb.

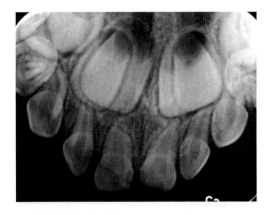

Figure 14.8 Root fracture of maxillary right primary central incisor. Courtesy of American Academy of Pediatric Dentistry members' library.

- *Follow-up*
  - If the coronal fragment is not mobile/displaced, follow up in one week.
  - If the coronal fragment is mobile/displaced:
    a. If fragment can be just repositioned, follow up in 8 weeks and then each year until exfoliated.
    b. If splinted, follow up in 2 weeks to remove splint and then 6 weeks, then each year until exfoliated.
    c. If extracted, follow up in 1 year and each year to monitor for the eruption of the permanent successor.
- *Complications*—None.
- *Criteria for success*—coronal fragment remains intact until tooth fully exfoliates and permanent successor erupts to replace it. If the coronal fragment is extracted and the root portion remains, the root portion resorbs normally as the permanent successor erupts into position.

Alveolar Fracture

- *Diagnosis*—clinically the alveolar segment is mobile and occlusal interference is evident (Figure 14.9).
- *Treatment*—reposition the segment so the teeth are in proper alignment and splint for 4 weeks.
- *Follow-up*
  - Monitor the teeth in the fracture line in 1 week.

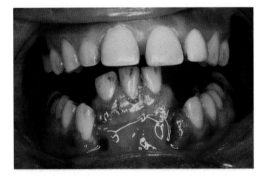

Figure 14.9 Mandibular alveolar fracture, permanent dentition. Courtesy of American Academy of Pediatric Dentistry members' library.

- Splint removal at 3–4 weeks, continue to monitor the teeth in the fracture line.
- In 6–8 weeks, continue to monitor the teeth in the fracture line.
- Follow up each year until teeth exfoliate.
  a. *Complications*—signs of an apical lesion or inflammatory root resorption of the primary anterior teeth. Sign of disturbances in the eruption of the permanent successors.
  b. *Criteria for success*—normal occlusion with no signs or symptoms associated with the primary incisors or disturbances in the eruption of the permanent successors.

Movement

Concussion

- *Diagnosis*—the concussion injury results in an impact directly to the periodontal ligament without causing any mobility to the tooth. Clinically the tooth presents with normal mobility and no bleeding. The patient may experience some discomfort when the tooth is touched. Radiographically normal periodontal ligament space.
- *Treatment*—rarely needed. An adjustment of the occlusion may be necessary if the patient experiences sensitivity.
- *Follow-up*—observe in 1 week and then again in 6–8 weeks.
- *Complications*—tooth becomes dark and may or may not require RCT. Root development does not continue in the immature primary tooth.
- *Criteria for success*—continued root development of the immature primary teeth.

Subluxation

- *Diagnosis*—clinically the tooth has increased mobility, without displacement from the socket; bleeding may be present in the gingival sulcus (Figure 14.10). Radiographically, normal periodontal ligament space and no abnormalities.

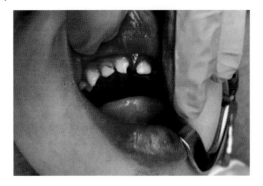

Figure 14.10 Maxillary right primary central incisor with enamel–dentin fracture with pulpal involvement and maxillary left primary central incisor with subluxation. Courtesy of Dr. Carol Caudill, VCU Department of Pediatric Dentistry.

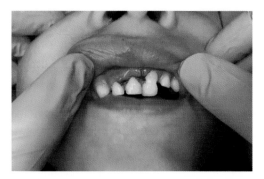

Figure 14.11 Lateral luxation of maxillary right primary lateral incisor and maxillary right primary central incisor. Extrusive luxation of maxillary left primary central incisor. Courtesy of Dr. Carol Caudill, VCU Department of Pediatric Dentistry.

- *Treatment*—No treatment. Advise the patient to brush with soft brush and nonalcohol chlorhexidine for one week. Instruct the patient not to incise on the anterior teeth; food should be cut up and chewed with the posterior teeth, for 2 weeks.
- *Follow-up*—1 week and then 6–8 weeks. Watch for crown discoloration; if it occurs, monitor for pathologic changes.
- *Complications*—primary tooth does not continue to develop, or it becomes dark in color with associated periapical pathology.
- *Criteria for success*—continued root development in the immature primary anterior tooth. Dark discoloration of crown is transient or becomes yellow in color, which would indicate pulp canal calcification/obliteration, requiring no treatment.

Extrusive Luxation

- *Diagnosis*—the tooth appears elongated, since it has been partially displaced from the socket (Figure 14.11 and see later Figure 14.17a). The tooth may be excessively mobile and radiographically there is an increase in the periodontal ligament space.
- *Treatment*—for a minor extrusion, as long as there is no interference with the occlusion the tooth can be left to spontaneously align. For severe extrusion, especially if

the primary tooth has a fully formed root, extraction is the treatment of choice.
- *Follow-up*—if the tooth is left in place, it should be monitored for discoloration and the possibility of infection. Follow-up occurs at 1 week, 6–8 weeks, 6 months, and 1 year.
- *Complications*—the primary tooth does not continue to develop or it becomes dark in color, with associated periapical pathology.
- *Criteria for success*—continued development of the primary tooth. Transient discoloration that disappears or turns yellow, indicating pulp canal obliteration/calcification.

Lateral Luxation

- *Diagnosis*—the tooth is displaced labially (Figure 14.12) or lingually (Figure 14.13 and see later Figure 14.18) without mobility. Displacement occurs more frequently in a palatal direction with the root in a labial direction. Radiographically, there will be an increased periodontal ligament space.
- *Treatment*—if there is no occlusal interference, no treatment is necessary. If, however, there is minor interference with the occlusion, it is possible to gently reposition the tooth. This should be done as soon as possible, since if it is delayed, a clot can form, making it more difficult to reposition the

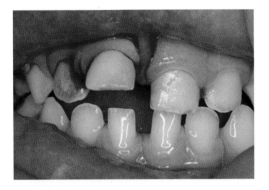

Figure 14.12 Labial luxation of maxillary right primary central incisor. Courtesy of American Academy of Pediatric Dentistry members' library.

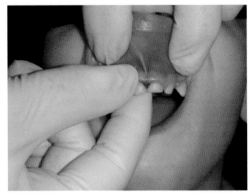

Figure 14.14 Manual repositioning of laterally luxated maxillary right primary central incisor.

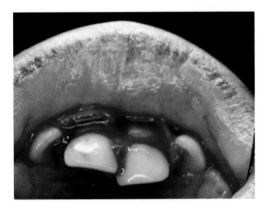

Figure 14.13 Lingual luxation of maxillary right and left primary central incisors. Courtesy of American Academy of Pediatric Dentistry members' library.

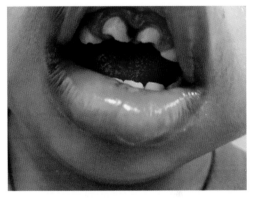

Figure 14.15 Intrusion luxation of maxillary right and left primary central incisors. Courtesy of Dr. Jennifer Waters, VCU Department of Pediatric Dentistry.

tooth (Figure 14.14). If the interference is severe, the tooth should be extracted.

- *Follow-up*—1 week, 2–3 weeks, 6–8 weeks (with radiograph), 1 year (with radiograph).
- *Complications*—the primary tooth does not continue to develop, or it becomes dark in color, with associated periapical pathology.
- *Criteria for success*—continued development of the primary tooth. Clinical and radiographic signs of normal periodontium. Transient discoloration may occur.

Intrusive Luxation

- *Diagnosis*—clinically, the teeth appear to be submerged (Figures 14.15 and 14.16).

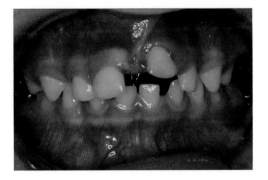

Figure 14.16 Intrusion of maxillary left primary cental incisor.

Intrusion of a primary tooth can result in serious damage to the permanent successor. The tooth is intruded, with the root either being displaced labially and possibly through the labial bone, or lingually where it may impinge on the developing permanent successor. An occlusal radiograph will show the position of the displaced tooth.

- *Treatment*—if the root tip is positioned labially, the tooth will spontaneously reposition itself. If the root tip is positioned lingually toward the permanent tooth bud, the primary tooth must be extracted to allow the permanent tooth bud the opportunity to develop normally.

  Follow-up—1 week, 3–4 weeks with radiograph, 6–8 weeks, 6 months with radiograph, and 1 year with radiograph.

- *Complications*—tooth is locked into position. Persistent discoloration. Radiographic signs of periapical pathology. Damage to the permanent successor; this should be discussed as a possibility so the guardian is not surprised later when and if the permanent tooth erupts with visible defects.

- *Criteria for success*—tooth spontaneously repositions, with no transient discoloration. Permanent successor erupts normally.

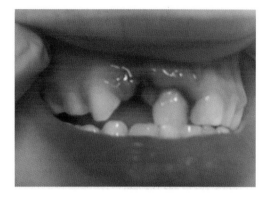

Figure 14.18 Avulsion of maxillary right primary lateral incisor, Lingual luxation of maxillary right primary central incisor. Courtesy of Dr. Carol Caudill, VCU Department of Pediatric Dentistry.

Avulsion

- *Diagnosis*—tooth is completely out of the socket (Figures 14.7b and 14.18). A radiograph is necessary to confirm that the tooth is not completely intruded.

- *Treatment*—**do not replant avulsed primary teeth** due to the risk of damaging the permanent successor tooth bud.

- *Follow-up*—1 week, 6 months with radiograph, and 1 year with radiograph.

- *Complications*—damage to the permanent tooth bud.

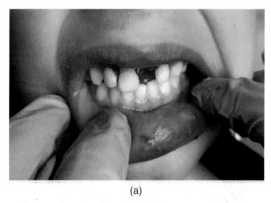

(a)

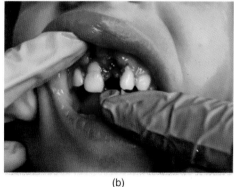

(b)

Figure 14.17 (a) Extrusive luxation of maxillary right primary central incisor and left primary lateral incisor, interfering with occlusion. (b) Avulsion of maxillary left central incisor. Courtesy of Dr. Carol Caudill, VCU Department of Pediatric Dentistry.

The Effect of Primary Tooth Trauma on the Permanent Successor

The distance between the permanent tooth germ and the periapical region of the primary tooth is less than 3 mm and it may be of hard tissue or consist only of fibrous connective tissue. Some of the more common sequelae to the permanent teeth following trauma to the primary predecessors are enamel discoloration, enamel hypoplasia, crown or root dilacerations, odontoma-like malformations, tooth-germ sequestration, partial or total interruption of root formation, and eruption disorders (de Fatima Guedes de Amorim *et al.*, 2011). In a study performed by de Fatima Guedes de Amorim *et al.* (2011), 148 children with traumatic dental injury to the primary anterior teeth were followed until the eruption of the permanent successors. What the authors discovered was that there was a significant association between age at the time of injury and the appearance of sequelae to the permanent teeth, and that a greater prevalence of sequelae occurred in children who experienced trauma between the ages of 1 and 3. This is of particular concern, since luxation injuries occur most often in children between 1 and 3 years of age and are typically due to the child becoming more ambulatory and experiencing more falls (Andersson *et al.*, 2012). The younger the child at the time of traumatic injury, the greater the sequelae to the permanent teeth (Riberio do Espirito Santo Jacomo & Campos, 2009). The high risk of sequelae in this younger age group (1–3 years) may be due to incomplete bone and permanent tooth-germ mineralization (Selliseth, 1970). Permanent tooth enamel discoloration and hypoplasia were more common in children who experienced trauma between age 1 and 2. A recurrence of trauma (reinjury to the same tooth) was an aggravating factor in permanent

tooth sequelae and led to an increased complexity of treatment (de Fatima Guedes de Amorim *et al.*, 2011).

In a retrospective study of 174 permanent teeth following trauma to their predecessors, the authors looked at the prevalence of various post-trauma sequelae in the permanent successors. Of the 174 permanent teeth, 89 (51.1%) presented with development disturbance and 85 (46.08%) demonstrated no sequelae. The most common sequelae were discoloration of the enamel and/or enamel hypoplasia at 46.08% followed by disturbances in eruption at 17.97% and root dilacerations at 15.73%. Intrusions of primary teeth were the type of injury most commonly associated with sequelae in the permanent successors (Riberio do Espirito Santo Jacomo & Campos, 2009). In a study performed by Skaare *et al.* (2015), intrusion injuries followed by avulsions are most often reported to cause mineralization disturbances, whereas luxation and subluxation cause deficiencies less frequently. More specifically, the proportion of permanent teeth with enamel defects caused by luxation injures were as follows (Skaare *et al.*, 2015):

- Concussion 8%.
- Subluxation 18%.
- Extrusion 8%.
- Lateral luxation 41%.
- Intrusion 38%.
- Avulsion 47%.

Parental Information Concerning Permanent Tooth Avulsion

It is advisable to provide parents with the necessary information to aid them in the event that their child suffers a traumatic injury that results in an avulsed permanent tooth.

As a provider, the following information can be printed onto a refrigerator magnet for at-home easy access.

Office Name: _____ **Emergency Contact Number**: _____

In the event that your child has traumatically lost their front permanent tooth (child is 7–8 years of age or older):

1. Remain calm.
2. Assess your child's level of consciousness—are they feeling lightheaded or dizzy? If your child is lightheaded or dizzy, take them to the emergency department.
3. Look for the avulsed permanent tooth.
4. Once located, placed the tooth in cold milk. If milk is not available and the child is young, they can spit into a cup and the tooth can be transported in the cup of saliva. If it is an older child, they can hold the tooth between their lower lip and teeth or on the side between the cheek and teeth to keep the tooth moist with saliva.
5. **Do not store the tooth in tap water**.
6. Try to be seen by a dentist within an hour or as soon as possible to have the tooth replanted and splinted.

References

Andersson, L., Andreasen, J.O., & Day, P. (2012) Guidelines for the management of traumatic dental injuries: 3. Injuries in the primary dentition. *Dental Traumatology*, 28, 174–182.

Atabek, D., Alacam, A., Aydintug I., & Konakoğlu, G. (2014) A retrospective study of traumatic dental injuries. *Dental Traumatology*, 30, 154–161.

Camp, J.H. (2008) Diagnosis dilemmas in vital pulp therapy: treatment for the toothache is changing, especially in young, *immature teeth*. *Pediatric Dentistry*, 30, 197–205.

Colak, I., Markovic, D., Petrovic, B., Peric, T., & Milenkovic, A. (2009) A retrospective study of intrusive injuries in primary dentition. *Dental Traumatology*, 25, 605–610.

de Fatima Guedes de Amorim, L., Estrela, C., & da Costa, L.R.R. (2011) Effects of traumatic dental injuries to primary teeth on permanent teeth – a clinic follow-up study. *Dental Traumatology*, 27, 117–121.

Goettems, M.L., Thurow, L.B., Noronha, T.G., da Silva, I.F., Jr., Kramer, P.F., *et al.* (2020) Incidence and prognosis of crown discoloration in traumatized primary teeth: a retrospective cohort study. *Dental Traumatology*, 36, 393–399.

Holan, G. (2006) Long-term effect of different treatment modalities for traumatized primary incisors presenting dark coronal discoloration with no other signs of injury. *Dental Traumatology*, 22, 14–17.

Holan, G. & Fuks, A.B. (1996) The diagnostic value of coronal dark-gray discoloration in primary teeth following traumatic injuries. *Pediatric Dentistry*, 18, 224–227.

McTigue, D.J. (2013) Overview of trauma management for primary and young permanent teeth. *Dental Clinics of North America*, 57, 39–57.

Ribierio do Espirito Santo Jacomo, D. & Campos, V. (2009) Prevalence of sequelae in the permanent anterior teeth after trauma in their predecessors: a longitudinal study of 8 years. *Dental Traumatology*, 25, 300–304.

Selliseth, N.E. (1970) The significance of traumatized primary incisors on the development and eruption of permanent teeth. *Report of the Congress European Orthodontic Society*, 46, 443–459.

Skaare, A.B., Maseng Aas A., & Wang, N.J. (2015) Enamel defects on permanent successors following luxation injuries to primary teeth and carers' experiences. *International Journal of Paediatric Dentistry*, 25, 221–228.

Soxman, J.A., Nasif, M.M., & Bouquot, J. (1984) Pulpal pathology in relation to discoloration of primary anterior teeth. *Journal of Dentistry for Children*, 51, 282–284.

15

Pulpal Treatment in Young Permanent Incisors Following Traumatic Injuries

Joe H. Camp

Pulp Capping and Pulpotomy

Preservation of vitality in young permanent immature teeth is imperative to allow completion of root formation in order to have the strongest root possible. If injury occurs, resulting in pulpal necrosis before dentinogenesis is completed, retention of the tooth is compromised by diminished root length and thinness of dentin. The thinner dentinal walls of the root lead to increased root fracture. The decrease in root length results in a lower root-to-crown ratio and may lead to tooth mobility, with resultant loss of attachment apparatus.

In a 4-year study, Cvek (1992) reported a significant increase in cervical root fractures in endodontically treated immature teeth. Dependent on the stage of development, fractures ranged from 77% in teeth with the least root development to 28% with the most developed roots (Figures 15.1a–d and 15.2a–c).

Direct pulp capping (Figure 15.3a–c) and pulpotomy attempt to preserve pulpal vitality by the application of a medicament or dental material to the exposed pulp. Pulpotomy differs from pulp capping only in that additional pulp tissue is removed before placement of the pulp-capping agent. The success rates of these procedures following injury in the young teeth are high (Cvek & Lundberg, 1983; Fuks *et al.*, 1987). While there is much disagreement on these vital procedures versus pulpectomy and root canal filling, there is almost universal agreement that these procedures are indicated in teeth with immature apices.

In young fractured teeth with pulp exposure, Cvek (1978) and Cvek and Lundberg (1983) have shown that inflammation and/or infection will be confined to the surface 2–3 mm. The underlying tissue will respond favorably to pulpotomy. Neither the exposure size nor time between injury and treatment up to 90 days is critical for healing when only the superficial layers of pulp are removed. It is usually not necessary or desirable to remove all the coronal pulp tissue. This partial pulpotomy is commonly referred to as a Cvek pulpotomy (Cvek, 1993) (Figures 15.4a–f and 15.5a–i).

Many medicaments and materials have been used for pulp capping and pulpotomy. Traditionally, calcium hydroxide ($Ca(OH)_2$) has been the most widely used agent of choice. However, additional recent research has shown mineral trioxide aggregate (MTA) to be more biologic while producing better results (Abedi *et al.*, 1996; Pitt Ford *et al.*, 1996). MTA has become the agent of choice (Figures 15.6a–c and 15.7a–e).

Healing is directly related to the capacity of the capping agent and restoration to provide a biologic seal against bacterial leakage, while simultaneously forming a dentinal bridge. MTA provides a biologically active substrate to which cells are attached. Calcium released from the MTA reacts with phosphate in the tissue fluid to produce hydroxyapatite (Sarkar *et al.*, 2002).

Handbook of Clinical Techniques in Pediatric Dentistry, Second Edition. Edited by Jane A. Soxman.
© 2022 John Wiley & Sons, Inc. Published 2022 by John Wiley & Sons, Inc.

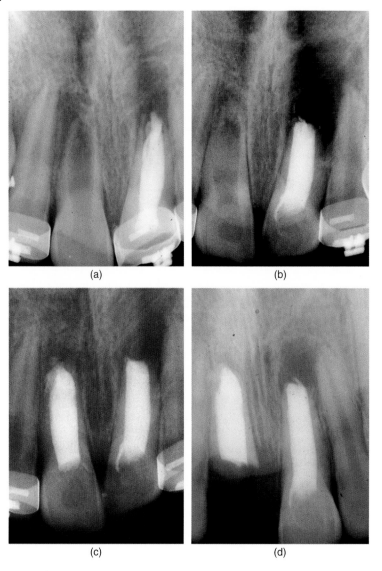

(a)

(b)

(c)

(d)

Figure 15.1 Fractured root of the maxillary right central incisor following successful apexification with calcium hydroxide and filling of root canal with guttapercha. (a) Preoperative radiograph. Unsuccessful previous root canal treatment with guttapercha in the left central incisor. (b) Successful apexification of the right incisor. The left incisor has root canal filled with guttapercha followed by an apical curettage. (c) Radiograph at 18 months. The right central has been filled with guttapercha. The lesion at the apex of the left incisor is healing. (d) Fracture of the thin root of the right central incisor 3 months later. The left incisor continues to heal apically.

In the Cvek pulpotomy, only tissue judged to be inflamed is removed. Removal of tissue is accomplished with an abrasive diamond or round carbide bur using high speed and copious water spray. All fibers of the pulp coronal to the amputation must be removed, otherwise hemorrhage will persist. After tissue removal is completed, the site is washed with sterile water or saline to remove all debris. Blowing air on the pulp is contraindicated because it will cause damage to the tissue from desiccation.

Hemorrhage control is obtained by light pressure on the pulp with a dampened cotton pellet. Hemostasis should be achieved in 1–2 min (Figures 15.4b, c and 15.5c). If bleeding persists, an additional 1–2 mm of pulpal tissue is removed. Hemostatic agents are contraindicated. A cotton pellet wetted with sodium hypochlorite (NaOCl) may be applied to help in hemorrhage control. The application of NaOCl to pulp tissue is hemostatic, but does not cause tissue damage. It does not inhibit pulpal healing, odontoblastic cell formation,

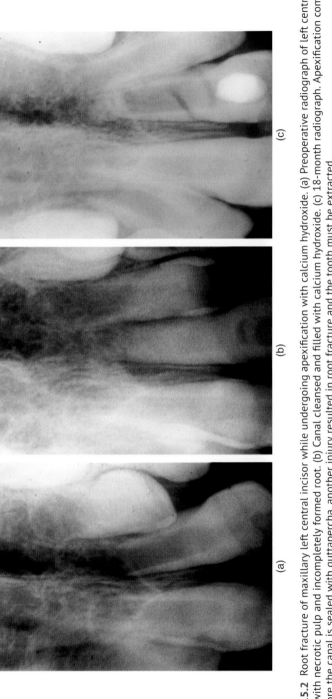

Figure 15.2 Root fracture of maxillary left central incisor while undergoing apexification with calcium hydroxide. (a) Preoperative radiograph of left central incisor with necrotic pulp and incompletely formed root. (b) Canal cleansed and filled with calcium hydroxide. (c) 18-month radiograph. Apexification completed, but before the canal is sealed with guttapercha, another injury resulted in root fracture and the tooth must be extracted.

(a)

(b)

(c)

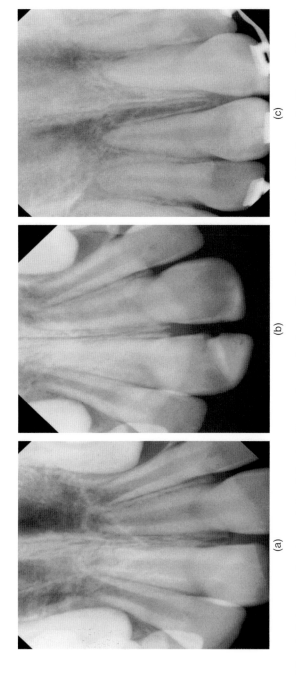

Figure 15.3 Apical closure and root completion following direct pulp capping in maxillary right central incisor. (a) Radiograph of fractured left incisor with pulp exposure. Note the immature roots. (b) Radiograph of mineral trioxide aggregate pulp capping covered with composite resin. (c) Radiograph 4.5 years after pulp capping showing dentinal bridging and completed root formation.

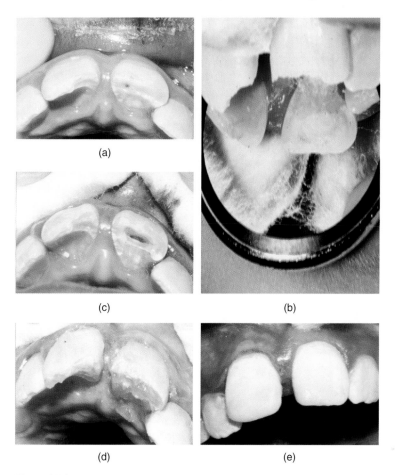

(a)

(c)

(b)

(d)

(e)

Figure 15.4 Cvek pulpotomy with mineral trioxide aggregate (MTA) on a maxillary right central incisor. (a) Clinical appearance of pulp exposure 4 days after injury. The right incisor has a pulp exposure and the left incisor has a minor dentin fracture. (b) Three millimeters of the pulp has been removed with a clean amputation, washed, and a wetted cotton pellet placed against the pulp to control hemorrhage. (c) The amputation site after cotton is removed. Note the lack of hemorrhage. (d) The pulp has been capped with 1.5 mm of white MTA. A thin layer of light-cured composite has been placed over the MTA and cured to protect it during sealing of the tooth. (e) The two central incisors are etched. (f) Sealing of the incisors with bonded composite restorations. A definitive well-contoured restoration will be placed in 8 weeks after healing has occurred.

or dentinal bridging (Akimoto *et al.*, 1998). Pulp capping will not be successful unless hemorrhage is controlled.

A 1–2-mm layer of MTA is placed directly over the exposure site. Because MTA requires 4–6 hours to set, it is covered with a thin layer of flowable light-cured composite resin or glass ionomer. Care should be exercised in covering only the MTA in order to have the maximum surface of dentin and enamel to etch for placement of the permanent restoration.

Research (Tsujimoto *et al.*, 2013) has demonstrated that placement of resin over wet, unset MTA does not alter the composition, setting, or action of the material. The tooth may then be etched and the final restoration placed.

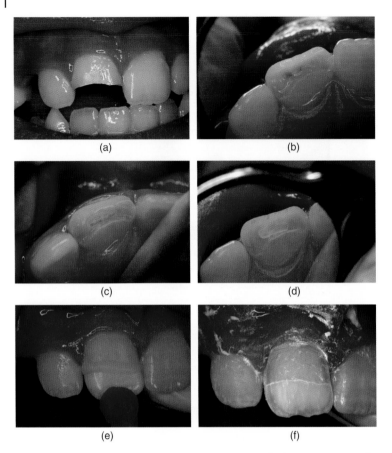

(a)

(b)

(c)

(d)

(e)

(f)

Figure 15.5 Cvek pulpotomy with calcium hydroxide (Ca(OH)$_2$) and restoration of crown on traumatically injured maxillary central incisor. (a) Facial views of fractured incisor. (b) Incisal view of tooth revealing pulp exposure. (c) Pulp chamber after 2 mm diamond bur preparation and hemostasis. (d) Ca(OH)$_2$ placed in prepared chamber. (e) Fractured coronal segment reattached with resin-modified glass ionomer cement. (f) Facial enamel preparation for placement of direct-bonded resin-based composite veneer. (g) Self-etching resin bonding agent applied. (h) Restored tooth after 26 months, immediately following routine prophylaxis. (i) Two radiographic views, 26 months after Cvek pulpotomy. Courtesy of Dr. Ted Croll, Case Western Reverse School of Dental Medicine.

Apexification and Apical Plug

Once the pulp has become necrotic, all deposition of dentin ceases. If this occurs before closure of the root, the tooth is left with an open apex and possibly a shortened root. Conventional endodontic procedures cannot be performed.

Apexification, generally with Ca(OH)$_2$ alone or in combination with other drugs to stimulate apical closure, was the accepted treatment for many years. Following apical closure with cementum, the canal was filled with guttapercha (Figure 15.1c). Although highly successful, this technique left a root highly susceptible to fracture, varying from 28% to 77% after 4 years (Cvek, 1992). The thinner the root dentin, the more likely the root was to fracture (Figures 15.1 and 15.2). Therefore, treatments oriented toward preserving vitality, pulp capping, and pulpotomy should be attempted if possible. If these conservative treatments fail, more radical endodontic treatments can still be performed.

Figure 15.5 (*Continued*)

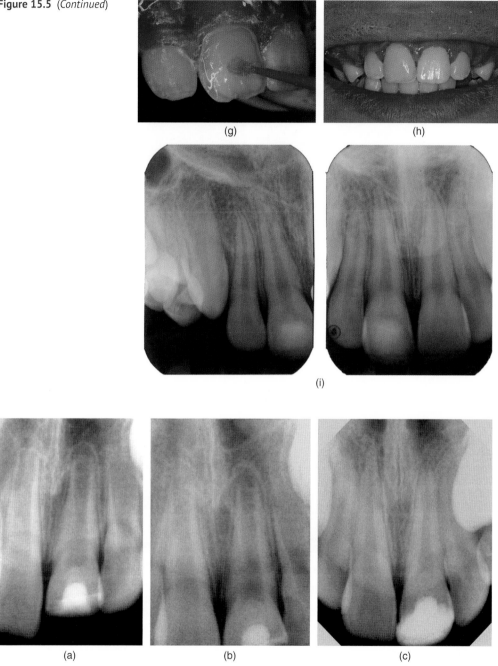

(g)

(h)

(i)

(a)

(b)

(c)

Figure 15.6 Cvek pulpotomy with mineral trioxide aggregate on a maxillary left central incisor with an open apex. (a) Radiograph 3 months after pulpotomy. Note the dentin bridge. (b) Radiograph 6 months after pulpotomy. The dentin bridge has thickened. (c) Radiograph 3.5 years after Cvek pulpotomy. The root formation is completed and the apex closed. The dentin bridge has thickened, but the root is free of abnormal calcification.

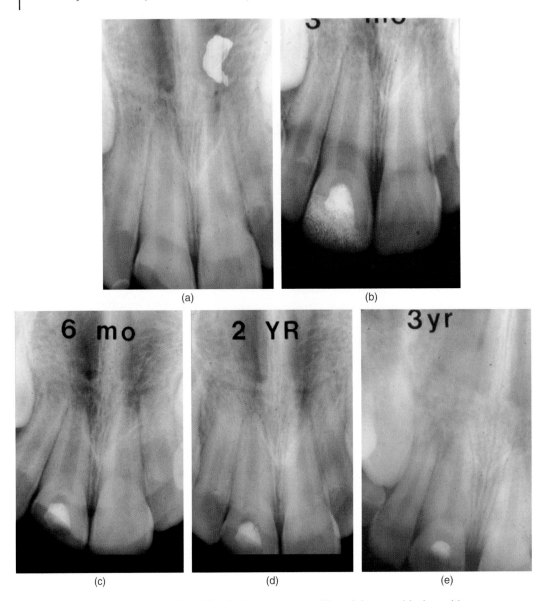

Figure 15.7 Cvek pulpotomy with calcium hydroxide on a maxillary right central incisor with an open apex. (a) Preoperative radiograph of fractured incisor with pulp exposure. (b) Radiograph at 12 weeks showing dentin bridge. (c) Radiograph at 6 months. Note the dentin bridge has not thickened any further. (d) Radiograph at 2 years. Root formation is completed. (e) Radiograph at 3 years. The canal is not calcified.

While apexification with pastes was highly successful, the treatment required 1–2 years to form the apical barrier. Alternative treatments with artificial barriers in the canal to allow immediate obturation of the canal were developed.

MTA, introduced in 1996 (Tittle *et al.*, 1996) as an apical barrier against which to pack a root filling, has become the standard. Subsequent research showed that MTA induced apical hard tissue formation, while causing less inflammation than previously used materials (Figures 15.8a–d and 15.9a–c).

After placement and setting of an apical plug of several millimeters of MTA, the canal can be obturated (Figure 15.8b). MTA is

Figure 15.8 Apical plug with mineral trioxide aggregate (MTA). (a) Preoperative radiograph of immature root, necrotic pulp, and periapical lesion. (b) Apical plug of 4 mm MTA. (c) Remainder of canal filled with bonded composite resin. (d) Radiograph at 3.5 years. Complete closure of apex with cementum and healing of periapical lesion. Patient is undergoing orthodontics.

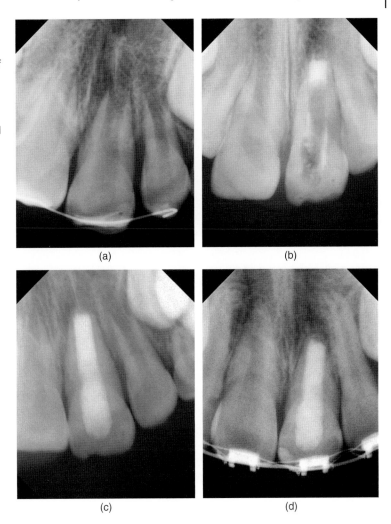

(a)

(b)

(c)

(d)

cementoconductive and stimulates cementogenesis at the apex with cementoblasts attached to the material (Figures 15.8d and 15.9c). Complete closure of the apex creates a biologic seal (Torabinejad *et al.*, 1997).

Apical Barrier Technique with Mineral Trioxide Aggregate

Following endodontic access, the tooth length is established with radiographs, as apex locators are not reliable in teeth with open apices (Berman & Fleischman, 1984; Hulsman & Pieper, 1989).

The use of the rubber dam is mandatory. The canal is cleansed and disinfected as in any root canal procedure. The use of NaOCl to dissolve necrotic tissue is essential. By using a small-diameter needle and keeping the tip 5–6 mm from the apex while injecting slowly, there is no danger of apical extrusion of the liquid.

An acidic pH, as occurs with suppuration, adversely affects the physical properties and hydration of MTA and weakens its microhardness (Lee *et al.*, 2004). If suppuration is present, the canal must be medicated with $Ca(OH)_2$ and sealed to allow resolution of the drainage. At a subsequent appointment

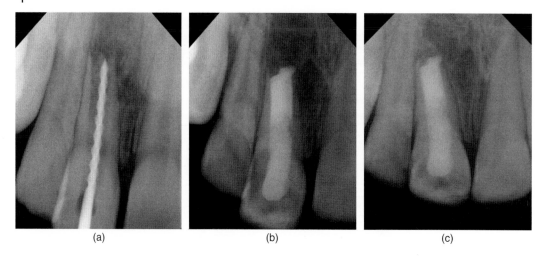

(a)   (b)   (c)

Figure 15.9 Apical plug with mineral trioxide aggregate (MTA). (a) Radiograph at time of treatment, with endodontic file in canal to establish tooth length. Immature root with large periapical lesion. (b) Apical plug of MTA and remainder of canal bonded with composite resin. (c) Radiograph at 2.25 years. Apical lesion is healed and apex closed with cementum.

in several weeks, the canal is re-entered and thoroughly cleansed of the Ca(OH)$_2$ medication, before placing the apical plug of MTA as described in the following section.

Once the canal is thoroughly cleansed and disinfected, it may be dried with paper points and the apical plug of MTA placed. Placement of the MTA in the pulp chamber is easily done with the small end of an amalgam carrier. The MTA is carefully packed to the apex with *measured* pluggers. Care must be taken if using metal blunt-ended pluggers to prevent overfill. While care is exercised to avoid an overfill of MTA, overfills are not a disaster and do not have to be removed surgically, as MTA is osteogenic. Any overfill will stimulate osteogenesis and will become encased in bone (Figure 15.10a–d).

The author has found that the use of a very large paper point turned in reverse makes an effective plugger for condensation. Small increments are placed in the chamber and condensed to the apex. As the end of the paper point becomes softened by moisture, it is discarded and a new one used. Small increments are easily condensed, whereas large amounts will block the canal and prevent condensation. Depth control is monitored by radiographs.

Placement of large amounts of MTA may lead to blockage of the canal before the material reaches the proper depth. Small increments of MTA can be achieved by filling the small end of an amalgam carrier, then partially extruding and removing part of the MTA plug before placing the remainder in the canal. If the canal becomes clogged with MTA before reaching the proper depth at the apex, the mass is easily loosened with a large endodontic reamer or file. If this happens, it may be necessary to remove a portion of the MTA from the canal and then continue condensation (Figure 15.11a–d).

A 4 mm plug of MTA has been shown to be significantly more effective than lower amounts in preventing dye leakage (Valois & Costa, 2004). Therefore, the apical 4 mm is filled with the plug of MTA (Figure 15.8b). The entire canal is not filled with MTA, as a bonded composite will be placed in the remainder of the canal, as described later, to strengthen the root.

All excess MTA is removed from the canal walls. To remove the residue of MTA on the lateral walls of the root, the canal can be scrubbed with large damp paper points, or the cotton-tipped applicators used to apply

Figure 15.10 Healing of a gross overfill of mineral trioxide aggregate (MTA) in an immature maxillary left central incisor. (a) Preoperative radiograph of central incisor with open apex and large periapical lesion. (b) Radiograph of accidental gross overfill of MTA while placing the apical plug. (c) Lesion on left central incisor is healing, and canal has been filled with guttapercha incisal to the MTA plug. The right central incisor has developed an apical lesion. (d) Radiograph of central incisors at 3 years. The apical lesion on the left central incisor with MTA overfill is completely healed, with the overfill surrounded by bone. The right central incisor has been filled with guttapercha and is healing.

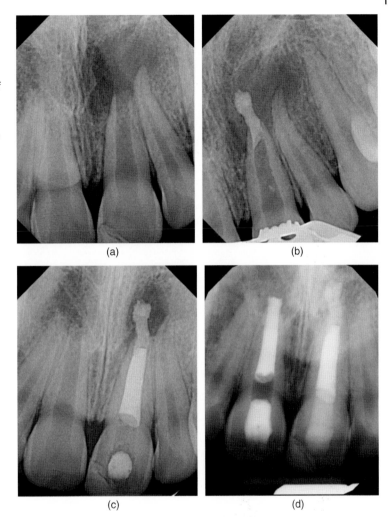

(a)

(b)

(c)

(d)

bonding agents in the composite technique. This is done so that the remainder of the canal can be strengthened with composite resin bonded to the dentinal walls.

Once the canal is cleaned of excess MTA and the apical plug determined by radiograph to be satisfactory, a wetted cotton pellet is placed in the canal until the MTA sets. The cotton pellet is pulled away from the MTA, so cotton fibers will not be incorporated into the material as it sets. Other dry pellets are placed in the chamber and the coronal access is sealed with temporary cement such as IRM® (Dentsply Caulk, Konstanz, Germany) or Cavit® (3M ESPE, St. Paul, MN, USA). This must be left for a minimum of 6 hours as the MTA sets.

Another appointment is made to complete bonding of the remainder of the canal to strengthen the root.

Strengthening the Root

The MTA is allowed to set for a minimum of 6 hours. When the patient returns, the tooth is re-entered and all the temporary cement and cotton pellets are removed. Verification of set of the MTA is done by probing against it with an endodontic file. The canal is thoroughly irrigated and dried with paper points. An acid-etch gel is placed in the canal to etch the dentinal walls. After thoroughly rinsing and drying, a

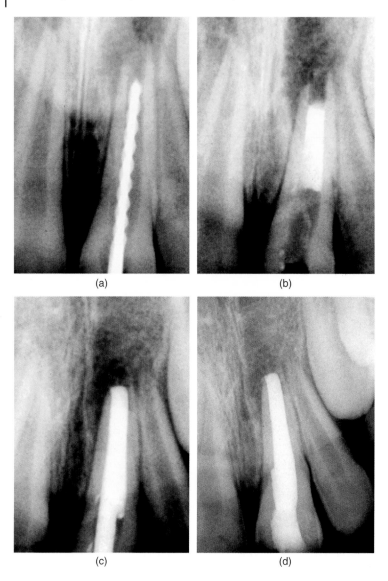

(a)

(b)

(c)

(d)

Figure 15.11 Reworking of apical plug of mineral trioxide aggregate (MTA) short of correct length. (a) Radiograph of maxillary central incisor with open apex. Endodontic file in place to determine tooth length. (b) Radiograph showing MTA plug canal short of proper depth. The MTA is loosened with a large endodontic file and condensed to the proper depth. (c) MTA plug condensed to proper depth and remainder of canal being filled with guttapercha. (d) Radiograph 1 year later. The apical lesion is nearly healed.

bonding agent is placed on the dentinal walls and cured. It is not necessary to avoid contact of the MTA with the acid-etchant or the bonding agent, as it causes no deleterious effects to the apical plug (Tsujimoto *et al.*, 2013).

The canal is then filled incrementally with 2 mm layers of any microfilled condensable composite (Figure 15.8c). Radiographic examination of the first increment of composite will help to avoid voids in the canal filling. The small amount of condensable composite is packed into place with blunt-ended pluggers

or large paper points reversed to use the larger end. Each increment of 2 mm of composite is cured. Curing times are four times the recommended curing time for the curing light to insure complete set of the composite. The light easily reaches the composite owing to the wide access and the large canal.

The first increment of composite is the most difficult to place without a void. Once the first increment is placed, a radiograph is recommended to ascertain that it is in contact with the MTA and has no voids. If this is not the case, it should be removed and a new increment placed and X-rayed again. Once the first composite is cured in place, it is rare to have a void in the other increments. The canal should *not* be filled with a self-curing flowable composite, as voids will definitely be trapped. Also, the large volume of composite will shrink away from the dentinal walls as polymerization occurs. The increments of condensable composite should fill only 2 mm to avoid shrinkage of the material. The material is placed in the tooth and cured until the root canal, pulp chamber, and access opening are obliterated (Figures 15.8c and 15.9b). Unless part of the crown is missing, this is the permanent restoration of the tooth.

Research (Hernandez *et al.*, 1994; Katebzadeh *et al.*, 1998) has shown that the use of newer dentinal bonding techniques will strengthen endodontically treated teeth to levels close to that of intact teeth. Utilization of this technique has virtually eliminated root fractures in these immature roots.

Regenerative Endodontics

Reports of nonvital immature teeth with open apices and suppuration have demonstrated ingrowth of pulp-like tissue and complete root formation, both in length and thickness of dentin, after treatment with a triple antibiotic paste (Iwaya *et al.*, 2001; Banchs & Trope, 2004).

The root canal is endodontically accessed and disinfected with copious irrigation with full strength NaOCl for 10–15 minutes. No instrumentation is performed on the canal. After carefully drying the canal, a paste of ciproflaxin, metronidazole, and minocycline is mixed and placed in the canal. A paper point or lentulo spiral can be used to place the paste. The canal is sealed with a temporary filling.

The paste is left in place for several weeks. The canal is re-entered and the antibiotic paste is washed out with NaOCl and dried. The periapical tissues are instrumented with endodontic files through the apex to create hemorrhage into the canal. After the canal becomes filled with blood, it is allowed to clot.

The clot is carefully removed to the cervical line. The remaining clot is covered with several millimeters of MTA and the tooth closed with a temporary filling. After hardening of the MTA, the tooth is permanently sealed with a resin-bonded composite.

The clot serves as a scaffold for pulp regeneration. Over a period of 1–2 years, calcified tissue resembling dentin radiographically is deposited in the canal and is contiguous with the dentinal walls.

Minocycline stains dentin green. Clindamycin has been shown to be an acceptable substitute for minocycline. Therefore, clindamycin should be used as a substitute for minocycline to prevent staining of the dentin (McTigue *et al.*, 2013).

References

Abedi, H.R., Torabinejad, M., Pitt Ford, T.R., & Backland, L.K. (1996) The use of mineral trioxide aggregate cement (MTA) as a direct pulp-capping agent. *Journal of Endodontics*, 22, 199 (abstract).

Akimoto, N., Momoi, Y., Kohno, A., Suzuki, S., Otsuki, M., *et al.* (1998) Biocompatibility of Clearfil Liner Bond 2 and Clearfil AP-X system to non-exposed and exposed primate teeth. *Quintessence International*, 29, 177–188.

Banchs, F. & Trope, M. (2004) Revascularization of immature permanent teeth with apical periodontitis: new treatment protocol? *Journal of Endodontics*, 30, 196–200.

Berman, L.H. & Fleischman, S.B. (1984) Evaluation of the accuracy of the neosono-D electronic apex locator. *Journal of Endodontics*, 10, 164–167.

Cvek, M. (1978) A clinical report on partial pulpotomy and capping with calcium hydroxide in permanent incisors with complicated crown fractures. *Journal of Endodontics*, 4, 232–237.

Cvek, M. (1992) Prognosis of luxated non-vital maxillary incisors treated with calcium hydroxide and filled with guttapercha. A retrospective clinical study. *Endodontics and Dental Traumatology*, 8, 45–55.

Cvek, M. (1993) Results after partial pulpotomy in crown fractured teeth 3–15 years after treatment. *Acta Stomatologica Croatica*, 27, 167–173.

Cvek, M. & Lundberg, M. (1983) Histological appearance of pulps after exposure by a crown fracture, partial pulpotomy, and clinical diagnosis of healing. *Journal of Endodontics*, 9, 8–11.

Fuks, A.B., Chosack, A., Klein, H., & Edelman, E. (1987) Partial pulpotomy as a treatment alternative for exposed pulps in crown-fractured permanent incisors. *Endodontics and Dental Traumatology*, 3, 100–102.

Hernandez, R., Bader, S., Boston, D., & Trope, M. (1994) Resistance to fracture of endodontically treated premolars restored with new generation dentin bonding systems. *International Endodontic Journal*, 27, 281–284.

Hulsman, M. & Pieper, K. (1989) Use of an electronic apex locator in the treatment of teeth with incomplete root formation. *Endodontics and Dental Traumatology*, 5, 238–241.

Iwaya, S., Ikawa, M., & Kubata, M. (2001) Revascularization of an immature permanent tooth with apical periodontitis and sinus tract. *Dental Traumatology*, 17, 185–187.

Katebzadeh, N., Dalton, B.C., & Trope, M. (1998) Strengthening immature teeth during and after apexification. *Journal of Endodontics*, 24, 256–259.

Lee, Y.L., Lee, B.S., Lin, F.H., Lin, A.Y., Lan, W.-H., & Lin, C.-P. (2004) Effects of physiological environments on the hydration behavior of mineral trioxide aggregate. *Biomaterials*, 25, 787–793.

McTigue, D.J., Subramanian, K., & Kumar, A. (2013) Management of immature permanent teeth with pulpal necrosis: a case series. *Journal of Pediatric Dentistry*, 35, 55–60.

Pitt Ford, T.R., Torabinejad, M., & Abedi, H.R. (1996) Mineral trioxide aggregate as a pulp-capping material. *Journal of the American Dental Association*, 127, 1491–1494.

Sarkar, N.K., Saunderi, B., Moiseyevai, R., Berzins, D.W., & Kawashima, I. (2002) Interaction of mineral trioxide aggregate (MTA) with a synthetic tissue fluid. *Journal of Dental Research*, **81**, A-391 (abstract # 3155).

Tittle, K.W., Farley, J., Linkhardt, M., & Torabinejad, M. (1996) Apical closure induction using bone growth factors and mineral trioxide aggregate. *Journal of Endodontics*, 22, 1998 (abstract #41).

Torabinejad, M., Pitt, F.T., McKendry, D., Abedi, H.R., Miller, D.A., & Kariyawasam, S.P. (1997) Histological assessment of mineral trioxide aggregate as a root-end filling in monkeys. *Journal of Endodontics*, 23, 225–228.

Tsujimoto, M., Tsujimoto, Y., Ookuba, A., Shiraishi, T., Watanabe, I., *et al.* (2013) Timing for composite resin placement on mineral trioxide aggregate. *Journal of Endodontics*, 39, 1167–1170.

Valois, C.R. & Costa, E.D. (2004) Influence of the thickness of mineral trioxide aggregate on sealing ability of root-end fillings in vitro. *Oral Surgery, Oral Medicine, Oral Pathology, Oral Radiology, Endodontology*, 97, 180–111.

16

Reattachment of Permanent Incisor Enamel Fragments

Jane A. Soxman

Uncomplicated crown fracture occurs more often than any other traumatic dental injury. The International Association of Dental Traumatology advocates reattachment of coronal fragments as the preferable method to restore uncomplicated crown fracture (Madhubala *et al.*, 2019). Reattachment of an intact enamel fragment for both uncomplicated and complicated crown fractures provides a restoration that is less expensive, rapidly performed, and esthetic, with an identical match in original shape, occlusal alignment, natural translucency, surface finish, and unique coloration (Martos *et al.*, 2017). This is considered to be interim treatment that does not preclude any future treatment, as no tooth structure is removed or modified. Fracture of permanent incisors is more likely to occur with incompetent lip posture and significant overjet (Bauss *et al.*, 2008). Overjet equal to or above 6 mm increased the incidence of incisor fracture fourfold in a study by Schatz *et al.* (2013). Anticipatory guidance is provided to prepare the patient and parents/guardians for this event. Orthodontic treatment to retract the maxillary permanent incisors should be initiated as soon as all four incisors are erupted (Figure 16.1).

After an incisor fracture, the enamel fragment should be immediately located and stored in water or a damp paper towel to avoid desiccation, resulting in an opaque appearance and poor bonding strength (Sharmin & Thomas, 2013) (Figure 16.2). Rehydration of a fragment in distilled water for 15 minutes or a humidification chamber was shown to provide greater fracture resistance after reattachment in uncomplicated crown fractures (Madhubala *et al.*, 2019). The humidification chamber designed by the authors provided the stronger attachment. In another study, rehydrating a fragment after 24 hours of dry time by soaking in water for 15 minutes before bonding provided enough moisture to significantly increase bonding strength (Poubel *et al.*, 2017). If a lip laceration has simultaneously occurred, the laceration should be explored for the tooth fragment (Figure 16.3). A lower occlusal radiograph may be obtained to rule out the presence of a fragment embedded in the lip.

Procedure

Occlusal, periapical, and eccentric shift shots of the fractured incisor may be obtained to evaluate for root fracture or displacement. Simple reattachment of tooth fragments with complete fragment adaptation is the most successful treatment (Garcia *et al.*, 2018). The use of local anesthesia should not be necessary. The fragment may be reattached with both uncomplicated and complicated fractures. If the fracture has resulted in a borderline pulp exposure, a pulp capping agent, such as calcium hydroxide compound or white mineral trioxide aggregate (MTA), should be applied, followed by glass ionomer before

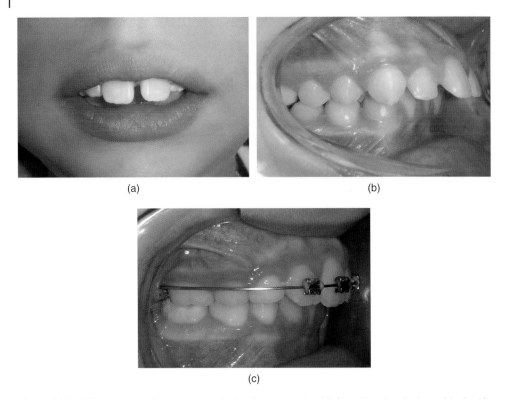

(a)

(b)

(c)

Figure 16.1 (a) Incompetent lip posture with significant overjet. (b) Class II malocclusion with significant overjet. (c) Overjet reduced with Phase I orthodontic intervention.

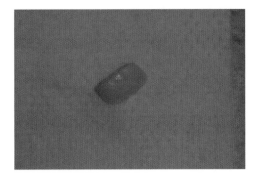

Figure 16.2 Desiccated enamel fragment.

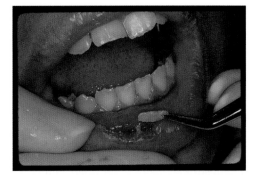

Figure 16.3 Enamel fragment being removed from lower lip laceration.

bonding. A pulpal exposure with a complicated fracture, seen within hours of the exposure and where complete hemostasis is achieved, may be treated conservatively with pulp capping. However, partial pulpotomy generally improves prognosis. If complete hemostasis cannot be achieved or more time has passed, a partial pulpotomy should be performed before reattachment.

If pulp capping with calcium hydroxide followed by glass ionomer is performed, bonding the fragment may no longer be possible due to the layers of material on the incisor now impeding the "fit" between the fragment and the incisor. A trough could be prepped in the fragment to accommodate the capping agent and glass ionomer, but the reattachment is compromised. Ultimately, in this case, a composite restoration will most likely be required.

Successful reattachment using only a bonding agent has been reported (Martos *et al.*, 2012; Giudice *et al.*, 2012). Andreasen *et al.* (1993) reported that reattachment with a bonding resin provides only half the original strength of the intact tooth. Bonding with flowable composite and composite resin has been successfully performed, providing from 2–7 years of function. Garcia *et al.* (2018) found an increase in bond strength between the tooth fragment and dentin with use of an intermediate material.

A fracture sloping to the cervical enhances the bond with increased area for bonding (Figure 16.4). The use of an anterior Parkell dry-field mouth prop greatly facilitates the procedure (Figure 16.5). The incisor and enamel fragment are individually decontaminated

with 0.2% chlorhexidine, conventionally etched with 37% phosphoric acid, and thoroughly rinsed with water (Figures 16.6–16.8, and 16.9). The use of a bevel, dentinal groove preparation, and chamfers does not enhance the retention of the fragment (Giudice *et al.*, 2012; Garcia *et al.*, 2018; de Sousa *et al.*, 2018). A bonding agent is applied to both

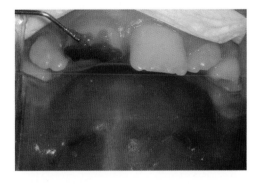

Figure 16.6 37% phosphoric acid applied to central incisor.

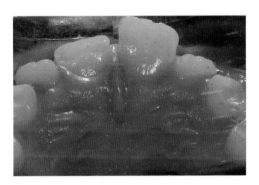

Figure 16.4 Fracture sloping to cervical.

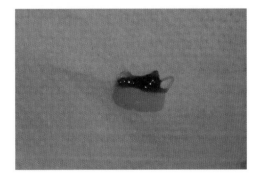

Figure 16.7 37% phosphoric acid applied to fragment.

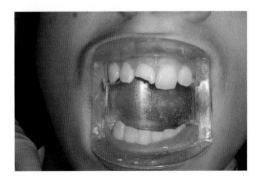

Figure 16.5 Parkell dry-field mouth prop.

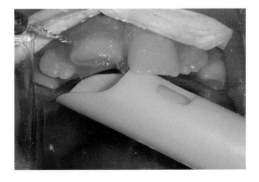

Figure 16.8 Central incisor rinsed.

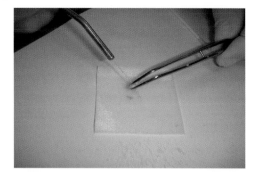

Figure 16.9 Fragment rinsed.

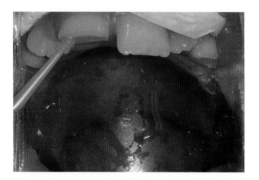

Figure 16.10 Bonding agent applied to central incisor.

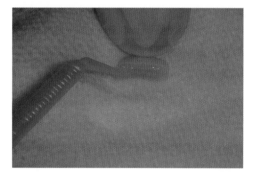

Figure 16.11 Bonding agent applied to fragment.

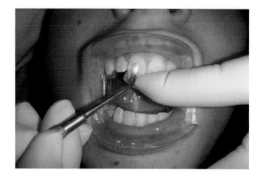

Figure 16.12 Excess composite removed with flat instrument.

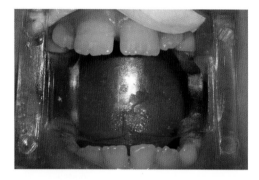

Figure 16.13 Fragment reattached to maxillary central incisor.

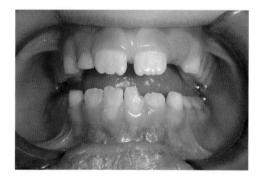

Figure 16.14 Class II fracture mandibular central incisor.

the incisor and the fragment and light-cured (Figures 16.10 and 16.11). A thin layer of composite resin may be applied to either the incisor and the fragment or both for enhanced retention (Cameron *et al.*, 2008). After matching the fragment to the coronal portion of the tooth, a flat instrument may be used to remove any excess composite from the facial and lingual surfaces (Figure 16.12). The bonded fragment is light-cured on the facial and lingual surfaces. The incisor is rapidly restored without discomfort and with an excellent esthetic result (Figure 16.13).

Reattachment of mandibular incisor enamel fragments may present a challenge due to their small size (Figure 16.14). The use of a holder

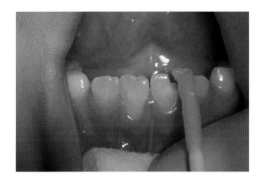

Figure 16.15 Pic-n-Stic carrying enamel fragment.

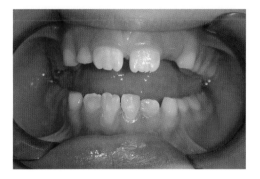

Figure 16.16 Fragment reattached to mandibular central incisor.

with an adhesive tip (Pic-n-Stic™, Pulpdent, Watertown, MA, USA) (Figure 16.15), rope, or

sticky wax facilitates carrying the fragment to the incisor (Figure 16.16).

Repeated trauma and nonphysiologic use of the incisor are the primary reasons for fragment failure (Macedo & Ritter, 2009). The patient is advised not to eat hard foods, not to bite his or her fingernails, and to notify the dentist about thermal discomfort, masticatory pain, or discoloration. Follow-up for evaluation of pulp vitality, along with periapical radiographs in 6–8 weeks and in 1 year, is recommended (Cameron *et al.*, 2008). If orthodontic treatment is in progress or anticipated in the future, the orthodontist should be informed of the traumatic incident and the periapical radiographs shared. Orthodontic movement post traumatic injury may result in pulpal changes; patient and parents/guardians should be informed of this possibility. A current periapical radiograph to evaluate radicular pathology or health should be obtained before commencing orthodontic movement. Parents/guardians should be informed that the bonded enamel fragment can be separated from the tooth during removal of the orthodontic bracket at the completion of orthodontic treatment.

References

Andreasen, F.M., Steinhardt, U., Bllle, M., & Munksgaard, E.C. (1993) Bonding of enamel-dentin crown fragments after crown fracture. An experimental study using bonding agents. *Dental Traumatology*, 9, 111–114.

Bauss, O., Freitag, S., Rohling, J., & Rahman, A. (2008) Influence of overjet and lip coverage on the prevalence and severity of incisor trauma. *Journal of Orofacial Orthopedics*, 69, 402–410.

Cameron, A., Widmer, R., Abbott, P., Heggie, A.C., & Raphael, S. (2008) Trauma management. In: Cameron, A.C. & Widmer, R.P. (eds.), *Handbook of Pediatric Dentistry*, 3rd edn. London: Mosby; 115–167.

de Sousa, A.P.B.R., Franca, K., & de Lucas Rezende, L.V.M. (2018) In vitro reattachment techniques: a systematic review. *Dental Traumatology*, 34, 397–310.

Garcia, F.C.P., Poubel D.L.N., Almeida J.C.F., Toledo, I.P., Poi, W.R., *et al.* (2018) Tooth fragment reattachment techniques—a systematic review. *Dental Traumatology*, 34, 135–143.

Giudice, L.G., Lapari, F., Lizio, A., Cervino, G., & and Cicciù, M. (2012) Tooth fragment reattachment technique on a pluri traumatized tooth. *Journal of Conservative Dentistry*, 5, 80–83.

Macedo, G.V. & Ritter, A.V. (2009) Essentials of rebonding tooth fragments for the best functional and esthetic outcomes. *Pediatric Dentistry*, 31, 110–116.

Madhubala A., Tewari, N., Mathur, V.P., & Bansal, K. (2019) Comparative evaluation of fracture resistance using two rehydration protocols for fragment reattachment in uncomplicated crown fractures. *Dental Traumatology*, 35, 199–203.

Martos, J., Koller, C.D., Silveira, L.F.M., & Cesar-Neto, J.B. (2012) Crown fragment reattachment in anterior-fractured tooth: a five-year follow-up. *European Journal of General Dentistry*, 1, 112–115.

Martos, J., Pinto, K.V.A., Miguelis, T.M.F., & Xavier, C.B. (2017) Management of an uncomplicated crown fracture by re-attaching the fractured fragment-case report. *Dental Traumatology*, 33, 485–489.

Poubel, D.L.N., Almeida, J.C.F., Dias Ribeiro, A.P., Maia, G.B., Martinez, J.M.G., & Garcia, F.C.P. (2017) Effect of dehydration and rehydration intervals on fracture resistance of reattached tooth fragments using a multimode adhesive. *Dental Traumatology*, 33, 451–457.

Schatz, J.-P., Hakeberg, M., Ostine, E., & Kiliaridis, S. (2013) Prevalence of traumatic injuries to permanent dentition and its association with overjet in a Swiss child population. *Dental Traumatology*, 29, 110–114.

Sharmin, D.D. & Thomas, E. (2013) Evaluation of the effect of storage medium on fragment reattachment. *Dental Traumatology*, 27, 99–102.

17

Ectopic Eruption of Maxillary First Permanent Molars

Ari Kupietzky and Jane A. Soxman

A smooth transition from the primary to the permanent dentition is of the utmost importance in managing a pediatric dental patient. Ectopic eruption (EE) of the maxillary first permanent molar is a common occurrence in the developing mixed dentition and is many times diagnosed first by the pediatric dentist.

EE is defined as a tooth erupting with a mesioangular eruption path. EE may be suspected if one of the two maxillary first permanent molars erupts and the contralateral permanent molar fails to erupt. Additionally, if clinically the mesial marginal ridge of the first permanent molar is beneath the distal prominence of the second primary molar, EE is suspected (Figure 17.1) (AAPD, 2019–2020). The impaction results in premature resorption of the distobuccal root of the neighboring primary molar (Figures 17.2a,b). Early correction of ectopically erupting maxillary first permanent molars is an integral part of interceptive orthodontics and is crucial for the proper development of a stable occlusion. If left untreated, EE may result in various complications, including early loss of the second primary molar, space loss, and impaction of second premolars. Future corrective treatment may be complicated, lengthy, costly, and may include the distalizing and uprighting of the permanent molar by use of headgear and fixed or removable appliances, with subsequent long-term space maintenance (Figure 17.3).

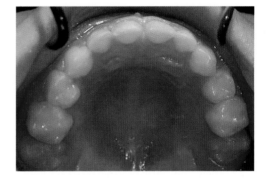

Figure 17.1 Clinical photograph showing mesial marginal ridge of the first permanent molar impacted beneath the distal prominence of the second primary molar.

Treatment of EE includes a broad spectrum of procedures, including observation with follow-up, elastomer separation, disking the distal of the adjacent second primary molar, the distal brass wire separation, fixed or removable appliance therapy, or extraction of the second primary molar and subsequent space regaining followed by space maintenance.

Treatment modalities may be divided into two categories: interproximal wedging and distal tipping. The former type of treatment has traditionally been used in cases of minimal to intermediate impaction of the first permanent molar on the distal aspect of second primary molar. When the impactions are severe, distal tipping techniques with or without second primary molar extraction have been indicated. Distal tipping techniques

Handbook of Clinical Techniques in Pediatric Dentistry, Second Edition. Edited by Jane A. Soxman.
© 2022 John Wiley & Sons, Inc. Published 2022 by John Wiley & Sons, Inc.

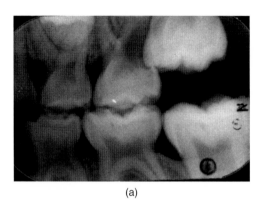
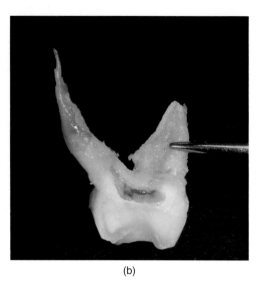

(a)   (b)

Figure 17.2 (a) Bitewing radiograph showing impacted maxillary first permanent molar, causing premature resorption of the adjacent primary molar. (b) Extracted second primary molar with distobuccal root resorption.

use fixed or removable appliances (examples include Humphrey appliance, sectioned wire with open coil spring, slingshot-type appliances, hemisection of adjacent primary tooth, and others).

This chapter presents step-by-step procedures for treatment of EE with orthodontic separators/elastomers and a brief description of more complicated treatment modalities.

Identification

EE of the maxillary first permanent molar usually presents between the ages of 5 and 7 years with bitewing or panoramic radiographic examination (AAPD, 2019–2020). The position of the unerupted first permanent molars on bitewing or panoramic radiographs should be noted and documented in the patient's chart, for example "first permanent molar in good position or not visualized" (Figure 17.4).

Observation

In many cases other than severe impaction, a conservative approach is suggested. Spontaneous self-correction occurs in 66% of cases by age 7 or 71% by age 9 (Figures 17.5 and 17.6a, b) (AAPD, 2019–2020). Progression may result in pulpal exposure of the second primary molar in 14.3% of EEs (Barberia-Leache *et al.*, 2005). The parent/guardian and child are advised to notify the dentist if there is discomfort, sinus tract, and/or mobility of the second primary molar during the observation period.

Elastomer Separators

The simplest method for correction uses a sequence of elastic separators. The technique can be used to resolve many of these impactions efficiently and effectively, with minimal patient discomfort (Cerny, 2003).

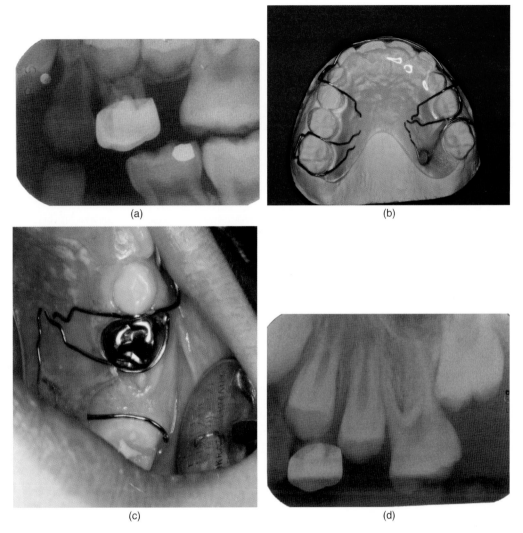

(a) (b)

(c) (d)

Figure 17.3 (a) If left untreated, EE may result in complications such as early loss of the second primary molar, space loss, and impaction of second premolars. (b) A removable appliance is used to distalize the permanent first molar and allow proper eruption of the second premolar. (c) Space has been regained allowing eruption of the blocked-out tooth. (d) The periapical radiograph demonstrates eruption of the second premolar.

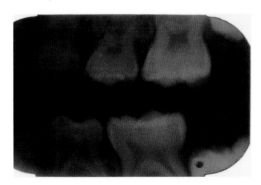

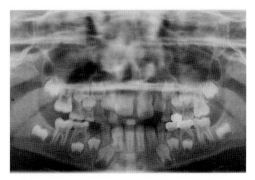

Figure 17.4 Bitewing radiograph showing unerupted maxillary left first permanent molar in a good position.

Figure 17.5 Panoramic radiograph showing impaction of maxillary right first permanent molar and spontaneous correction of ectopic maxillary left first permanent molar.

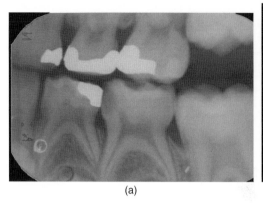 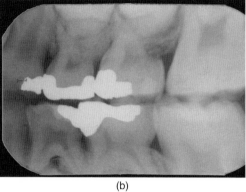

(a)   (b)

Figure 17.6 In many cases other than severe impaction, a conservative approach is suggested. (a) The unerupted maxillary first permanent molar in the bitewing radiograph was followed. (b) The molar erupted 6 months later without intervention. Source: Kupietzky (2000).

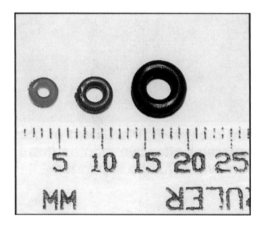

Figure 17.7 Elastomers of variable sizes: green (standard)−3 mm diameter, 0.75 mm thick; blue (standard)−4 mm diameter, 1 mm thick; black (jumbo)−6 mm diameter, 2 mm thick. Source: Reproduced with permission from Cerny (2003).

Conventional elastomeric ring separators come in two sizes: green—3 mm diameter, 0.75 mm thick; blue—4 mm diameter, 1 mm thick (Figure 17.7). These sizes are easy to fit and effective at moving teeth apart as much as 1 mm. However, in more severe impactions, a larger and thicker elastomer has been suggested (Cerny, 2003).

Separators (elastomers) may be placed using separator pliers or floss (Figure 17.8a–e). When used in sequence with the smaller orthodontic separators, "jumbo separators," 6 mm diameter × 2 mm thick, can move teeth apart as much

as 2 mm, which is often enough to free many partially impacted molars (Figure 17.9a–f). The jumbo separators should be soaked in hot water for 2–3 minutes before fitting. This makes them more pliable and less susceptible to fracture. Care should be taken not to over-stretch the separator while attempting to place it between the two teeth. Stretching the separator by no more than one-third of its diameter allows easy placement, with little distortion and deactivation. Patients should be instructed to continue routine tooth brushing, but not to floss or use toothpicks around the separators. Separators should be radiopaque for identification, since submersion into the gingiva can occur. Notation is made in the dental record when the separator is removed to monitor removal (Figure 17.10a, b).

The Brass Wire Technique

The brass wire technique is a fairly simple procedure and can be used successfully in moderately and occasionally even in severely impacted molar cases. The technique was first described by Levitas (1964) over 50 years ago.

1. A bitewing radiograph should be taken before placement of the brass wire to determine the position of the marginal ridge and interproximal contact area of the molars (Figures 17.11a and 17.12a).

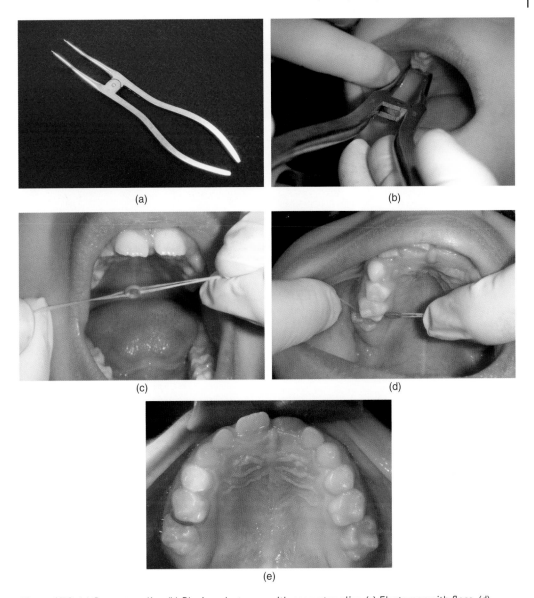

Figure 17.8 (a) Separator plier. (b) Placing elastomer with separator plier. (c) Elastomer with floss. (d) Placing elastomer with floss. (e) Deimpacted maxillary first permanent molar.

2. Local anesthesia may be required dependent on the severity of the impaction and the temperament of the patient. It may include infiltration of the buccal and palatal papillae.

3. A brass wire is placed between the contact area of the impacted first permanent molar and the adjacent primary molar with the use of a Mathieu plier or mosquito needle holder. Placement is from the palatal tissue distal to the primary molar out toward the buccal. The brass wire can be purchased as single preformed loops (0.020 or 0.025 in., Ortho Organizers, San Marcos, CA, USA) or can be prepared from a coil of wire (Malin, Brookpart, OH, USA) by flattening out one end with a Howe utility plier. The flat end facilitates insertion from palatal to buccal

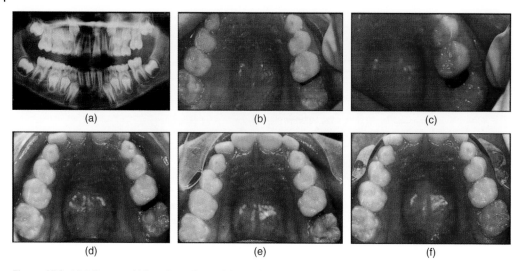

(a)   (b)   (c)

(d)   (e)   (f)

Figure 17.9 (a) A 9-year-old female patient with partially impacted upper left first molar. (b) Placement of blue separator. (c) Placement of jumbo separator 1 week later. (d) Jumbo separator 2 months later. (e) After removal of jumbo separator. (f) Six weeks after separation. Source: Reproduced with permission from Cerny (2003).

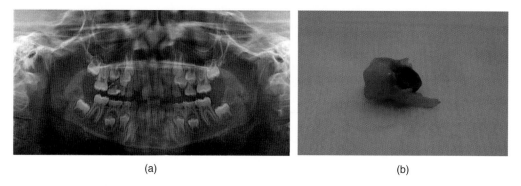

(a)   (b)

Figure 17.10 (a) Panoramic radiograph showing subgingival separator (elastomer). (b) Extracted maxillary second primary molar with attached separator (elastomer).

(Figure 17.13). Leave extra extension for twisting.

4. The other end of the wire is then bent over the marginal ridge area and twisted with the buccal end. The wire is tightened until snug. The excess wire is cut, and the twisted end is tucked into the proximal area to minimize irritation of the buccal mucosa. The clinician should standardize the direction of the twist for future tightening without unraveling (Figure 17.14).

5. The separator must encircle the area of contact. Its prolonged activation acts to separate the contacting molars. A bitewing radiograph should be taken after wire placement to confirm its correct position, especially in moderate to severe impaction cases (Figures 17.11b and 17.12b).

6. An initial attempt should be made to place a 0.028 in. wire. If unsuccessful, a thinner wire (0.020 in.) may be used, to be replaced with the thicker wire at a future visit. If unsuccessful, two other wedging techniques may be attempted. One method uses metal separators of various diameters (Hirayama & Chow, 1992; Kim & Park, 2005), the other uses a clinical aid consisting of a catheter to

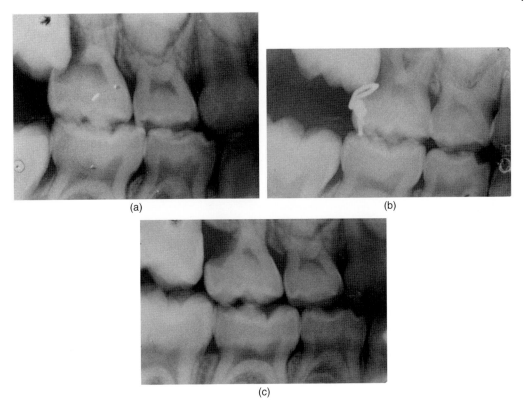

(a)   (b)

(c)

Figure 17.11 (a) Right bitewing radiograph taken at pretreatment. (b) Radiograph taken at placement of brass wire. Note thickness of 0.020 in. wire, compared to 0.028 in. wire in Figure 17.12. (c) Radiograph taken at 3 months after removal of brass wire. Source: Kupietzky (2000).

place the wire interproximally (Huang & Childers, 1995).

7. The patient should be seen at 3–4-week intervals for wire tightening. Careful supervision is important. The wire may induce infection and early loss of the primary molar. However, proper oral hygiene is adequate in most cases to prevent any inflammation or infection.

8. Tightening of the wire is tolerated by most patients, but some may complain of mild pain and discomfort. Pediatric patient management techniques should be used. Many orthodontists refer these cases to the pediatric dentist because of difficulty in managing young children through these types of procedures.

9. The wire may be removed when the permanent molar is deimpacted and will actually slip through the contact area during routine activation. A bitewing (Figures 17.11c and 17.12c) and periapical radiograph (Figure 17.12d) may be taken to assess the stability of the primary molar and its ability to act as a space maintainer. The patient should be seen 3 months later to assess the primary molar. Primary molars may function for many years, although they sustained severe root resorption and even coronal resorption without any symptoms. In the event that the second primary molar is lost prematurely due to mobility or infection, space can be maintained with a simple band-and-loop appliance. Figures 17.15 and 17.16 present treatment and post-treatment clinical views of the radiographs in Figures 17.11 and 17.12.

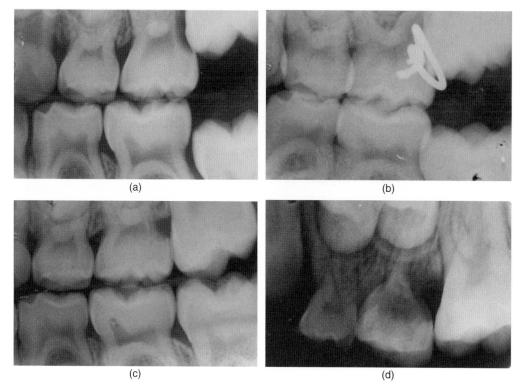

(a)

(b)

(c)

(d)

Figure 17.12 (a) Left bitewing radiograph taken at pretreatment. (b) Radiograph taken at placement of brass wire. Note thickness of 0.028 in. wire, relative to 0.020 in. wire in Figure 17.11. (c) Radiograph taken at 3 months after removal of brass wire. (d) Periapical radiograph taken 6 months after treatment. No symptoms were present. Primary second molar was stable and functioning well as a "space maintainer." Source: Kupietzky (2000).

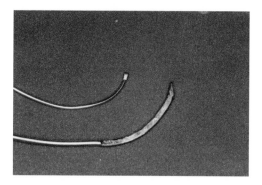

Figure 17.13 Close-up view of brass wire. The brass wire can be purchased as a single preformed loop (0.020 or 0.025 in. thickness; Ortho Organizers) or can be prepared from a coil (0.028 in., Malin) of wire by flattening out one end with a Howe utility plier. The flat end facilitates insertion from palatal to buccal. Leave extra extension for twisting. Two thicknesses are shown (0.020 and 0.028 in.). Source: Kupietzky (2000).

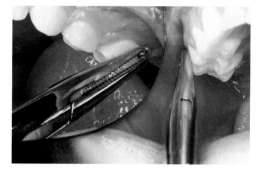

Figure 17.14 The clinician should standardize the direction of the twist of the brass wire for future tightening without unraveling.

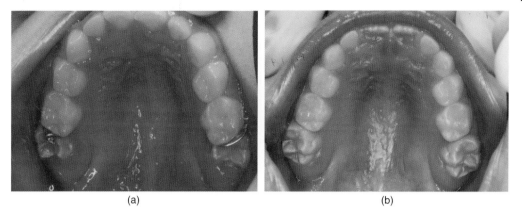

(a)   (b)

Figure 17.15 (a) Occlusal view of the 6-year-old patient shown in Figures 17.11 and 17.12, demonstrating bilateral ectopically erupting first permanent molars. Brass wire placement is shown. On the patient's right side, a 0.020 in. wire was placed (Malin). On the left side, a 0.028 in. preformed wire was used (Ortho Organizers), after attempts to place the thicker wire failed. At a later visit, the wire was replaced with the 0.028 in. wire. (b) Post-treatment occlusal view.

Figure 17.16 The brass wire is placed between the contact area of the impacted first permanent molar and the adjacent primary molar with the use of a Mathieu plier or Mosquito needle holder. Placement is from the palatal tissue distal to the primary molar, out toward the buccal. (a) Occlusal view before treatment. (b) Occlusal view after treatment.

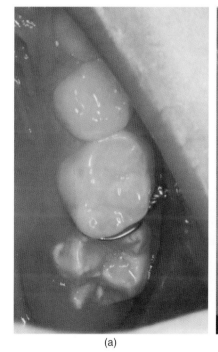 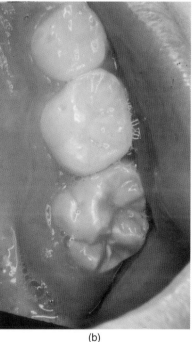

(a)   (b)

Disking of the Adjacent Maxillary Second Primary Molar

A wooden wedge is placed on the distal of the adjacent second primary molar, and a 169 L carbide bur at high speed is used to disk the distal of the second primary molar. Infiltration into the papilla with a small amount of local anesthesia may be necessary. This procedure will not result in caries or sensitivity, but may deimpact the maxillary first permanent molar (Figure 17.17a–d).

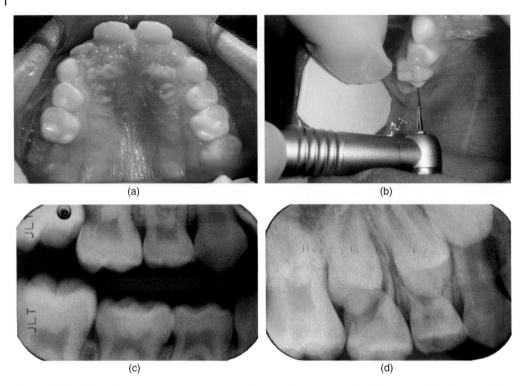

(a)

(b)

(c)

(d)

Figure 17.17 (a) Maxillary right first permanent molar ectopic eruption. (b) 169 L bur to disk the distal of the maxillary second primary molar. (c) Periapical radiograph with ectopic eruption of maxillary right first permanent molar, before disking distal of maxillary right second primary molar. (d) Correction of ectopic eruption of maxillary right first permanent molar, after disking distal of maxillary right second primary molar.

Spring Separator

A spring separator may also be used to deimpact the permanent molar (Figure 17.18a–c).

Distal Tipping Techniques

When the degree of impaction or inaccessibility of the first permanent molar prevents separation, active appliance therapy is indicated to deimpact the tooth. In extreme situations, the second primary molar may be extracted, and following eruption of the permanent molar, space regaining and distalization are mandated. followed by space maintenance until eruption of the second premolar (Figure 17.3).

Appliances may be either the fixed segmental type or a removable acrylic appliance. The former usually consists of a band cemented to the second primary molar, with an active spring soldered to the band engaging the occlusal surface of the permanent molar or bonded button attached to the tooth. The Halterman appliance (Halterman, 1982) consists of a reverse band and loop incorporating a distal spur. A chain elastic is placed from the spur to a bonded button on the ectopically erupting permanent molar (Figure 17.19).

In cases of extreme mobility of the primary second molar, the appliance may extend to the contralateral side for proper anchorage (Figure 17.20). An alternative unilateral application is a modified Halterman appliance consisting of a bonded acrylic appliance to

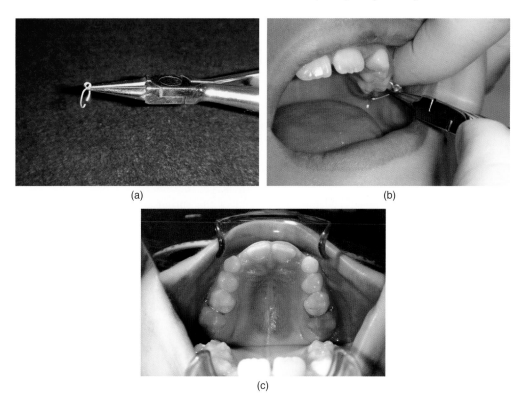

(a)

(b)

(c)

Figure 17.18 (a) Spring separator. (b) Inserting spring separator. (c) Spring separators to deimpact the right and left maxillary permanent molars.

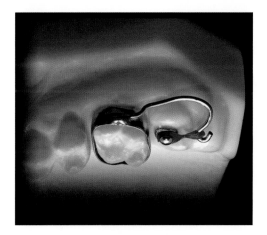

Figure 17.19 Halterman appliance.

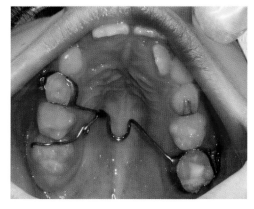

Figure 17.20 In cases of extreme mobility of the primary second molar, the appliance may extend to the contralateral side for proper anchorage.

both the first and second primary molars, affording more stability and fixation of the second primary molar (Figure 17.21).

The ectopic spring-loaded distalizer (QC Orthodontics Lab, Fuquay-Varina, NC, USA)

offers another choice for appliance use with ectopically erupting maxillary first permanent molars (Figure 17.22a, b). This appliance requires good cooperation. The extension wrapping around the distobuccal cusp must

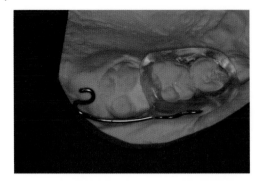

Figure 17.21 A modified Halterman appliance consisting of a bonded acrylic appliance to both the first and second primary molars affords more stability and fixation of the second primary molar. A button is bonded onto the occlusal table of the permanent molar and a chain is attached.

be secured with flowable composite before cutting the elastic chain. After the elastic chain is removed, the distalizing spring activates (Figure 17.22c–j).

Removable appliances may also be used to distalize an ectopically erupting first permanent molar (Figure 17.23a, b). The removable appliance is designed with typical retention clasps and a palatal finger spring, which reaches the occlusal table of the blocked molar. An acrylic button is attached to the distal end of the spring and contacts the occlusal surface of the molar. Other methods include bonding either a button or a composite extension to the molar to engage the activated spring.

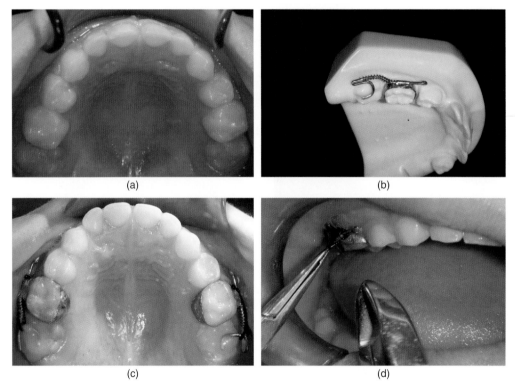

(a)

(b)

(c)

(d)

Figure 17.22 (a) Bilateral ectopic eruption of maxillary first permanent molars. (b) Ectopic spring-loaded distalizer appliance. (c) Appliance delivered and flowable composite placed to secure extension over distobuccal cusp tip. (d) Black chain elastic cut to activate spring. (e) Black chain elastic removed. (f) 3 months after delivery and activation. (g) 9 months after delivery. (h) 11 months after delivery. (i) Appliance removed 12 months after delivery. (j) 1 year after appliance removed.

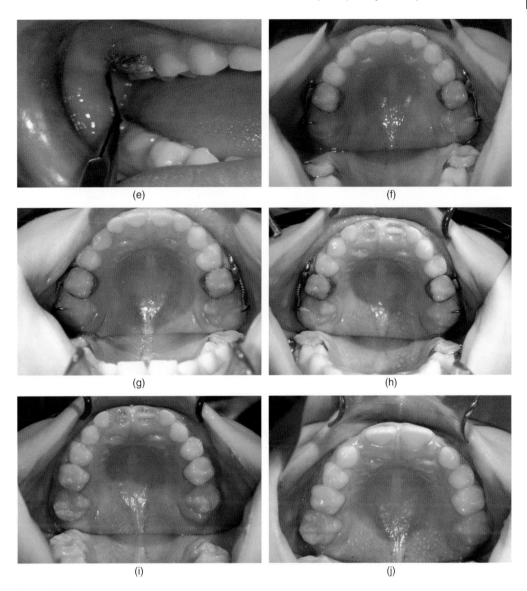

Figure 17.22 (*Continued*)

Space Control

With EE, space control is a more appropriate term than space maintenance, as unavoidable space loss will occur in almost every case due to the mesial eruption path of the maxillary first permanent molar. The maxillary second premolar will be blocked out (Figure 17.24). If the maxillary second primary molar is prematurely lost before full eruption of the maxillary

first permanent molar, the appliance of choice is the band and loop. The first primary molar is banded, and the loop extends distally to the mesial of the partially erupted first permanent molar. When the first permanent molar is adequately erupted for banding, or the first primary molar is mobile and near exfoliation, the appliance may be changed to a transpalatal for unilateral loss of a second primary molar, or a Nance appliance for bilateral loss of second

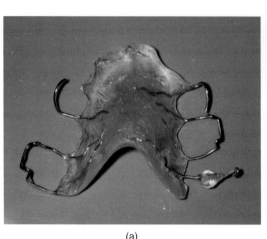
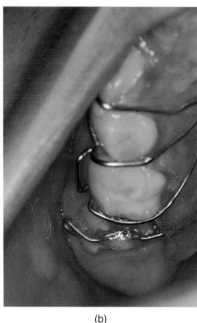

(a)   (b)

Figure 17.23 (a) The removable appliance is designed with typical retention clasps and a palatal finger spring that reaches the occlusal table of the blocked molar. (b) An acrylic button is attached to the distal end of the spring and contacts the occlusal surface of the molar.

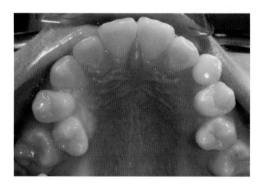

Figure 17.24 Maxillary second premolar blocked out and erupted on palate due to space loss.

primary molars. The parent/guardian should be informed of the possible requirement for a second appliance to maintain the space for the second premolar.

Summary

EE signifies a disturbance in the normal eruption of the permanent dentition, with the maxillary first permanent molars most often affected. The diagnosis of EE is typically made during radiographic examination. Clinical experience indicates that maxillary first permanent molars, with the mesial marginal ridge locked beneath the distal prominence of the second primary molar, require one of the forms of intervention discussed in this chapter for correction in order to permit normal eruption. Timely identification and intervention are mandatory. If left untreated, EE may result in various sequelae, including early loss of the second primary molar, space loss, and impaction of second premolars.

Note

Selected texts and figures have been adapted with permission from Dr. Kupietzky's previous work:

Kupietzky, A. (2000) Correction of ectopic eruptions of permanent molars utilizing the brass wire technique. *Pediatric Dentistry*, **22**, 408–412. Figures 17.6, 17.9, 17.11, and 17.12.

References

American Academy of Pediatric Dentistry. (2019–2020) *Management of the developing dentition and occlusion in pediatric dentistry. The Reference Manual of Pediatric Dentistry.* Chicago, IL: American Academy of Pediatric Dentistry; 362–386.

Barberia-Leache, E., Suarez-Clua, M.C., & Saavedra-Ontiveros, D. (2005) Ectopic eruption of the maxillary first permanent molar: characteristics and occurrence in growing children. *Angle Orthodontics*, 75, 610–615.

Cerny, R. (2003) Jumbo separators for partial molar impactions. *Journal of Clinical Orthodontics*, 37, 33–35.

Halterman, C.W. (1982) A simple technique for the treatment of ectopically erupting permanent first molars. *Journal of the American Dental Association*, 105, 1031–1033.

Hirayama, K. & Chow, M.H. (1992) Correcting ectopic first permanent molars with metal or elastic separators. *Pediatric Dentistry*, 14, 342–343.

Huang, W. & Childers, N.K. (1995) Clinical aid in placing brass wires to treat ectopically erupting permanent first molars. *Pediatric Dentistry*, 17, 122–123.

Kim, Y.H. & Park, K.T. (2005) Simple treatment of ectopic eruption with a triangular wedging spring. *Pediatric Dentistry*, 27, 143–145.

Levitas, T.C. (1964) A simple technique for correcting an ectopically erupting maxillary first permanent molar. *Journal of Dentistry for Children*, 31, 16–18.

18

Ectopic Eruption of Maxillary Permanent Canines
Jane A. Soxman

The maxillary permanent canine normally erupts at the age of 11–12 years (AAPD, 2019–2020a). Ectopic eruption of a maxillary permanent canine should be a consideration with asymmetric canine eruption, and congenital absence or microdontia of the permanent lateral incisor (Liuk *et al.*, 2013; AAPD, 2019–2020b). Figure 18.1a shows a congenitally missing maxillary right permanent lateral incisor, microdontia of a maxillary left permanent lateral incisor, and mild ectopic eruption of a maxillary left permanent canine. Figure 18.1b shows ectopic eruption of a maxillary right permanent canine with a congenitally missing maxillary right permanent lateral incisor and

microdontia of a maxillary left permanent lateral incisor. Digital palpation to determine the status of the maxillary permanent canines should be routinely performed. The canine bulge should be palpable high in the alveolar process above the primary canine by the age of 9–10 years if dental and chronologic ages are synonymous. At the age of 11–12 years, the absence of the canine bulge indicates a significantly higher possibility of palatal displacement (Chalakkal *et al.*, 2011; AAPD, 2019–2020b).

If the canine bulge is not palpated or the canine appears to be in an abnormal position with mesial inclination on palpation, radiographic examination with a panoramic or

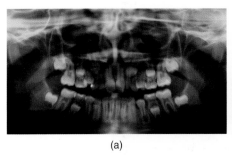
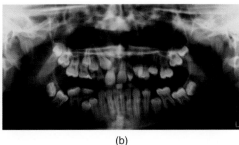

(a)   (b)

Figure 18.1 (a) Panoramic radiograph showing congenitally missing maxillary right permanent lateral incisor, microdontia of maxillary left permanent lateral incisor, and ectopic eruption of maxillary left permanent canine. (b) Panoramic radiograph showing ectopic eruption of maxillary right permanent canine with congenitally missing maxillary right permanent lateral incisor and microdontia of maxillary left permanent lateral incisor.

Handbook of Clinical Techniques in Pediatric Dentistry, Second Edition. Edited by Jane A. Soxman.
© 2022 John Wiley & Sons, Inc. Published 2022 by John Wiley & Sons, Inc.

periapical radiograph is indicated. Periapical radiographs are more specific than panoramic to show buccal-lingual position and root resorption. Cone beam computer tomography (CBCT) provides more accurate information than panoramic, occlusal, or periapical radiographs (Tsolakis *et al.*, 2018) (Figure 18.2a–c).

Abnormal inclination of the canine, mesially angled toward or superimposed over the root of the permanent lateral incisor or premolar, signals the need for immediate intervention to avoid root resorption, which can rapidly occur (Fricker *et al.*, 2008) (Figures 18.3–18.5a, b, and 18.6).

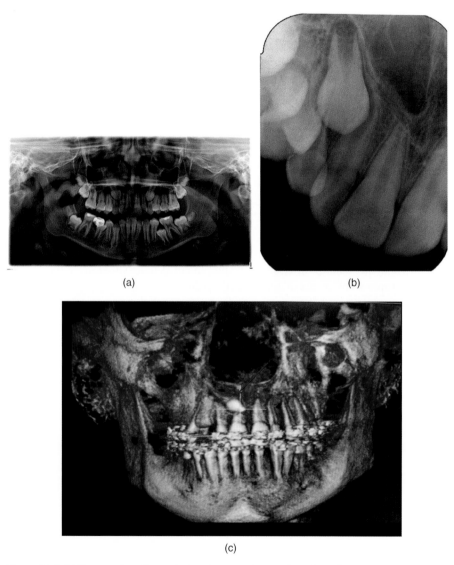

(a)

(b)

(c)

Figure 18.2 (a) Panoramic radiograph showing ectopic eruption of maxillary right permanent canine. (b) Periapical radiograph showing maxillary right permanent canine palatal to maxillary right permanent lateral incisor with no apparent root resorption. (c) Cone beam computer tomography showing ectopic eruption of maxillary right permanent canine with root resorption of maxillary right permanent central incisor.

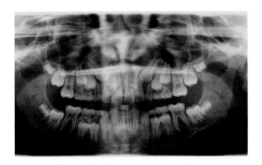

Figure 18.3 Panoramic radiograph showing bilateral ectopic position of maxillary permanent canines.

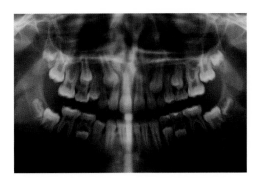

Figure 18.4 Panoramic radiograph showing abnormal inclination of the maxillary right permanent canine superimposed over the root of the maxillary right permanent lateral incisor.

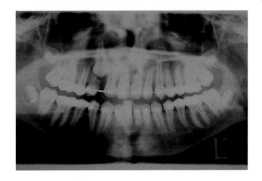

Figure 18.6 Panoramic radiograph showing root resorption of the maxillary right first premolar due to ectopic eruption of the maxillary right permanent canine.

An over-retained maxillary primary canine may indicate ectopic position of a permanent maxillary canine or a congenitally missing permanent successor (Figures 18.7a, b and 18.8a, b).

Intervention

Timely intervention will promote normal eruption, with spontaneous uprighting and distal movement of the crown for both palatally or centrally positioned permanent canines (Bonetti *et al.*, 2011). Extract the primary canines after the permanent lateral incisors

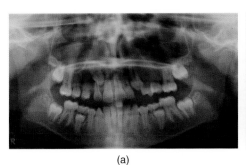

(a)

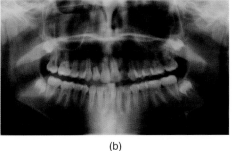

(b)

Figure 18.5 (a) Panoramic radiograph showing ectopic position of maxillary right permanent canine. (b) Panoramic radiograph showing root resorption of maxillary right permanent lateral incisor resulting from ectopic eruption of maxillary right permanent canine.

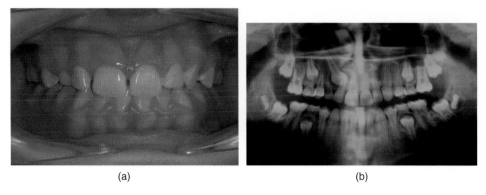

(a)   (b)

Figure 18.7 (a) Photograph showing over-retained maxillary right primary canine. (b) Panoramic radiograph showing ectopic position of maxillary right permanent canine with over-retained maxillary right primary canine.

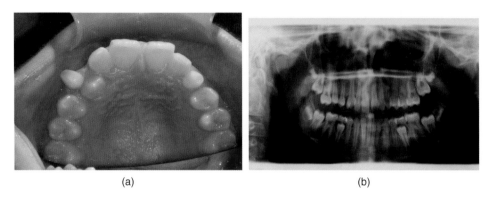

(a)   (b)

Figure 18.8 (a) Upper occlusal photograph of over-retained maxillary right primary canine causing palatal displacement of maxillary right permanent canine, and also showing retention of maxillary left primary canine. (b) Panoramic radiograph showing maxillary left primary canine with congenitally missing maxillary left permanent successor.

are fully erupted. With the normal sequence of eruption, the maxillary first premolars erupt before the permanent canines. Maxillary premolars typically erupt when one-half to three-fourths of the root has formed (Terlaji & Donly, 2001). With a minimum of one-half root formation of the first premolar, the first primary molar is also extracted. Extraction of the first primary molar before one-half root formation of the premolar may delay eruption of the premolar (Shapira *et al.*, 1998). Adding extraction of the maxillary first primary molar significantly improves the eruption path for the permanent canine (Figure 18.9a, b). Improvement of intraosseous position and uneventful eruption occurred in 97.3% of

cases when extraction of the maxillary first primary molar was combined with extraction of the maxillary primary canine (Bonetti *et al.*, 2011).

Unilateral or bilateral extraction is a case-by-case decision determined by the amount of arch length deficiency. If the ectopic canine is unilateral, with no arch length deficiency, extraction is limited to the primary canine and first primary molar on the affected side. In the presence of moderate to significant arch length deficiency, bilateral extractions are indicated (Figure 18.10) (personal communication with Dr. Vincent Kokich).

Baccetti *et al.* (2008) found that after removal of the primary canines, normal eruption of a

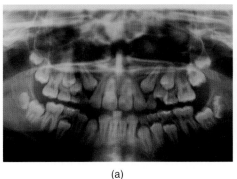
(a)

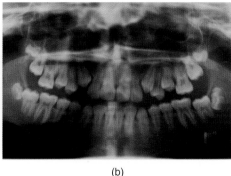
(b)

Figure 18.9 (a) Panoramic radiograph showing bilateral ectopic position of the maxillary permanent canines. (b) Panoramic radiograph showing uprighting of maxillary right and left permanent canines 1 year after extraction of maxillary right and left primary canines and maxillary right first primary molar.

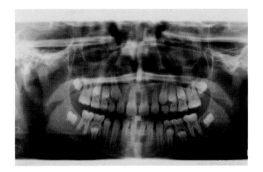

Figure 18.10 Panoramic radiograph showing indication for unilateral extraction of maxillary right primary canine and maxillary right first primary molar, instead of bilateral extraction of primary canines and primary first molars due to no arch length deficiency.

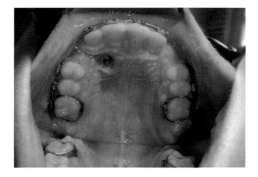

Figure 18.11 Occlusal photograph showing exposure of palatally impacted maxillary permanent canine.

palatally displaced canine was increased from 35% to 65%. Adding cervical pull headgear increased the chance for intraosseous uprighting and normal eruption to 87.5%. Another study found that rapid palatal expansion, after extraction of primary canines in the late mixed dentition, combined with a transpalatal arch, promoted normal eruption of palatally displaced canines (Sigler *et al.*, 2011).

In the case of microdontia or a missing permanent lateral incisor, the absence of guidance for a normal eruption path often results in palatal impaction (Soxman, 2019). Although timely extraction of the primary canine and first primary molar is performed, exposure and orthodontic force may still be required to bring a horizontally impacted maxillary permanent canine into its proper position in the maxillary arch (Figure 18.11).

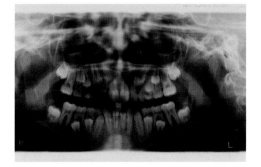

Figure 18.12 Panoramic radiograph showing distally displaced mandibular premolars with ectopic position of maxillary permanent canines.

Distally displaced mandibular premolars are a valuable developmental risk indicator associated with palatally displaced maxillary canines. Observation of bitewing and periapical radiographs may provide an opportunity for earlier diagnosis (Baccetti *et al.*, 2010) (Figure 18.12). Another risk factor is a unilateral or bilateral cross-bite in individuals with a narrow maxilla due to a decrease in space available (Arboleda-Ariza *et al.*, 2018).

References

American Academy of Pediatric Dentistry. (2019–2020a) Resources: dental growth and development. *The Reference Manual of Pediatric Dentistry*, Chicago, IL: American Academy of Pediatric Dentistry; 505.

American Academy of Pediatric Dentistry. (2019–2020b) Management of the developing dentition and occlusion. *The Reference Manual of Pediatric Dentistry*. Chicago, IL: American Academy of Pediatric Dentistry; 362–378.

Arboleda-Ariza, N., Schilling, J., Arriola-Guillen, L.E., Ruíz-Mora, G.A., Rodríguez-Cárdenas, Y.A., & Aliaga-Del Castillo, A. (2018) Maxillary transverse dimensions in subjects with and without impacted canines: a comparative cone-beam computed tomography study. *American Journal of Orthodontics and Dentofacial Orthopedics*, 154, 495–503.

Baccetti, T., Leonardi, M., & Armi, P. (2008) A randomized clinical study of two interceptive approaches to palatally displaced canines. *European Journal of Orthodontics*, 30, 381–385.

Baccetti, T., Leonardi, M., & Gliuntini, V. (2010) Distally displaced premolars: a dental anomaly associated with palatally displaced canines. *American Journal of Orthodontics and Dentofacial Orthopedics*, 138, 318–322.

Bonetti, G.A., Zanarini, M., Incerti Parenti, S., Marini, I., & Gatto, M.R. (2011) Preventive treatment of ectopically erupting maxillary canines by extraction of deciduous canines and first molars: a randomized clinical trial. *American Journal of Orthodontics and Dentofacial Orthopedics*, 139, 316–323.

Chalakkal, P., Thomas, A.M., & Chopra, S. (2011) Displacement, location, and angulation of unerupted permanent maxillary canines and absence of canine bulge in children.

American Journal of Orthodontics and Dentofacial Orthopedics, 139, 345–350.

Fricker, J., Kharbanda, O.P., & Dando, J. (2008) Orthodontic diagnosis and treatment in the mixed dentition. In: Cameron, A.C. & Widmer, R.P. (eds.), *Handbook of Pediatric Dentistry*, 3rd edn. London: Mosby; 341–377.

Liuk, I.W., Olive, R.J., Griffin, M., Monsour, P. (213) Maxillary lateral incisor morphology and palatally displaed canines: a case-controlled cone-beam volumetric tomography study. *American Journal of Orthodontics and Dentofacial Orthopedics*, 143, 522–526.

Shapira, Y., Kuftinec, M.M., & Stom, D. (1998) Early diagnosis and interception of potential maxillary canine impaction. *Journal of the American Dental Association*, 129, 1450–1454.

Sigler, L.M., Baccetti, T., & McNamara, J.A., Jr. (2011) Effect of rapid maxillary expansion and transpalatal arch treatment associated with deciduous canine extraction on the eruption of palatally displaced canines: a 2-center prospective study. *American Journal of Orthodontics and Dentofacial Orthopedics*, 139, e235–e244.

Soxman, J.A. (2019) Anomalies of tooth eruption. In: Soxman, J.A., Wunsch, P.B., & Haberland, C.M. *Anomalies of the Developing Dentition*. Cham: Springer *Nature*; 45–73.

Terlaji, R.D. & Donly, K.J. (2001) Treatment planning for space maintenance in the primary and mixed dentition. *Journal of Dentistry for Children*, 68, 109–114.

Tsolakis, A.I., Kalavritinos M., Bitsanis, E., Sanoudos, M., Benetou, V., *et al.* (2018) Reliability of different radiographic methods for the localization of displaced maxillary canines. *Ameican Journal of Orthodontics and Dentofacial Orthopedics,* 153, 308–314.

19

Infraocclusion of Mandibular Primary Molars

Jane A. Soxman

When the occlusal surface of a primary molar is 1 mm or more below the occlusal plane of the adjacent teeth, the primary molar is deemed to be submerged or infraoccluded (Hvaring *et al.*, 2014). Submerging is usually the first clinical indication of an ankylosed primary molar (Figures 19.1 and 19.2). With normal development, adjacent teeth continue to erupt, and vertical bone height of the alveolar bone continues to increase, creating an impression of submerging the affected primary molar. Ankylosis results from a fusion between the root's cementum and/or dentin with the surrounding alveolar bone during the course of eruption, resulting in cessation of eruption of the primary molar and proximal alveolar bone growth. Interruption in the integrity of the periodontal ligament (PDL) impedes eruptive forces in the ankylosed tooth. This eruptive disturbance may occur prior to emergence or after the primary molar is in occlusion. Incidence may occur with a familial pattern but etiology is not known. An association is sometimes found with congenitally missing permanent successor (Studen-Pavloich & Viera, 2018). Other theories causing infraocclusion include ankylosis, trauma, and infection (Aristidis & Boutiou, 2016).

Since only a small area of the root is affected, detection with a radiograph may be difficult (Tieu *et al.*, 2013). A conventional radiograph may or may not show loss of the PDL (AAPD, 2019–2020). Cone beam tomography provides greater detail (Aristidis & Boutiou, 2016). An increase in the occurrence of dental anomalies associated with infraocclusion has been reported. One study reported an increased incidence of distal angulation of the mandibular second premolar, microdontia of maxillary permanent lateral incisors, palatally displaced canines, and tooth agenesis (Shalish *et al.*, 2010). Other consequences of infraocclusion in the developing dentition include tilting of adjacent teeth, supraeruption of opposing teeth in the maxillary arch, ectopic eruption, or impaction of the permanent successor (Aristidis & Boutiou, 2016). The prevalence of infraocclusion in mandibular primary molars is 10-fold higher than in the maxilla. The presence or absence of a permanent successor is a primary factor influencing the treatment plan.

Submerged with Permanent Successor

In most cases, exfoliation of the infraoccluded primary molar occurs at the appropriate time without intervention. If a submerged primary molar is maintaining arch length, is preventing mesial shift of the first permanent molar, or is not impeding eruption of the permanent successor, the tooth may be maintained until normal exfoliation or until the contralateral primary molar exfoliates (Fricker *et al.*, 2008). If the contralateral primary molar has exfoliated, its permanent successor has erupted,

Handbook of Clinical Techniques in Pediatric Dentistry, Second Edition. Edited by Jane A. Soxman.
© 2022 John Wiley & Sons, Inc. Published 2022 by John Wiley & Sons, Inc.

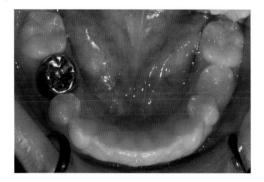

Figure 19.1 Submerging mandibular second primary molar occlusal view.

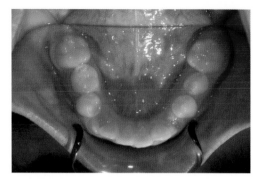

Figure 19.3 Submerged mandibular right second primary molar with contralateral second premolar erupted.

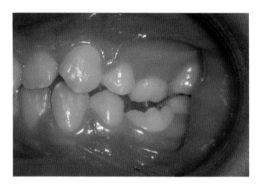

Figure 19.2 Submerging mandibular second primary molar buccal view.

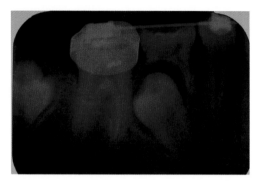

Figure 19.4 Periapical radiograph showing ectopic eruption of permanent successor.

and the infraoccluded primary molar is not mobile, extraction of the infraoccluded primary molar is indicated (Figure 19.3). A periapical radiograph may be obtained to determine the root length of the primary molar and to confirm the presence or position of the succedaneous premolar. If the premolar is erupting with a mesial or distal path of eruption, the mesial or distal root of the mandibular primary molar may not resorb, causing infraocclusion and over-retention of the mandibular primary molar (Figures 19.4 and 19.5). Crown build-up to preserve space, preventing tipping of adjacent teeth and supraeruption of the tooth in the opposite arch, may be performed (Dias *et al.*, 2012). With continued retention after loss of the contralateral primary molar, extraction of the retained primary molar is indicated. Distal eruption of the succeeding premolar is

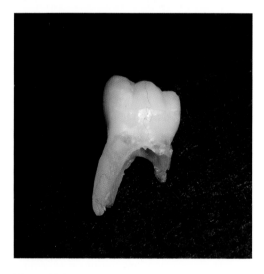

Figure 19.5 Extracted infraoccluded mandibular second primary molar with lack of distal root resorption.

a complication that also occurs and warrants consideration of timely extraction and appropriate space management (Tieu *et al.*, 2013). Root development of the permanent successor may be delayed, with delayed root resorption of an ankylosed primary molar. If the decision is made not to extract the ankylosed primary molar, both root formation and eruption of the permanent successor, along with root resorption of the ankylosed primary molar, should be periodically evaluated (Nazif *et al.*, 1986).

Late extraction of primary molars with severe infraocclusion may result in risk to alveolar bone development. To protect vertical alveolar bone growth between mandibular first permanent molars and second premolars, earlier extraction is indicated in the presence of a marked marginal ridge discrepancy, resulting in tipping of adjacent teeth, space loss, and ectopic position of the premolar (Dias *et al.*, 2012). Vertical or oblique bone loss, apparent on radiographic examination, signals extraction of the ankylosed primary molar to maintain marginal alveolar bone height (Figure 19.6). After early extraction, a vertical bony defect may be present, but continued eruption of the adjacent teeth will promote growth of the bone and tissue to their normal levels, eliminating the alveolar defect (Kokich & Kokich, 2006).

Sectioning ankylosed primary molars for extraction maintains alveolar bone and prevents root fracture (see the procedure for extracting an ankylosed primary molar in Chapter 13).

Submerged with Congenitally Missing Permanent Successor

In the absence of ankylosis, primary molars without permanent successors may function for many years before exfoliation, preserving alveolar bone height and width (Sletten *et al.*, 2003; Sabri, 2004). If a periapical radiograph shows flat bone levels between the submerged primary molar and adjacent teeth, the

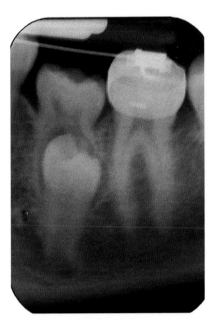

Figure 19.6 Periapical radiograph showing vertical bone loss of infraoccluded mandibular left second primary molar.

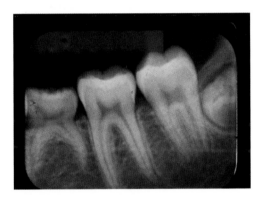

Figure 19.7 Periapical radiograph showing submerged mandibular second primary molar with level interproximal bone and congenitally missing successor.

tooth may be maintained, preserving alveolar bone until facial growth is complete, and an implant can be placed (Kokich & Kokich, 2006) (Figure 19.7). In this case, the mesial and distal surfaces of the mandibular primary molar can be disked to achieve premolar width. The mesiodistal width at the cementoenamel junction measured on a bitewing or periapical

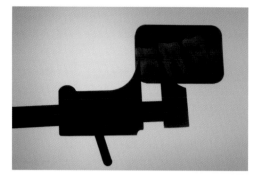

Figure 19.8 Measuring cementoenamel junction on periapical radiograph with Boley gauge.

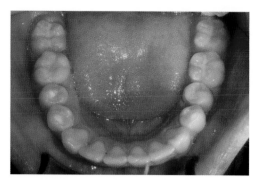

Figure 19.10 Reshaped mandibular second primary molar to premolar morphology.

radiograph provides a good guideline for the amount of reduction, as does comparison to the contralateral side (Figure 19.8). The average width of the mandibular second premolar is 7.5 mm (Kokich & Kokich, 2006); 7 mm has also been recommended as the width to attain (Sabri, 2004). This size can be marked with a pencil or marking pen on the occlusal of the primary molar to provide a guide for reduction. After administration of local anesthesia and rubber dam placement, a carbide fissure or diamond bur may be used to remove interproximal enamel, avoiding pulpal exposure. The bur is maintained in a vertical position (Figure 19.9). A layer of composite may be added on the mesial and distal surfaces to prevent caries. The occlusal surface is built up with composite to achieve a level occlusal plane, preventing supereruption of the tooth in

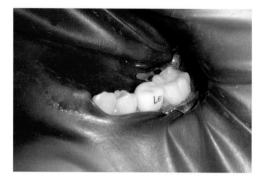

Figure 19.11 Zirconia crown on mandibular second primary molar. Note the "prime" notation for a more narrow mesial–distal size crown. Size removed with a spoon or rubber point after cementation.

the upper arch (Figure 19.10). Alternatively, a stainless-steel, preveneered, or zirconia crown may be placed (Figure 19.11).

Because the roots of the primary molar diverge beyond the width of the crown, there may be unwarranted concern that the space cannot be closed adequately with interproximal reduction. The socket wall of the adjacent permanent teeth moves closer, and is eventually in contact with the roots of the primary molar, causing root resorption. Bone replaces the roots, creating an ideal site for a future implant (Kokich & Kokich, 2006).

With vertical bone loss, extraction is indicated (Figure 19.12). An orthodontic consultation will assist in determining whether to maintain or close the space after extraction. If the decision is to maintain the space for a

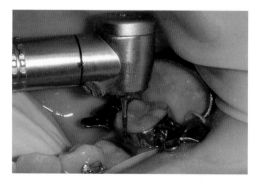

Figure 19.9 Interproximal reduction on distal of second primary molar.

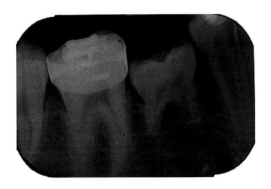

Figure 19.12 Periapical radiograph of infraoccluded mandibular second primary molar with congenitally missing permanent successor.

future restoration, the orthodontic goals will include establishing the appropriate amount of space for an implant and the preservation of the alveolar ridge.

Delaying extraction of an ankylosed primary molar, until after orthodontic treatment, will often result in a vertical defect in the alveolar bone, especially if there has been significant vertical development of the surrounding alveolar ridge. Bone grafting most likely will be necessary, increasing treatment costs and difficulty placing an implant (Sabri, 2004).

The timing for extraction in a growing child is critical. If early extraction is performed due to observed early submerging, the alveolar ridge usually moves occlusally, with eruption of adjacent teeth as the periosteum is stretched over the extraction site. Vertical crestal bony defects are prevented. Early extraction of the ankylosed mandibular second primary molar is preferred over late (Sabri, 2004).

If substantial bone resorption with significant buccolingual narrowing of the alveolar ridge and loss of vertical height occur after extraction, the first premolar may be orthodontically moved into the extraction site. This movement will provide a suitable ridge for a single-tooth implant for the first premolar after facial growth is complete. An osseointegrated implant is biologically conservative and the first choice for a congenitally missing mandibular premolar. An implant can be placed after vertical facial growth is complete, confirmed by serial cephalometric superimpositions. On an average, girls' facial growth may occur until the age of 17 years and boys' until the age of 21 years (Kokich & Kokich, 2006).

With early extraction, the width of the alveolar ridge may be reduced by 30% over 7 years. Although the ridges may still be wide enough for an implant, the implant must be placed toward the lingual, because the ridge resorbs more on the facial side. The consequence is that the occlusion on the buccal and lingual cusps of the implant's crown must be altered to avoid fracture of the abutment or the implant crown (Kokich & Kokich, 2006).

Appropriate management of infraoccluded mandibular primary molars is mandatory to preserve the alveolar bone and for future orthodontic and possible prosthetic considerations. Interdisciplinary collaboration is mandatory. Orthodontists should be given the opportunity to prepare and maintain alveolar bone throughout the mixed dentition. Inappropriate management will negatively impact orthodontic treatment, creating significant challenges, if the advantages and disadvantages of the approaches are not understood (Tieu *et al.*, 2013). Appropriate and timely management of infraoccluded primary molars will reduce treatment costs and prevent negative consequences that could last a lifetime.

References

American Academy of Pediatric Dentistry. (2019–2020) Management of the developing dentition and occlusion in pediatric dentistry. *The Reference Manual of Pediatric Dentistry.* Chicago, IL: American Academy of Pediatric Dentistry; 362–378.

Aristidis, A. & Boutiou, E. (2016) Etiology, diagnosis, consequences and treatment of infraoccluded primary molars. *Open Dental Journal*, 10, 714–719.

Dias, C., Closs, L.Q., Fontanella, V., & Borba de Araujo, F. (2012) Vertical alveolar growth in subjects with infraoccluded mandibular deciduous molars. *American Journal of Orthodontics and Dentofacial Orthopedics*, 141, 81–86.

Fricker, J., Kharbanda, O.P., & Dando, J. (2008) Orthodontic diagnosis and treatment in the mixed dentition. In: Cameron, A.C. & Widmer, R.P. (eds.), *Handbook of Pediatric Dentistry*, 3rd edn. London: Mosby; 341–377.

Hvaring, C.L., Ogaard, B., Stenvik, A., & Birkeland, K. (2014) The prognosis of retained primary molars without successors: infraocclusion, root resorption and restorations in 111 patients. *European Journal of Orthodontics*, 36, 26–30.

Kokich, V.G. & Kokich, V.O. (2006) Congenitally missing mandibular second premolars: clinical options. *American Journal of Orthodontics and Dentofacial Orthopedics*, 130, 437–444.

Nazif, M., Zullo, T., & Paulette, S. (1986) The effects of primary molar ankylosis on root resorption and the development of permanent successors. *Journal of Dentistry for Children*, 53, 115–118.

Sabri, R. (2004) Management of congenitally missing second premolars with orthodontics and single-tooth implants. *American Journal of Orthodontics and Dentofacial Orthopedics*, 125, 634–642.

Shalish, M., Peck, S., Wasserstein, A., & Peck, L. (2010) Increased occurrence of dental anomalies associated with infraocclusion of deciduous molars. *Angle Orthodontist*, 80, 440–445.

Sletten, D.W., Smith, B.M., Southard, K.A., Casko, J.S., & Southard, T.E. (2003) Retained deciduous mandibular molars in adults: a radiographic study of long-term changes. *American Journal of Orthodontics and Dentofacial Orthopedics*, 124, 625–630.

Studen-Pavloich, D. & Viera, A.M. (2018) Dental development, morphology, eruption and related pathologies. In: Nowak, A.J. & Casamassimo P.S. (eds.), *The Handbook of Pediatric Dentistry,* 5th edn. Chicago, IL: American Academy of Pediatric Dentistry; 16-44.

Tieu, L.D., Walker, S.L., Major, M.P., & Flores-Mir, C. (2013) Management of ankylosed primary molars with premolar successors. *Journal of the American Dental Association*, 144, 602–611.

20

Space Maintenance

Jane A. Soxman

Space maintenance may be necessary after premature tooth loss in the primary and mixed dentitions to preserve arch length, width, and perimeter (AAPD, 2019–2020a). Space loss is considered to be one of the major contributors to malocclusion in the permanent dentition, along with ectopic eruption or impaction of premolars (Simon *et al.*, 2012; Dean, 2012). Some space loss, with a decrease in arch length occurring in the first 6 months after premature tooth loss, is to be expected during the time of active eruption of the permanent dentition (Bell *et al.*, 2011). For cases in which space loss has already occurred, such as with ectopic eruption of maxillary first permanent molars or space loss due to interproximal caries before extraction, appliances are used for space control. Preservation of the tooth with restoration or delaying extraction should be considered, understanding that the natural tooth is the best space maintainer. If orthodontic treatment is to begin within 6 months of primary molar loss or the permanent successor is near eruption, a space maintainer may not be necessary.

Criteria for space maintainers are (Alexander *et al.*, 2015):

- Dental age when the tooth was lost.
- The tooth that was lost.
- Tooth loss from maxilla or mandible.
- Presence or absence of the permanent successor.
- Occurrence of space loss prior to loss of tooth.
- Arch length requirements for the permanent successors.
- Cooperation and oral health status of child.

Sequence of Eruption

Sequence of eruption, which may vary, should be considered when treatment planning for a space maintainer in the early and late mixed dentition. In the mandible, the first permanent molars erupt first, followed by the central incisors, lateral incisors, canines, first premolars, and second premolars. In the maxilla, the first permanent molars are followed by the central incisors, lateral incisors, first premolars, second premolars, and, last, the canines. This sequence of eruption in the maxilla will be a consideration when managing ectopic eruption of the maxillary permanent canines (AAPD, 2019–2020b).

Dental Age

Dental age and chronologic age may differ. Typically, the permanent first molar erupts at the age of 5.5–7 years, and mandibular incisors erupt at the age of 6–7 years, but if eruption

Handbook of Clinical Techniques in Pediatric Dentistry, Second Edition. Edited by Jane A. Soxman.
© 2022 John Wiley & Sons, Inc. Published 2022 by John Wiley & Sons, Inc.

does not occur until the age of 8 or 9 years, the child is dentally delayed. This delay typically follows throughout the eruption of the permanent dentition. Conversely, if the permanent dentition erupts earlier than usual, the child is dentally ahead (AAPD, 2019–2020b).

Alveolar Bone Covering Permanent Successor

The amount of alveolar bone covering the permanent successor should also be considered. About 6 months is necessary for the permanent successor to move through 1 mm of bone, which can be determined with a bitewing or periapical radiograph (Simon *et al.*, 2012).

Root Development of Permanent Successor

Root length of the permanent successor should be evaluated. Premolars typically erupt when one-half to three-fourths of the root has formed (Terlaji & Donly, 2001). If the primary molar is extracted due to an abscess, the permanent successor may erupt more rapidly than expected with less root formation.

Time Elapsed Since Loss of Primary Tooth

Space maintainers should be inserted within a few weeks after an extraction. Space loss usually occurs within 6 months after premature loss of a primary molar (Simon *et al.*, 2012). Space loss typically occurs more rapidly in the maxilla than in the mandible. Inform parents/guardians that if too much time elapses before insertion, space closure may occur and the space maintainer will no longer fit. Another impression and laboratory fee for fabrication of a revised space maintainer will be necessary. If possible, obtain a photograph

or radiograph of the site to document space loss before inserting the appliance.

Space Maintenance Appliances

Fixed appliances are preferable to removable, avoiding loss, breakage, choking, and noncompliance with wear. The band and loop or crown and loop are used for premature loss of a maxillary or mandibular first primary molar. For premature loss of a second primary molar, the Nance or transpalatal arch appliances are used in the maxillary arch and the lower lingual holding arch (passive lingual arch) is used in the mandible. Actual examples of appliances can be used for a more detailed explanation, along with a mixed-dentition typodont (Kilgore International, Coldwater, MI, USA) (Figure 20.1).

Problems with Space Maintainers

Space maintainers require follow-up. Parents/guardians should be informed of the need to immediately notify the practice if the space maintainer becomes loose, is dislodged from the tooth, is broken, or is interfering with the eruption of a permanent tooth (Figure 20.2). If the primary molar banded for the appliance exfoliates, a second appliance may be indicated

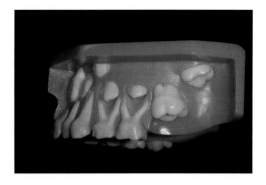

Figure 20.1 Mixed-dentition typodont (Kilgore International).

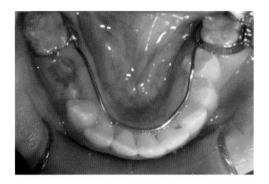

Figure 20.2 Lingual arch wire interfering with eruption of mandibular second premolar.

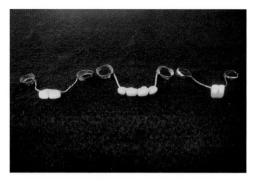

Figure 20.3 Maxillary and mandibular pedo partials for premature loss of primary incisors.

to maintain space for a second premolar. Fixed appliances may increase the incidence of caries on the banded molar or adjacent teeth in children with high caries risk (Fricker *et al.*, 2008). Poor oral hygiene can result in decalcification at the cervical margin of the band. Cementing bands with glass ionomer cement may reduce the risk of decalcification and caries. Removing the appliance to perform prophylaxis may be advisable every 6 months. A portion of the appliance may impinge on the gingival tissues after a period. Any complaint of discomfort by the child should be reported to the practice. Documentation in the patient's chart of provision of this information to parents is advisable. Mean survival times for space maintainers are reported as between 26 and 27 months. The main reasons for failure were cement loss, split bands, eruption interference, bent wire, and solder breakage (Fathian *et al.*, 2007). A lingual arch wire with a long arm has a significantly higher chance of solder breakage. Some insurance companies provide a code to recement an appliance.

Primary Incisors

After eruption of the primary canines, premature loss of one or more primary incisors due to trauma or caries results in negligible space loss (Fricker *et al.*, 2008). Space maintenance is necessary only for aesthetic concerns or parental

desire (Simon *et al.*, 2012; Kupietzky, 2001). If the primary canines have erupted and are in occlusion, space loss is unlikely (Dean & Law, 2018).

If a digit-sucking habit is of enough intensity, the space for the erupting permanent incisor may be reduced (AAPD, 2019–2020a). With a significant overjet due to a parafunctional habit, fabrication of a partial denture (pedo partial) should be delayed until cessation of the habit. A fixed partial denture can be fabricated for both the maxilla and the mandible with one or more denture teeth (Figure 20.3). If primary molar bands are not available when the impression is obtained or if the child cannot cooperate for banding, banding can be performed on the plaster model by the laboratory fabricating the appliance.

First Primary Molar

If the maxillary or mandibular first permanent molars are fully erupted and in good occlusion, and if the permanent incisors are erupted, space maintenance may not be necessary (Dean & Law, 2018). In addition, if the child is younger than 4 years, and a periapical radiograph shows the first permanent molar to be a few millimeters below the alveolar bone or with less than one-half root formation, placement of a space maintainer may be delayed until closer to the anticipated time of eruption of the first permanent molar. Alexander *et al.* (2015) found an association between the first permanent molar occlusion and facial form. During a nine-month observation period, space loss occurred in both the maxilla and the mandible in patients with a Class I or end-on molar occlusion and a leptoprosopic (long and narrow) facial form. In the same observation period, patients with mesoprosopic/euryprosopic (normal/short or broad) facial forms and Class I occlusion, space loss occurred only in the mandible (Alexander *et al.*, 2015).

With loss of the first primary molar, before the eruption of the first permanent molar or when the first permanent molar is erupting, a fixed band and loop or crown and loop in the maxilla or mandible or a lingual arch wire in the mandible is necessary to avoid mesial drift of the second primary molar into the extraction site (Tunison *et al.*, 2008; Dean & Law, 2018) (Figure 20.4a, b). For premature loss of a first primary molar in the maxilla or the mandible, the second primary molar is banded, and the loop extends mesially to the distal of the primary canine (Figures 20.5 and 20.6).

Although a first permanent molar may be fully erupted in the maxilla, space loss has been shown to occur primarily as a result of distal drift of the primary canine into the extraction site and palatal movement of the maxillary incisors (Figure 20.7) (Lin *et al.*, 2007). This

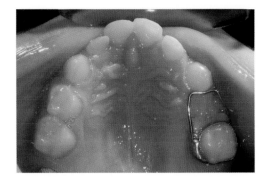

Figure 20.5 Band and loop for premature loss of maxillary first primary molar with unerupted first permanent molar.

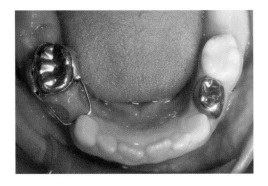

Figure 20.6 Band and loop for premature loss of mandibular first primary molar with partially erupted first permanent molar.

same distal movement of the primary canine may occur in the mandible (Tunison *et al.*, 2008).

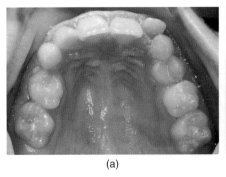
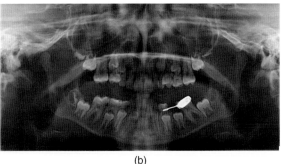

(a)   (b)

Figure 20.4 (a) Occlusal photograph showing space loss blocking out the maxillary right first premolar. (b) Panoramic radiograph showing maxillary right first premolar blocked out.

Figure 20.7 Distal drift of maxillary right primary canine into first primary molar extraction site.

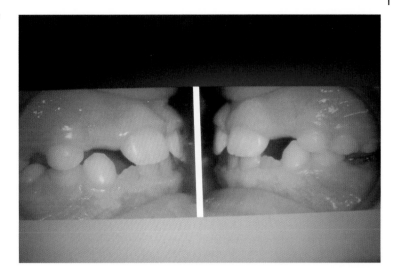

Second Primary Molar

Premature loss of a second primary molar always requires a space maintainer due to movement of the first permanent molar in both arches. In the maxilla, the first permanent molars bodily move mesially and rotate around the palatal root. Mesial and lingual tipping of the crown occurs in the mandible (Dean & Law, 2018). If the first permanent molar is fully erupted, it is banded and the appliance is fabricated with a loop extending to the distal of the first primary molar, or the first primary molar is banded with the loop extending distally to mesial of the first permanent molar (Figures 20.8 and 20.9). If the crown of the first permanent molar is not sufficiently erupted for banding, the first primary molar is instead banded, and the loop extends distally to the mesial of the partially erupted first permanent molar (Figure 20.10). When the crown of the first permanent molar is sufficiently erupted for banding, or when the first primary molar is near exfoliation, a Nance or transpalatal arch appliance replaces the band and loop in the maxillary arch. In the mandibular arch, a passive lingual arch appliance is recommended after eruption of the mandibular incisors for premature loss of a second primary molar (Figure 20.11).

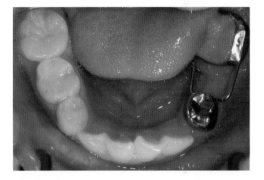

Figure 20.8 Band and loop with first permanent molar banded and loop extending mesially to distal of the first primary molar.

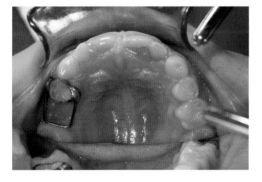

Figure 20.9 Band and loop with first primary molar banded and loop extending distally to mesial of the first permanent molar.

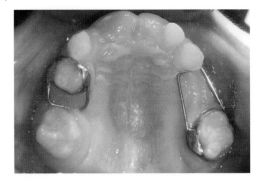

Figure 20.10 Band and loop with first primary molar banded and loop extending distally to the mesial of the partially erupted first permanent molar. This appliance is often necessary as an interim appliance with premature loss of the second primary molar due to ectopic eruption of the maxillary first permanent molar. Note that space loss has occurred due to ectopic eruption along with rotation of the first permanent molar on the long axis. A Nance appliance will be fabricated for this patient when the right and left maxillary first permanent molars are erupted adequately to band.

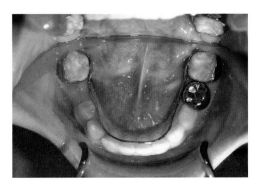

Figure 20.11 Passive lingual arch appliance for premature loss of mandibular second primary molar.

A distal shoe appliance is the appliance of choice in both the maxilla and mandible with an unerupted first permanent molar. Parents/guardians should be informed at the outset that a second appliance may be required if the second premolar is unerupted and the first primary molar is mobile or exfoliated, and that dental insurance may not cover the second appliance.

Band and Loop

The band and loop is most often used for unilateral space loss, but may be used bilaterally in the mandible before eruption of the mandibular permanent incisors. The primary or permanent molar is banded. A 0.036 in. round wire is used to make a loop that extends to the abutment tooth. The loop should be wide enough to permit eruption of the premolar, should that occur before removal of the appliance (Figures 20.12 and 20.13).

Transpalatal Arch/Palatal Arch Bar

The maxillary first permanent molars are banded and a 0.036 or 0.040 in. round wire is contoured to the posterior hard palate

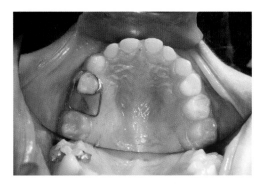

Figure 20.12 Band and loop with wide loop.

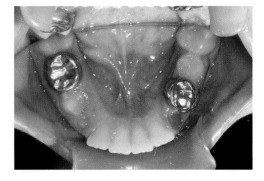

Figure 20.13 Mandibular second premolar erupting inside the loop of the band and loop.

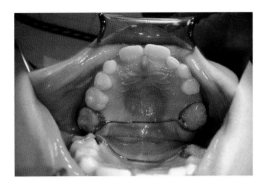

Figure 20.14 Transpalatal arch/palatal arch bar for premature unilateral loss of a maxillary second primary molar.

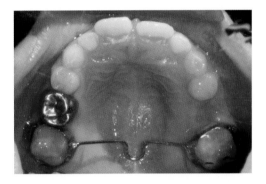

Figure 20.15 Transpalatal arch/palatal arch bar with an omega loop for premature unilateral loss of a maxillary second primary molar.

and soldered to the palatal side of the bands (Figure 20.14). This appliance prevents mesial tipping of the first permanent molar and is used only with unilateral loss of a second primary molar. The remaining second primary molar assists in reducing the tendency of the maxillary first permanent molar to rotate around its palatal root, causing space loss. An omega loop may be incorporated in the transpalatal bar for placing a light distal force, curtailing tipping and/or rotation of the first permanent molars (Terlaji & Donly, 2001) (Figure 20.15).

Nance Appliance

A Nance appliance is used for unilateral or bilateral loss of maxillary second primary

molars. The first permanent molars are banded, and a transpalatal wire, embedded in an acrylic button to provide resistance to mesial movement, contacts the palatal rugae (Figure 20.16a, b). Soft tissue irritation with food impaction under the acrylic button is a problem with this appliance (Dean & Law, 2018). Providing the patient with a Monoject™ syringe (Cardinal Health, Dublin, OH, USA) to irrigate the area may be helpful. If using for premature loss unilaterally of a second primary molar and if there is any concern regarding the possibility of early extraction of the contralateral second primary molar, the Nance appliance should be the appliance of choice.

Lower Lingual Holding Arch/Passive Lingual Arch

This is indicated for bilateral loss of the mandibular second primary molars after eruption of the permanent mandibular incisors, to avoid interference with their eruption (Dean, 2012). If a mandibular incisor is erupting to the lingual at the time of the delivery, waiting 2–3 weeks should be adequate time for the permanent incisor to spontaneously correct its position in the arch. If an over-retained primary incisor is causing lingual eruption of the permanent incisor, extraction should be performed (Figure 20.17a, b). (The struts on the distal of the primary canines should not have been included in the fabrication of the appliance. The struts impede the natural distal drift of the permanent incisors, which would create more space in the anterior.) This appliance may also be used to prevent lingual tipping of mandibular incisors after premature loss of the primary canines (Dean & Law, 2018). The mandibular first permanent or second primary molars are banded. A 0.036 or 0.040 in. round wire is soldered to the lingual surface of the molar bands. The wire should contact the lingual surface of all mandibular incisors. Struts may be placed on the distal of mandibular incisors with good

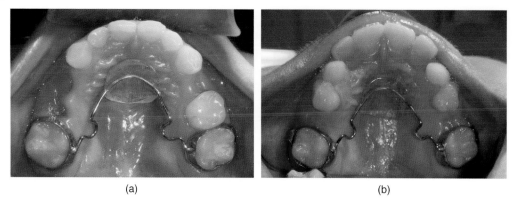

(a)   (b)

Figure 20.16 (a) Nance appliance for unilateral premature loss of a maxillary second primary molar. (b) Nance appliance for bilateral premature loss of maxillary second primary molars.

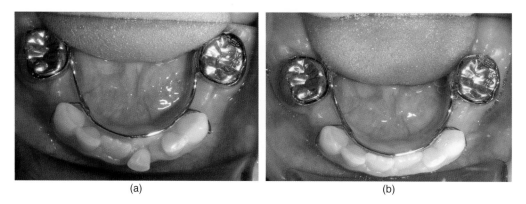

(a)   (b)

Figure 20.17 (a) Mandibular central incisor erupting in lingual position and lingual arch wire impeding eruption. (b) Lingual arch wire delivered 3 weeks later after spontaneous correction in arch of mandibular central incisor.

alignment to deter distal drift of the incisors (Figure 20.18a–c).

Distal Shoe

This appliance is used with premature loss of a second primary molar in the maxilla or mandible when the first permanent molar is unerupted (Dean & Law, 2018) (Figures 20.19 and 20.20a). The subgingival blade of the distal shoe guides the eruption path of the first permanent molar, preventing mesial drift that would result in blocking out the second premolar. A periapical radiograph is necessary to determine the position of the developing first permanent molar. A plaster or scanned model and periapical radiograph may be sent to the laboratory for appliance fabrication before extraction of the second primary molar. Delivering the appliance at the time of the extraction avoids an additional appointment, another injection of local anesthesia, and surgical incision for blade insertion. The first primary molar is banded or restored with a stainless-steel crown for attachment of a 0.036 or 0.040 in. round wire. The wire extends to a distal blade, placed subgingivally 1.0–1.5 mm below the marginal ridge of the unerupted permanent molar (Figure 20.20b). A periapical radiograph is obtained with try-in before cementation to evaluate the position

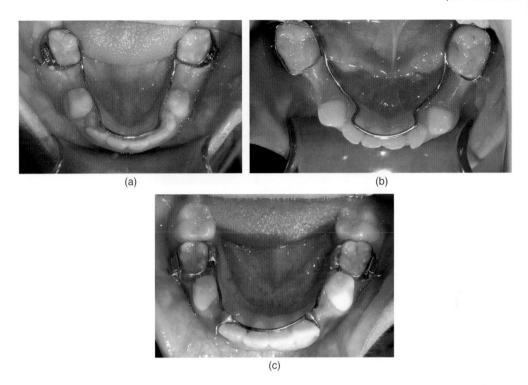

(a) (b)

(c)

Figure 20.18 (a) Lower lingual arch or passive lingual arch for premature loss of mandibular second primary molars. (b) Lower lingual arch for premature loss of right and left mandibular first primary molars with mandibular first permanent molars unerupted. (c) Lower lingual arch wire with struts on mandibular permanent lateral incisors to prevent lingual tipping and distal drift of the mandibular permanent lateral incisors.

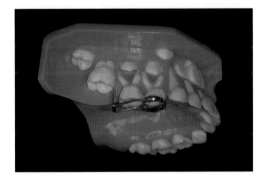

Figure 20.19 Distal shoe appliance on mixed-dentition typodont.

of the distal shoe blade in relation to the first permanent molar (Figure 20.20b). A Howe plier may be used to adjust the blade for correct alignment and another periapical radiograph to confirm the position is obtained

(Figure 20.20c). If necessary, the distal shoe blade may be shortened with a carbide bur at high speed. The subgingival blade guides the path of eruption of the first permanent molar (Figure 20.20d). The patient is monitored clinically and radiographically to assess the integrity of the appliance, gingival health, and the eruption path of the permanent first molar (Brill, 2002) (Figure 20.20e). Upon eruption of the first permanent molar (Figure 20.20f), the blade may be removed and the loop remains, creating a band-and-loop appliance. Otherwise, a transpalatal appliance may be utilized to avoid mesial tipping of the maxillary first permanent molar and mesial movement resulting in space loss for the second premolar. The distal shoe may also be used in the mandible (Figure 20.21a, b). Upon eruption of the first permanent molar, the distal shoe blade may

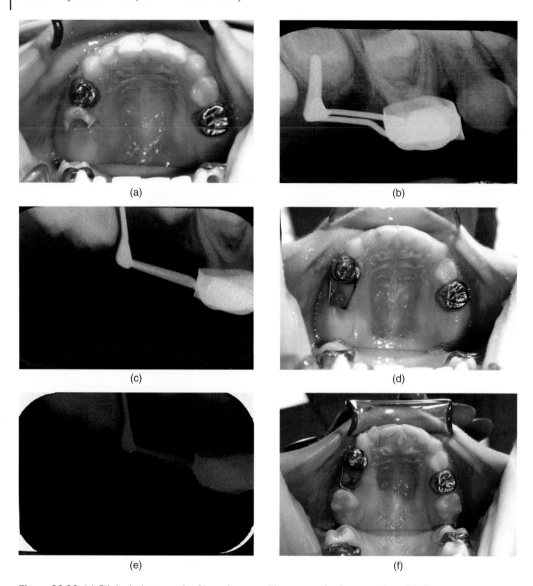

(a)   (b)

(c)   (d)

(e)   (f)

Figure 20.20 (a) Clinical photograph of hopeless maxillary second primary molar with first permanent molar unerupted. (b) Periapical radiograph to evaluate blade position with try-in. (c) Periapical radiograph after adjustment of blade alignment. (d) Clinical photograph of distal shoe 3 weeks after delivery. (e) Periapical radiograph showing first permanent molar being guided into the proper position by the blade of the distal shoe. (f) Clinical photograph showing first permanent molar successfully erupted.

be removed for the appliance to maintain the space, and a band and loop or a lingual arch wire can be fabricated. This appliance is not commonly used because of the requirement for conscientious follow-up and risk of infection with poor oral hygiene. The distal shoe is contraindicated in immunocompromised children (Simon *et al.*, 2012).

Banding and Impression for Appliance Fabrication

Stainless-steel bands, a band remover, and a bite stick to seat the bands are required for fitting molar bands (Figure 20.22). Stainless-steel bands without brackets or buccal tubes for

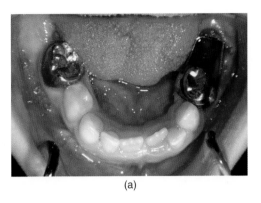

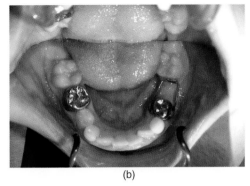

(a)   (b)

Figure 20.21 (a) Distal shoe in mandible immediately after delivery. (b) Distal shoe in mandible with first permanent molar erupted and appropriate time for removal.

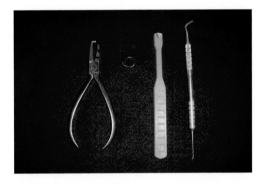

Figure 20.22 Band remover, stainless-steel band, bite stick, and band seater.

fabrication of space maintainers may be purchased. If the practice does not have the armamentarium for molar banding or the child cannot cooperate for banding, the molars can be banded by the laboratory on the plaster model. In some cases, placing an orthodontic separator between the first permanent molar and the second primary molar will open the contact, to facilitate seating the band. The separator remains in place for about a week. Measuring the molar to be banded with a Boley gauge may help to select the correct size for the band before try-in. A band seater and/or bite stick, or in some cases a tongue blade, may be used to have the patient seat the crown. If using a band seater or bite stick, step around the band for seating.

Impression material should be fast setting. Filling one-half of the tray with impression material or using a half-tray facilitates obtaining the impression for a band-and-loop space maintainer (Figure 20.23a, b). If the patient has a gag reflex, suggest that the he or she press a foot into the chair with a bent knee, while the impression is being taken (Figure 20.24). If a child is crying while the impression is being obtained, use compound instead of alginate to avoid possible aspiration of impression material.

The band remover is used to remove the band approaching from the buccal and palatal sides after taking the impression (Figure 20.25a, b). The band is seated in the impression, taking care to place the band in the proper occluso-cervical direction. Movement of the bands within the impression while pouring the plaster into the impression may result in an improper position of the band once the plaster sets. Placing staples to stabilize the band has been recommended (personal communication, Dr. Greg Psaltis). Staples may be bent or unbent (Figure 20.26). A Howe plier is used to bend the staples over the band (Figure 20.27a, b). Alternatively, a staple may be placed over the band and gently tapped down over it (Figure 20.28). The ends of the staples may be removed with wire cutters prior to fabricating the appliance (Figure 20.29).

An alternative to conventional alginate impressions and plaster models is three-dimensional scanning and digital models. Digital impressions were preferred by 51% of

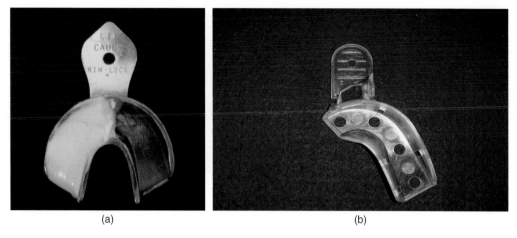

(a)   (b)

Figure 20.23 (a) One half of tray filled with impression material for band and loop. (b) Half impression tray.

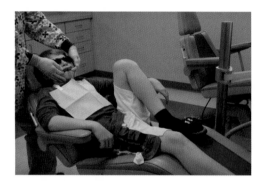

Figure 20.24 Bent knee to reduce gag reflex while taking impression.

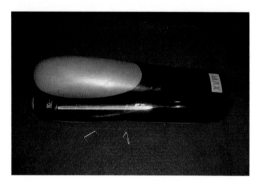

Figure 20.26 Stapler with bent and unbent staples.

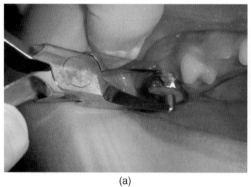

(a)

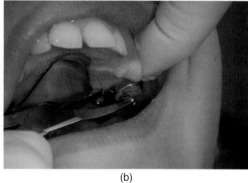

(b)

Figure 20.25 (a) Removing band from molar with band remover on buccal surface. (b) Removing band from molar with band remover on palatal surface.

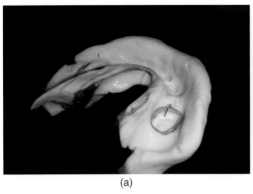
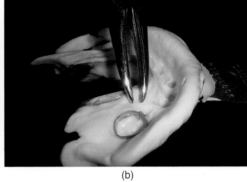

(a)   (b)

Figure 20.27 (a) Staple to secure band in impression. (b) Howe plier to bend staple over band.

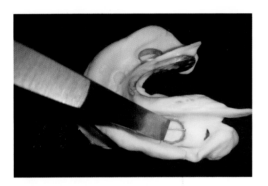
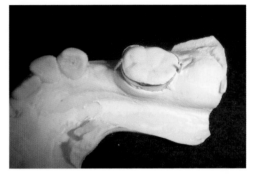

Figure 20.28 Unbent staple over band in impression being secured with opposite end of cotton plier.

Figure 20.29 Plaster model with banded primary molar and staple to secure band.

subjects in one study (Burhardt *et al.*, 2016). Scanning may be preferable for patients with a gag reflex that prohibits obtaining an alginate impression. Additionally, banding the teeth is not necessary. Laboratory fees are higher for fabricating space maintainers with digital impressions, because a fee is charged by the laboratory to create the scanned resin model and band the teeth.

Chairside Fabrication

Kits are available for customized chairside fabrication of the band-and-loop and distal shoe appliances (Denovo Dental, Baldwin Park, CA, USA; Space Maintainer Laboratories,

Chatsworth, CA, USA). Kits contain bands, precrimped/precontoured stainless-steel crowns, and blades for a distal shoe. No impression is required, no return visit with chair time, no wait time for return from laboratory, laboratory fees are eliminated, and the appliance can be fabricated and delivered during sedation or general anesthesia. The full fee for the appliance can be collected the same day. Immediate repair or replacement of the appliance is possible, and performing fabrication at the time of the extraction avoids space loss, with possible delay in delivery due to no-show or cancellation. The single negative feature is that the loops are too narrow to permit unimpeded eruption of the permanent tooth (Figure 20.30a, b).

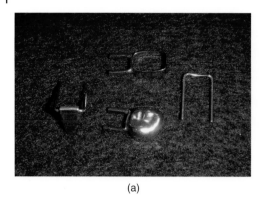
(a)

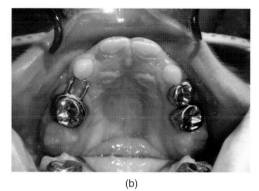
(b)

Figure 20.30 (a) Chairside space maintainers. (b) Chairside space maintainer after delivery.

After Appliance Delivery

Space maintenance requires supervision and parent/guardian compliance. The date of insertion and removal of appliances should be recorded in a designated place for regular review of patients with space maintainers. If the patient is no longer being seen in the practice, and the practice is unable to contact the parent/guardian by mail, phone, or email regarding the need for evaluation of the status of the space maintainer, a letter sent via certified mail with a return receipt is suggested for legal documentation of this notification.

Appliances may be removed once a year for prophylaxis and fluoride application to insure healthy tooth structure under and around the bands.

Timely and appropriate use of space maintenance or of space control will significantly influence the development of favorable arch form and decrease the incidence of malocclusion and future costs for orthodontic intervention, along with permitting normal eruption of the developing permanent dentition. Parental/guardian compliance with follow-up to monitor space maintainers is mandatory.

References

Alexander, S.A., Askari, M., & Lewis, P. (2015) The premature loss of primary first molars: space loss to molar occlusal and facial patterns. *Angle Orthodontics*, 85, 218–223.

American Academy of Pediatric Dentistry. (2019–2020a) Management of the developing dentition and occlusion in pediatric dentistry. *The Reference Manual of Pediatric Dentistry*. Chicago, IL: American Academy of Pediatric Dentistry; 362–378.

American Academy of Pediatric Dentistry. (2019–2020b) Resources: dental growth and development. *The Reference Manual of Pediatric Dentistry*. Chicago, IL: American Academy of Pediatric Dentistry; 505.

Bell, R.A., Dean, J.A., McDonald, R.E., & Avery, D.R. (2011) Managing the developing dentition. In: Dean, J.A., Avery, D.R., & McDonald R.E. (eds.), *Dentistry for the Child and Adolescent. Maryland Heights, MO*: Mosby Elsevier; 550–613.

Brill, W.A. (2002) The distal shoe maintainer: chairside fabrication and clinical performance. *Pediatric Dentistry*, 24, 561–565.

Burhardt, L., Livas, C., Kerdijk, W., van der Meer, W.J., & Ren, Y. 4 (2016) Treatment comfort, time perception, and preference for conventional and digital impression techniques: a comparative study in young patients. *American Journal of Orthodontics and Dentofacial Orthopedics*, **150**, 261–267.

Dean, J.A. (2012) Bilateral space management in the mixed dentition. In: Moursi, A.M. (ed.), *Clinical Cases in Pediatric Dentistry*. Oxford: Wiley Blackwell; 212–215.

Dean, J.A. & Law, C.S. (2018) Growth and development/management of the developing occlusion. In: Nowak, A.J. & Casamassimo, P.S. (eds.), *The Handbook of Pediatric Dentistry*, 5th edn. Chicago, IL: American Academy of Pediatric Dentistry; 191–225.

Fathian, M., Kennedy, D.B., & Nouri, M.R. (2007) Laboratory-made space maintainers: a 7-year retrospective study from private dental practice. *Pediatric Dentistry*, 29, 500–506.

Fricker, J., Kharbanda, O.P., & Dando, J. (2008) Orthodontic diagnosis and treatment in the mixed dentition. In: Cameron, A.C. & Widmer, R.P. (eds.), *Handbook of Pediatric Dentistry*, 3rd edn. London: Mosby; 341–377.

Kupietzky, A. (2001) The treatment and long-term management of severe multiple avulsions of primary teeth in a 19-month-old child. *Pediatric Dentistry*, 23, 517–521.

Lin, Y.-T., Lin, W.-H., & Lin, Y.-T.J. (2007) Immediate and six-month space changes after premature loss of a primary maxillary first molar. *Journal of the American Dental Association*, 138, 362–368.

Simon, T., Nwabueze, I., Oueis, H., & Stenger, J. (2012) Space maintenance in the primary and mixed dentitions. *Journal of the Michigan Dental Association*, 94, 38–40.

Terlaji, R.D. & Donly, K.J. (2001) Treatment planning for space maintenance in the primary and mixed dentition. *Journal of Dentistry for Children*, 68, 109–114.

Tunison, W., Flores-Mir, C., El Badrawy, H., Nassar, U., & El-Bialy, T. (2008) Dental arch space changes following premature loss of primary first molars: a systematic review. *Pediatric Dentistry*, 30, 297–302.

21

Interceptive Orthodontic Treatment in The Mixed Dentition
Jane A. Soxman

Early identification and timely corrective intervention for a malocclusion are essential in the mixed dentition for both short- and long-term benefits. Interceptive orthodontic treatment is for the correction of a minor malocclusion in which one to four teeth are involved and is typically performed in the mixed dentition stage of development. This early intervention does not preclude the possibility of a need for future comprehensive orthodontic treatment. The correction of maxillary anterior crossbite, maxillary posterior crossbite, and mandibular incisor crowding are discussed in this chapter for inclusion in pediatric and general practice.

Maxillary Anterior Crossbite

A permanent incisor may erupt palatally in the maxilla, resulting in a crossbite relationship in centric occlusion. Intervention is necessary if there is deviation on opening or closing, traumatic occlusion with attrition of the mandibular incisor(s), and/or periodontal complication with gingival recession and thinning of the labial alveolar plate (Figure 21.1) (Fricker *et al.*, 2008).

Tongue Blade

This correction is limited to partially erupted maxillary incisors without excessive overbite (Fricker *et al.*, 2008). A tongue blade is placed on the lingual near the incisal edge

of the incisor(s) in crossbite and torque with forward pressure is placed on the incisor(s) (Figure 21.2a, b). Alternatively, the child is told to close against the tongue blade while it is held against the chin. The tongue blade is held firmly in position until someone else counts out loud slowly to 50 or for about 1 minute. If this is repeated at least six times each day with half-hour intervals, correction will occur within a few days (Fricker *et al.*, 2008). Because the roots are still rather short, since not yet fully developed in length, there is some mobility that facilitates correction. The parent/caregiver should be present for this instruction. A bag of tongue blades is given to the child. His or her overbite acts as a retainer.

Two appliances that do not require compliance or concerns with loss of a removable appliance are anterior recurve or Z-springs and a reverse inclined plane.

Anterior Recurve or Z-Springs

An appliance with stainless-steel helical-loop finger springs incorporated from a lingual arch wire soldered to the bands of maxillary first permanent or second primary molars provides effective and reliable correction of maxillary permanent incisor crossbite. This fixed appliance offers increased stability and rigidity, controlling applied force to the lingual of the contacted incisor(s). One or more maxillary incisors in crossbite may be engaged (Figures 21.3a–d and Figure 21.4). A button

Handbook of Clinical Techniques in Pediatric Dentistry, Second Edition. Edited by Jane A. Soxman.
© 2022 John Wiley & Sons, Inc. Published 2022 by John Wiley & Sons, Inc.

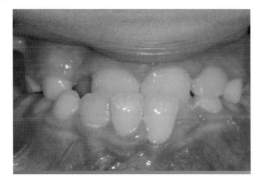

Figure 21.1 Clinical photograph of gingival recession caused by maxillary incisors in crossbite.

of composite may be placed on the lingual surface to make a retentive undercut to engage the spring and deter incisal movement of the spring. Occlusion should be checked after bonding the composite button to insure no interference. The spring is engaged gingival to the composite button in the cingulum. Forward pressure of the spring on the lingual surface of the tooth in crossbite corrects the tooth or teeth in crossbite. This fixed appliance applies continuous force and is not dependent on child or parent compliance. Correction typically occurs in 2–3 weeks. Because most children have a rather deep bite, the bite may be slightly opened to facilitate the correction; however, this may not be necessary. Upon delivery, bonded composite or the cement used for the

bands may be placed on the occlusal of the banded molars to open the bite (Figure 21.3c).

The child should be evaluated in 1–2 weeks after delivery. If correction has occurred and overbite is sufficient for retention, the appliance may be removed. If active treatment time extends to 4 weeks, the appliance should be removed to evaluate the spring, which may not be exerting the anticipated force due to overheating at the time of soldering the spring to the appliance (Bell, 2001).

Reverse Inclined Plane

An anterior crossbite may be the result of a forward shift of the mandible (Figure 21.5). Upper airway obstruction should be ruled out prior to use of the inclined plane, since the shift may be occurring to open the airway and relapse will occur. The mandibular first permanent molars or second primary molars are banded and an acrylic inclined plane is fabricated to fit over the mandibular incisors (Figure 21.6a). The inclined plane restricts forward repositioning of the mandible. Pressure placed on the palatal surface of the maxillary incisors pushes them labially (Figure 21.6b). Overbite retains the positive overjet after removal of the reverse inclined plane. An alternative is to place a layer of composite over the mandibular incisors to mimic the inclined plane's action.

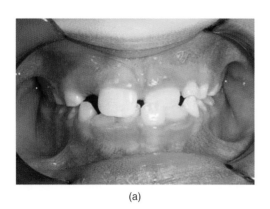

(a)

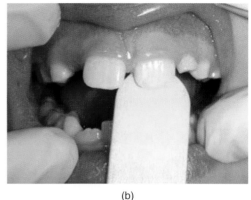

(b)

Figure 21.2 (a) Clinical photograph of maxillary left permanent central incisor in crossbite. (b) Tongue blade for crossbite correction.

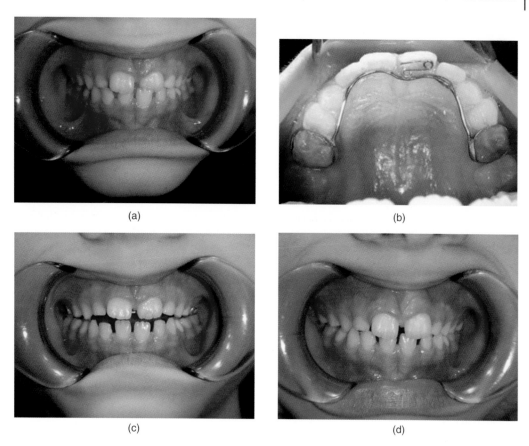

(a)

(b)

(c)

(d)

Figure 21.3 (a) Clinical photograph showing crossbite of maxillary left permanent central incisor. (b) Clinical photograph showing appliance to correct crossbite of maxillary permanent central incisor with build-up on primary molars to open bite. (c) Clinical photograph showing bite opened, facilitating crossbite correction. (d) Clinical photograph showing corrected left permanent central incisor.

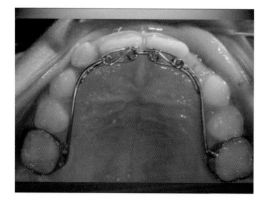

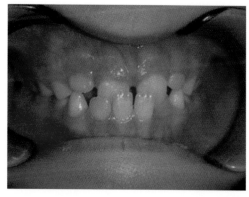

Figure 21.4 Clinical photograph showing appliance to correct crossbite of maxillary right and left permanent central incisors.

Figure 21.5 Clinical photograph of maxillary anterior crossbite prior to inclined plane.

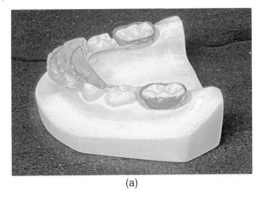
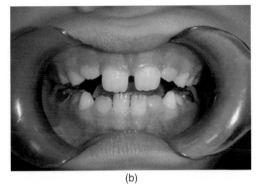

(a)   (b)

Figure 21.6 (a) Reverse inclined plane appliance. Source: Courtesy of QC Orthodontic Lab, Inc. (b) Clinical photograph showing reverse inclined plane after delivery.

If this option is chosen, to insure safe removal, the composite should be a different shade from the enamel to distinguish the two (Fricker *et al.*, 2008).

Maxillary Posterior Crossbite

A maxillary transverse deficiency can be corrected with expansion of the palate with a combination of orthopedic and orthodontic tooth movement (Figure 21.7). Rapid maxillary expansion (RME), slow maxillary expansion (SME), and surgically assisted maxillary expansion are expansion modalities for treatment. In this chapter, two appliances for RME and one appliance for SME are discussed.

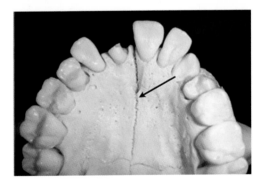

Figure 21.7 Photograph of the maxilla in mixed dentition showing the midpalatal suture.

Many different types and designs of RME and SME appliances are available. Personal preference determines the choice. Discussion with the dental laboratory will assist in this decision. The dental laboratory may band the teeth for fabricating the appliance.

Standard cephalometric analysis may not be necessary for diagnostic records (Allen *et al.*, 2003). However, facial and intraoral photographs, models (plaster or digitally scanned), and a panoramic radiograph should be obtained.

Skeletal gains are most successful in patients who have not peaked in skeletal growth. The increasing digitation of the palatal suture causes difficulty in achieving separation after puberty (Agarwal & Mathur, 2010). Cone beam computed tomography (CBCT) images may be obtained to determine the radiographic stages of midpalatal suture maturation. By age 6, normal palatal growth is close to completion. These stages are then classified according to the appearance of the suture line. A straight high-density sutural line with little or no inter-digitation and a sutural line with a scalloped appearance were most often observed up to 13 years of age. In girls, fusion of the palatine and maxillary regions of the midpalatal suture was complete after 11 years of age. Classification in stages with CBCT is deemed to have to potential to insure successful RME or unnecessary surgically assisted expansion for older adolescents and young adults (Angelieri *et al.*, 2013). Tonello *et al.* (2017) agreed that nonsurgical RME may be performed in patients over 15 years of age, documented with CBCT showing Stage C maturation with parallel, scalloped high-density lines that are close to each other and separated at some points by small low-density spaces.

Functional unilateral crossbite is typically the result of dental interference that produces a shift from centric relation to the crossbite side. The mandible itself is usually symmetric, but the functional shift, due to interference, improperly repositions the mandible, creating an asymmetric facial appearance when the teeth are in occlusion (Figure 21.8a, b). The condyles are positioned asymmetrically,

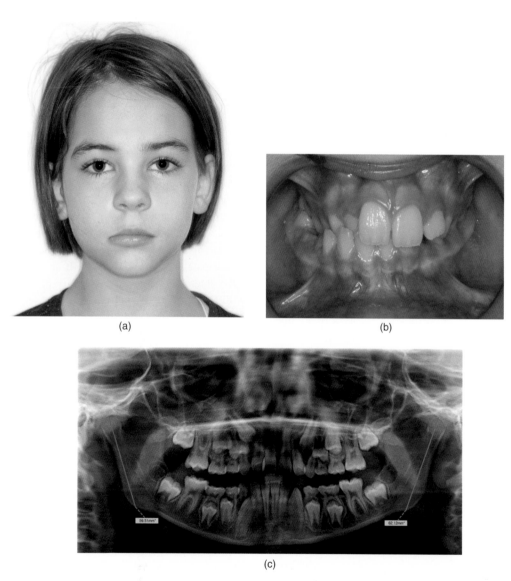

(a)

(b)

(c)

Figure 21.8 (a) Facial photograph showing shift of mandible to right caused by right posterior crossbite. (b) Intraoral photograph showing right posterior crossbite. (c) Panoramic radiograph of same patient showing shorter ramus on the right side.

with resulting asymmetric muscular function. The condyles on the crossbite side are positioned more superiorly and posteriorly in the glenoid fossa on the crossbite side. The joint space of the condyle on the noncrossbite side is increased. A panoramic radiograph may reveal a shorter ramus on the side in crossbite (Figure 21.8c). This functional crossbite produced significant asymmetry of the mandible in 7–10-year-old children. Maxillary expansion is considered to be the treatment of choice for patients in the mixed dentition, with the elimination of the positional and skeletal asymmetries present prior to treatment. Expansion resolves the transverse deficiency of the maxilla and permits a normal centric relationship (Pinto *et al.*, 2001).

Skeletal crossbite may result from different maxillomandibular presentations (Allen *et al.*, 2003):

- Narrow maxilla, normal mandible.
- Normal maxilla, wide mandible.
- Narrow maxilla, wide mandible.

Rapid Maxillary Expansion

RME, also termed rapid palatal expansion (RPE), is an orthopedic procedure to open the midpalatal suture, correcting maxillary dental and skeletal transverse discrepancies (Figure 21.7). Two designs of expansion appliances that are commonly used are the hyrax type (Figure 21.9) and the Haas type. The hyrax

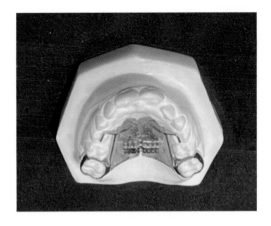

Figure 21.10 Haas expansion appliance. Source: Courtesy of QC Orthodontic Lab, Inc.

is also referred to as the hygienic expander, because the Haas is designed with an acrylic plate on the palate, making hygiene more of a challenge. The Haas screw is typically embedded in the acrylic plate. Heavy wires embedded in the acrylic plate are soldered to bands and course along the palatal surface of the primary molars. This design applies a lateral force to both the teeth and the walls of the palate (Figure 21.10). Both appliances open laterally using a key that is provided with the appliance (Figure 21.11). The key is placed in the screw and turned once or twice a day, opening the midpalatal suture. The hyrax functions similarly, but is easier to clean.

Expansion continues once or twice a day, with the maximum amount of expansion limited to the expander screw (Figure 21.12a, b) or

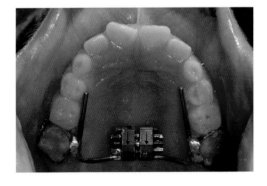

Figure 21.9 Hyrax expansion appliance.

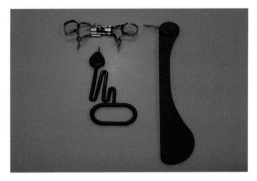

Figure 21.11 Hyrax expander and keys.

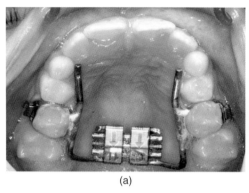

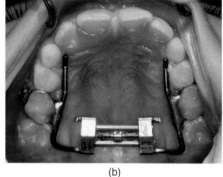

(a)   (b)

Figure 21.12 (a) Hyrax expansion appliance at delivery. (b) Hyrax expansion appliance after full activation.

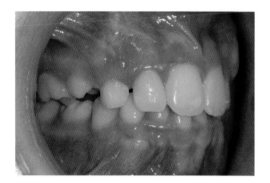

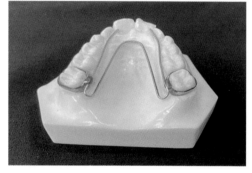

Figure 21.13 Brodie bite.

Figure 21.14 W-Arch expansion appliance.

until the lingual cusps of the maxillary molars are on the buccal cusps of the mandibular molars. In some cases, overexpansion may result in a Brodie bite, which should be avoided, with the maxillary premolar or molar lingual cusps totally labial to the buccal cusps of the mandibular premolar or molars (Figure 21.13). Autocorrection can be anticipated with normal relapse.

Slow Maxillary Expansion

As with RPE appliances, there are many choices for SME. The W-Arch is a commonly used fixed appliance that requires no involvement by the parent/caregiver (Figure 21.14). Initial and periodic activations are performed by the dentist. SME does not require turning a screw for expansion, so may be preferable for a child with a gag reflex or if parental/caregiver compliance is a concern. The lingual arch wire of the appliance should be fabricated to rest 1–1.5 mm away from the palatal soft tissue. Activation is performed in-office by opening the apices of the W-Arch. Proper force levels are achieved when the appliance is opened 3–4 mm wider than the passive width. This opening of the appliance should be performed prior to insertion. The expansion continues with opening the arch 2 mm per month or until the crossbite is overcorrected, as described with RPE (Agarwal & Mathur, 2010).

RME with anchorage to the maxillary first permanent molars may result in buccal displacement outside the alveolar process, damaging the periodontal support, reduction in buccal bone plate height and thickness, recession of the gingiva, fenestration, and finally root resorption. Anchorage to maxillary second primary molars was proposed as an alternative to reduce these side effects of RME.

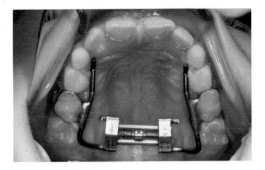

Figure 21.15 Hyrax expansion appliance with anchorage to maxillary second primary molars.

Ugolini *et al.* (2015) showed that anchorage to the maxillary second primary molars resulted in reduced molar angulation, with increased upper intercanine distance and more stable expansion in the anterior segment compared to anchorage to the maxillary first permanent molars. Another study supported anchorage to the second primary molars, finding no reduction in buccal bone plate thickness of the maxillary first permanent molars, except for mesial roots bilaterally (Figure 21.15) (Digregorio *et al.*, 2019).

The opening of the midpalatal suture is reported to be nonparallel and triangular, with a maximum opening anteriorly that gradually reduces posteriorly in the palate, resulting in a diastema between the maxillary central incisors. The diastema is self-corrective with elastic recoil of the transseptal fibers (Agarwal & Mathur, 2010). Parents/caregivers should be informed that a space between the central incisors will open during the expansion and that the space should spontaneously close within a few months after removal of the appliance (Figure 21.16a, b). Depending on clinician preference, retention time may vary from 3–5 months using the appliance as a retainer, or another type of retainer may be fabricated.

There are multiple benefits with RME. In addition to correcting dental and skeletal transverse discrepancies, studies have shown moderate evidence that RME in growing children increases nasal airway dimensions, improving breathing (Baratieri *et al.*, 2011). Children between 8 and 17 years of age were grouped as high risk and low risk for sleep-disordered breathing, determined with a Pediatric Sleep Questionnaire and an Obstructive Sleep Apnea Quality of Life Questionnaire. Children treated with RME showed an average improvement of 14% in quality of life scores in the high-risk group. The conclusion was that RME may positively impact the quality of life for children with a narrow maxilla and mild sleep-disordered breathing (Katyal *et al.*, 2013). Children with resistance otitis media with effusion (OME) showed similar effects with RME as with placement of ventilation tubes. Hearing threshold levels also improved. Prior to anesthesia and surgical intervention,

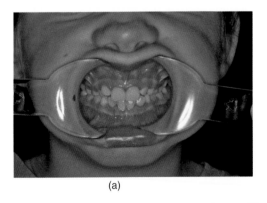

(a)

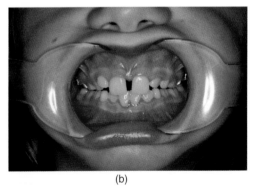

(b)

Figure 21.16 (a) Clinical photograph showing maxillary incisors prior to expansion. (b) Clinical photograph showing diastema between maxillary central incisors created by maxillary expansion.

RME should be the preferred intervention for children with resistance OME and palatal constriction, prior to anesthesia and placement of ventilation tubes (Klig *et al.*, 2016). Fagundes *et al.* (2017) reported similar findings with improvement of hearing in children with previous hearing impairment post RME. The expansion of the midpalatal suture in a pyramidal shape, with maximum expansion near the incisors, increases the width of the nasal cavity, improving breathing (Agarwal & Mathur, 2010). Nasal volume capacity is increased due to expansion of the external walls of the nasal cavity. The ability to breathe through the nose instead of the mouth occurred in 80% of patients after RME, with the additional positive effect of decreased halitosis (Erhamza & Ozdiler, 2018). RME has been shown to reduce or cease nocturnal enuresis due to significant positive effects on the pathophysiologic mechanisms associated with this condition (Al-Taal *et al.*, 2015). With attempts to cure nocturnal enuresis, children with normal transverse occlusion should also be considered as candidates for RME (Bazargani *et al.*, 2016).

Mandibular Incisor Crowding

Lower Lingual Holding Arch

The lower lingual holding arch (LLHA) is a well-documented method to preserve arch length by maintaining the leeway space in the mixed dentition during the transition from the late mixed to the permanent dentition (Figure 21.17a, b) (Hudson *et al.*, 2013). Leeway space is the result of the difference in the combined mesiodistal widths of the primary canines and primary molars compared with the combined mesiodistal widths of their permanent successors. Most of the difference is due to the width differential between the second primary molars and the second premolars.

The LLHA permits passive resolution of mild mandibular incisor crowding during the transition from the late mixed to the permanent dentition, with distal drift of the canines and premolars. The mandibular first permanent molars are banded, a stainless-steel wire is soldered to the lingual of each band, and extends around the arch on the lingual surface of the mandibular teeth. Up to 4.8 mm of leeway space becomes available during the replacement of the primary canines and molars to the permanent canines and premolars (Brennan & Gianelly, 2000). With the late mesial shift, the first permanent molars move mesially into the leeway space and the arch length is decreased. Timely placement of this appliance may also provide 2–4 mm of space relief for mandibular incisor crowding (Figure 21.18a, b). The wire in Figure 21.18b should be just above the cingulum, as shown in Figure 21.18c.

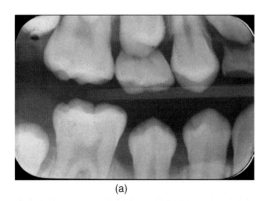

(a)

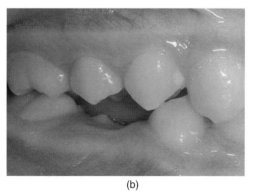

(b)

Figure 21.17 (a) Bitewing radiograph showing the leeway space after loss of the primary molars. (b) Intraoral photograph showing the leeway space.

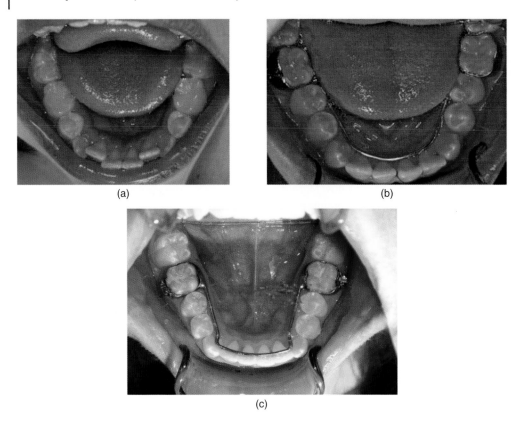

Figure 21.18 (a) Intraoral photograph showing mandibular incisor crowding at time of delivery of lower lingual holding arch (LLHA). (b) Intraoral photograph showing resolution of mandibular incisor crowding after distal drift of the mandibular canines and premolars into the leeway space. (c) LLHA in proper position at cingulum.

Chen *et al.* (2019) reported both resolution of mandibular incisor crowding and no significant arch length or perimeter changes greater than 1 mm. Another advantage of this appliance is the stability of the mandibular incisors (Sinclair & Little, 2009). Stability of the mandibular incisor alignment was reported 9 years post retention for 76% of patients treated only with a passive LLHA. Patients who were expanded more than 1 mm (0.5 mm per side) were sharply contrasting, with more relapse than those treated with passive lingual arches. This finding suggests that the passive lingual arch, providing arch length preservation, may be the more appropriate treatment, with the additional benefit of resolution of lower incisor crowding (Brennan & Gianelli, 2000).

The appliance should remain in place until the mandibular incisor crowding is resolved, after the canines and premolars have erupted and the mandibular second molars have erupted. Earlier removal may cause mesial movement of the first permanent molars, with eruptive pressure from the mandibular second molars. Since this appliance prevents mesial movement of the mandibular first molars, maintaining the leeway space, monitoring is necessary to evaluate possible impaction of the mandibular second permanent molars. Since the late mesial shift of the mandibular molars is inhibited, the first permanent molars may remain in a Class II relationship. Initial angulation of the mandibular second permanent molar, space–width ratio, and the sex and age of the patient were not found to have a significant effect on the eruption pattern of the mandibular second molars (Figure 21.19) (Rubin *et al.*, 2012).

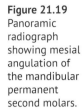

Figure 21.19
Panoramic radiograph showing mesial angulation of the mandibular permanent second molars.

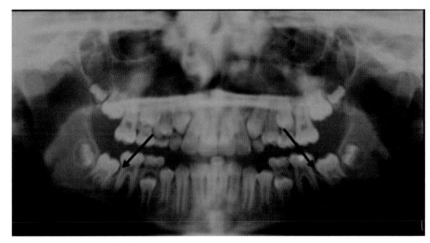

Note

Thanks to John F. Buzzatto, DMD, Diplomate American Board of Orthodontics, for his review of this chapter.

References

Agarwal, A. & Mathur, R. (2010) Maxillary expansion. *International Journal of Pediatric Dentistry*, 3, 139–146.

Allen, D., Rebellato, J., Sheats, R., & Ceron, A.M. (2003) Skeletal and dental contributors to posterior crossbites. *Angle Orthodontics*, 73, 515–524.

Al-Taal, N., Alfatlawi, F., Ransjo M., & Ayhan Basciftci, F. (2015) Effect of maxillary expansion on monosymptomatic primary nocturnal enuresis. *Angle Orthodontics*, 85, 102–108.

Angelieri, F., Cevidanes, L.H., Franchi, L., Gonçalves, J.R., Benavides, E., & McNamara, J.A., Jr., (2013) Midpalatal suture maturation: classification method for individual assessment before rapid maxillary expansion. *American Journal of Orthodontics and Dentofacial Orthopedics*, 144, 759–769.

Baratieri, C., Alves, M., Gomes de Souza, M.M., Tirre de Souza Araújo, M., & Cople Maia, L. (2011) Does rapid maxillary expansion have long-term effects on airway dimensions and breathing? *American Journal of Orthodontics and Dentofacial Orthopedics*, 140, 146–156.

Bazargani, F., Jonson-Ring, I., & Neveus, T. (2016) Rapid maxillary expansion in therapy-resistant enuretic children: an orthodontic perspective. *Angle Orthodontics*, 86, 481–486.

Bell, R. (2001) A simple fixed anterior crossbite appliance. American Academy of Pediatric Dentistry Annual Session.

Brennan, M.M. & Gianelli, A.A. (2000) The use of a lingual arch in the mixed dentition to resolve incisor crowding. *American Journal of Orthodontics and Dentofacial Orthopedics*, 117, 81–85.

Chen, C.-Y., Hsu K.-L.C., Marghalani, A.M., Dhar, V., & Coll, J.A. (2019) Systematic review and meta-analysis of passive lower lingual arch for resolving mandibular incisor crowding and effects on arch dimension. *Pediatric Dentistry*, 41, 9–19.

Digregorio, M.V., Fastuca, R., Zecca, P.A., Caprioglio, A., & Lagravère, M.O. (2019)

Buccal bone plate thickness after rapid maxillary expansion in mixed and permanent dentitions. *American Journal of Orthodontics and Dentofacial Orthopedics*, 155, 198–206.

Erhamza, T.S. & Ozdiler, F.E. (2018) Effect of rapid maxillary expansion on halitosis. *American Journal of Orthodontics and Dentofacial Orthopedics*, 154, 702–707.

Fagundes, N.C.F., Rabello, N.M., Maia, L.C., Normando, D., & Ribeiro Mello, K.C.F. (2017) Can rapid maxillary expansion cause auditory improvement in children and adolescents with hearing loss? A systematic review. *Angle Orthodontics*, 87, 886–896.

Fricker, J., Kharbanda O.P., & Dando, J. (2008) Orthodontic diagnosis and treatment in the mixed dentition. In: Cameron, A.C. & Widmer, R.P. (eds.), *Handbook of Pediatric Dentistry*, 3rd edn. London: Mosby; 341–377.

Hudson, A.P.G., Harris, A.M.P., Mohamed, N., & Joubert, J. (2013) Use of a passive lower lingual arch in the management of anterior crowding in the mixed dentition. *Journal of the South African Dental Association,* 68, 114, 116–119.

Katyal, V., Pamula, Y., Daynes, C.N., Martin, J., Dreyer, C.W., *et al.* (2013) Craniofacial and upper airway morphology in pediatric sleep-disordered breathing and changes in quality of life with rapid maxillary expansion. *American Journal of Orthodontics and Dentofacial Orthopedics*, 144, 860–871.

Klig, N., Yoruk, O., Kilig, S.C., Çatal, G., & Kurt, S. (2016) Rapid maxillary expansion versus middle ear tube placement: comparison of hearing improvements in children with resistance otitis media with effusion. *Angle Orthodontics*, 86, 761–767.

Pinto, A.S., Buschang, P.H., Throckmorton, G.S., & Chen, P. (2001) Morphological and positional asymmetries of young children with functional unilateral posterior crossbite. *American Journal of Orthodontics and Dentofacial Orthopedics*, 120, 513–520.

Rubin, R.L., Bacetti, T., & McNamara, J.A. (2012) Mandibular second molar eruption difficulties related to the maintenance of arch perimeter in the mixed dentition. *American Journal of Orthodontics and Dentofacial Orthopedics*, 141, 146–152.

Sinclair, P.M. & Little, R.M. (2009) Clinical implications of the University of Washington post-retention studies. *Journal of Clinical Orthodontics*, 43, 645–651.

Tonello, D.L., de Miranda Ladewig, V., Guedes, F.P., Ferreira Conti, A.C.C., Almeida-Pedrin, R.R., & Capelozza-Filho, L. (2017) Midpalatal suture maturation in 11-to-15-year-olds: a cone-beam computed tomographic study. *American Journal of Orthodontics and Dentofacial Orthopedics*, 152, 4–48.

Ugolini, A., Cerruto, C., Di Vece, L., Huanca Ghislanzoni, L., Sforza, C., *et al.* (2015) Dental arch response to Haas-type rapid maxillary expansion anchored to deciduous vs permanent molars: a multicentric randomized controlled trail. *Angle Orthodontics*, 85, 570–576.

22

Non-Nutritive Sucking and Parafunctional Habits
Jane A. Soxman

Prolonged pacifier and finger/thumb sucking have detrimental effects on both dentoalveolar and facial development. Protracted pacifier habits most often result in anterior open bite and bilateral Class II malocclusion, while protracted thumb and finger habits result in anterior open bite (Warren *et al.*, 2005). Frequency, intensity, and duration of the forces are considerations. Duration is considered to be most influential in the development of increased overjet, anterior open bite, and posterior crossbite. The use of pacifiers beyond the second or third year of life may result in a malocclusion that requires future orthodontic intervention. Thumb or finger sucking should be discontinued at the time of the eruption of the maxillary permanent incisors. Timely discontinuation or modification of non-nutritive sucking may prevent or significantly reduce malocclusion (AAPD, 2019–2020; Warren *et al.*, 2001, 2005).

Pacifier Habits

Parents/guardians are often unaware of the dramatic effects of prolonged pacifier use in the primary dentition (Figure 22.1). Both conventional and physiologic pacifiers have been shown to cause alterations in the dental arches and occlusion (Zardetto *et al.*, 2002). Pacifier use has been shown to reduce the incidence of sudden infant death syndrome, with a decrease in the auditory threshold during sleep and easier arousal (Soxman, 2007). Offering the pacifier between feedings provides a protective effect, with lower incidence of overweight and obesity at 9 and 15 months of age (Amer *et al.*, 2017). Otitis media is increased with bedtime pacifier use. Because the Eustachian tube is in a horizontal position in an infant or toddler, oral microbes easily enter the Eustachian tube with sucking on the pacifier in a supine position (Soxman, 2007).

A typodont of the primary dentition is helpful to demonstrate normal occlusion (Figure 22.2). A 2-year-old child may sit on the parent/guardian's lap for examination. The examiner offers a large mirror to the parent/guardian, places the child's teeth in centric occlusion, and retracts the lips to reveal the open bite and posterior crossbite (Figure 22.3). This visualization is typically astonishing to the parent/guardian and is all that is necessary for immediate cessation of the habit.

Piercing or trimming the pacifier nipple shorter, dipping the nipple in white vinegar, or immediate cessation, "cold turkey," may be recommended. Rocking, singing, or reading to the child at bedtime may be suggested as a substitute for the pacifier (Adair, 2003). The Fridababy Paci Weaning System™ (Frida, Miami, FL, USA) is proven to stop the pacifier habit in as few as 5 days. This patented system, which has passed all federal safety regulations, has five different nipples, with each nipple smaller and less satisfying than its predecessor (Figure 22.4e).

Handbook of Clinical Techniques in Pediatric Dentistry, Second Edition. Edited by Jane A. Soxman.
© 2022 John Wiley & Sons, Inc. Published 2022 by John Wiley & Sons, Inc.

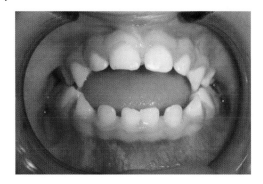

Figure 22.1 Anterior open bite with palatal constriction.

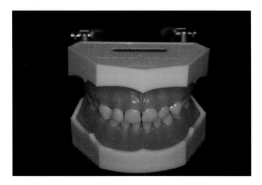

Figure 22.2 Typodont primary dentition, Kilgore International (Coldwater, MI, USA).

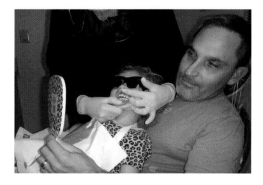

Figure 22.3 Showing occlusion with hand mirror.

Cessation of a pacifier habit at the age of 2 years satisfies the early physical and psychologic needs for sucking, while minimizing the risk for malocclusion (Warren *et al.*, 2001). Resolution of malocclusion may spontaneously occur in 6 months to 1 year

with discontinuation of the pacifier under age 3 years (Figure 22.4a, b) (Soxman, 2007). In the presence of accompanying crossbite, the open bite may resolve, but existing palatal constriction may or may not resolve without future palatal expansion (Figures 22.4c, d).

The midpalatal suture has not yet fused in a young child. The pressure exerted by the buccinator muscles on the maxillary primary molars during sucking causes palatal constriction. With the reduction in the width of the maxilla, the maxillary primary canines prematurely occlude with the mandibular canines, resulting in a functional crossbite (Figure 22.5a, b). The need for future crossbite correction with continuation of the habit is discussed, along with the need for immediate habit cessation (Soxman, 2007). The canine interference can be painlessly corrected with a cooperative child. A coarse diamond bur is used for incisal reduction of the right and left maxillary and mandibular primary canines, removing the incisal contacts and interference. No local anesthesia is necessary, as only enameloplasty is being performed (Figure 22.5c, d). Once the incisal edges are removed, centric occlusion can be achieved along with improved muscle balance and unrestricted growth (Figure 22.5e).

Finger/Thumb Sucking

Habit therapy with an appliance to reduce overjet and open bite should be instituted when the maxillary permanent incisors erupt (Fricker *et al.*, 2008). Significant overjet is associated with maxillary incisor fracture (Schatz *et al.*, 2013). With accompanying incompetent lip posture, the incidence of incisor fracture is compounded (Bauss *et al.*, 2008). First-phase orthodontic treatment may be performed after eruption of the permanent maxillary central and lateral incisors.

Taste aversion with hot-tasting or bitter-flavored preparations applied to the thumb or fingers may stop the habit (Fricker *et al.*,

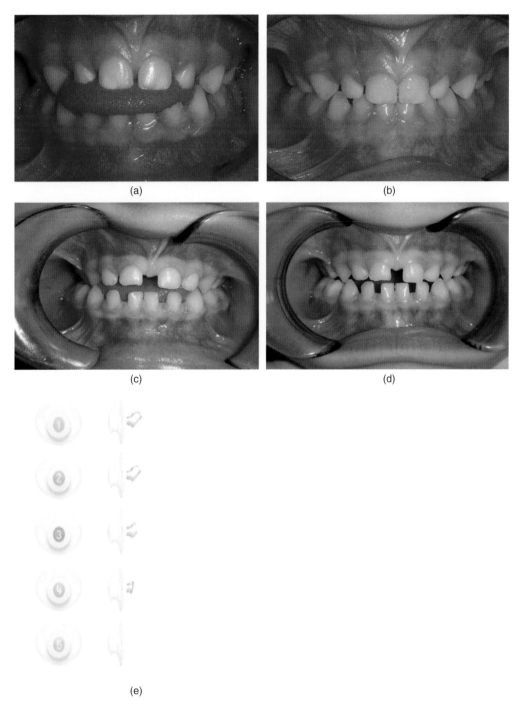

Figure 22.4 (a) Occlusion age 2 years 10 months during pacifier use. (b) Occlusion 6 months after cessation of pacifier habit. (c) Occlusion age 3 years 2 months during pacifier use. (d) Occlusion 6 months after cessation of pacifier habit with some residual palatal constriction. (e) Fridababy Paci Weaning System.

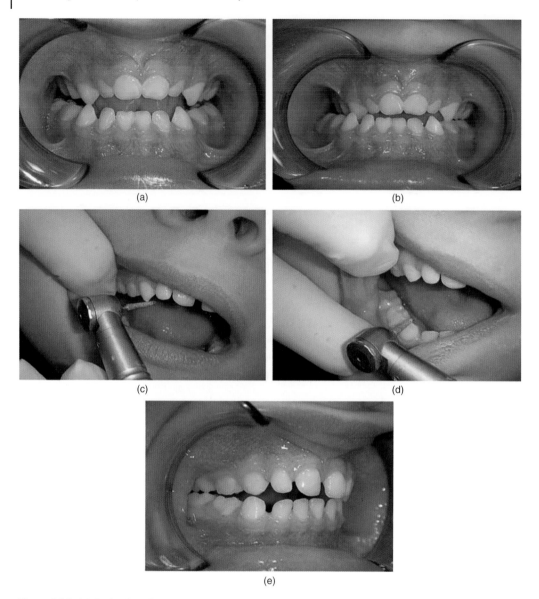

Figure 22.5 (a) Canine interference due to palatal constriction. (b) Functional crossbite due to canine interference. (c) Maxillary primary canine reduction with coarse diamond bur. (d) Mandibular primary canine reduction with coarse diamond bur. (e) Post primary canine reduction.

2008). For children older than 3 years, Mavala Stop (Mavala, Geneva, Switzerland) nail polish is applied to the finger(s) or thumb, with recommendation of daily application of a fresh coat. Mavala Stop is also recommended for persistent nail biting.

TGuard Aero™ (MED, Matthews, NC, USA) offers products for both thumb and finger sucking (Figures 22.6 and 22.7). Each product is available in three sizes: a small size for children aged 3 and 4 years, a medium size for ages 5 and 6 years, and a large size for ages 7 years and older. TGuards are made in the United States from a Food and Drug Administration (FDA)-listed, medical-grade material, which is bisphenol A (BPA) and phthalate free.

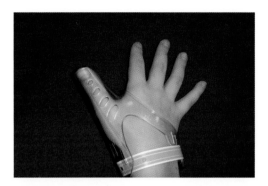

Figure 22.6 TGuard for thumb.

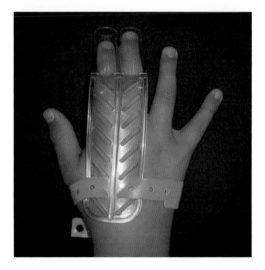

Figure 22.7 TGuard for adjacent fingers.

Each kit provides 60 bracelets with instalock clasps and a reward chart, with stickers. The bracelets can be removed only with scissors. The TGuard is worn when thumb/finger sucking typically occurs, such as while watching television or bedtime. The guards may also be used to temporarily curtail finger or thumb sucking, permitting chaffed skin to heal. No banding, impressions, or laboratory fees are required. The TGuard can be ordered on the Internet (www.tguard.com). The company states 90% success rates in about 3 weeks, with a money-back guarantee.

If alternative treatments such as a decorative band-aid on the finger/thumb, rewards, taste aversion, and TGuard are unsuccessful, fixed appliance therapy may be considered after the age of 4 years. Fixed appliances should be presented to the child as "reminders." The first follow-up visit is recommended in 2 weeks and then bimonthly. The seal with sucking is broken, and the pressure of the orbicularis oris muscle, which encircles the mouth, may assist to retract the maxillary incisors if sucking continues for a period after delivering the appliance.

The crib and bluegrass are popular appliances to correct a finger/thumb habit (Figures 22.8a, b and 22.9a, b). Orthodontic bands are fitted on the maxillary second primary molars or first permanent molars. If the practice does not have orthodontic bands, the laboratory fabricating the appliance can band the molars on the plaster model. An impression of both arches and a wax bite registration, taken in centric occlusion, for fabrication insure no interferences. A crib is fabricated with a palatal bar with a vertical fence-like portion on a 0.040 stainless-steel arch wire soldered to the bands. Fabrication of the bluegrass appliance is the same as for the crib, but this appliance uses beads or a Teflon roller for distraction. The child can turn the roller or beads with his or her tongue instead of sucking a finger or thumb. This appliance may require up to 36 weeks before habit cessation (Greenleaf & Mink, 2003).

Tongue Thrust

The tongue's normal resting posture is on the hard palate. The tongue may rest in a lower, forward position with hypertrophied tonsils, a constricted maxillary arch, macroglossia, or due to muscle memory after a prolonged pacifier-, thumb-, or finger-sucking habit. Swallowing with tongue thrust is of no clinical significance if the resting tongue posture is normal. To determine the presence of a tongue thrust, the patient's lower lip is retracted, and the patient is asked to swallow (Figure 22.10). The tongue will thrust forward through the

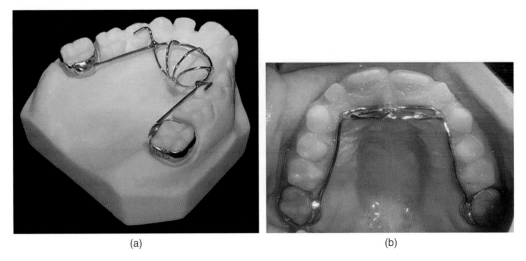

(a)   (b)

Figure 22.8 (a) Crib on laboratory model. Source: Courtesy of QC Orthodontics Lab, Inc. (b) Intraoral photograph of crib.

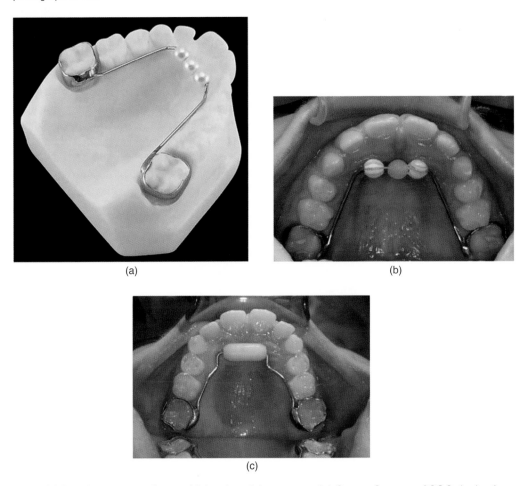

(a)   (b)

(c)

Figure 22.9 (a) Bluegrass appliance with beads on laboratory model. Source: Courtesy of QC Orthodontics Lab, Inc. (b) Intraoral photograph of bluegrass appliance with beads. (c) Intraoral photograph of bluegrass appliance with Teflon roller.

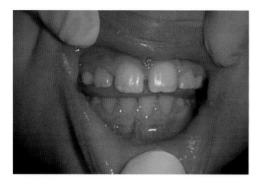

Figure 22.10 Demonstrating tongue thrust with upper and lower lip retracted as the patient swallows.

incisors during swallowing with a tongue thrust. If the tongue protrudes forward through the incisors at rest, an open bite with incisor displacement may occur (AAPD, 2019–2020).

Although success rates vary, an overextended crib may be used to close an anterior open bite, eliminate a tongue thrust, or reduce an anterior tongue position (Figure 22.11). The appliance may force the tongue to a more posterior and higher position. The appliance is worn for about 10 months. There is no agreement regarding the consistency of success with this appliance in changing tongue postures, but tongue adaptation may occur with the overextended crib. The existing morphology of the oral cavity appears to be more influential in tongue posture than the tongue

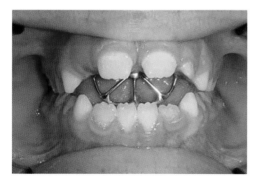

Figure 22.11 Overextended crib for tongue thrust and anterior tongue position.

molding the dental arches (Taslan *et al.*, 2010). A crib with a rake that has sharp projections, commonly known as a hay-rake, is also an option (Figure 22.12a, b). A similar appliance may be used in the mandible (Figure 22.12c). A removable appliance combining a Teflon roller to correct digit sucking, a slow palatal expander to correct posterior crossbite, and a crib to correct tongue thrust was developed by Kulkarni and Lau (Figure 22.13; Kulkarni & Lau, 2010). The fee to fabricate this as a removable appliance is very high; a modified fixed appliance is shown in this section.

Bruxing

Bruxing during sleep is often cited as a parental concern. Numerous contributory factors have been suggested such as allergies, upper airway obstruction, emotional stress, fatigue, malocclusion, and neurologic disabilities (Soxman, 2013; Marks, 1980; AAPD, 2019–2020). Insana *et al.* (2013) reported that almost 40% of preschoolers and 50% of first graders brux at least one night a week. In preschoolers, bruxing was associated with internalizing behaviors such as anxiety, depression, and withdrawal. Children who brux are also more likely to have reported health problems such as ear infections, frequent colds/flu, allergies, and constant rhinitis. Bruxing may be a sign of other medical/behavioral problems (Insana *et al.*, 2013). Gastric reflux may be suspected with a scalloped, rather than flat appearance of the occlusal surfaces in the mandibular primary molars. An association between gastroesophageal reflux and asthma in children has been suggested, but this has not been clearly shown (Thakkar *et al.*, 2010).

A history of allergies may suggest instituting environmental changes to remove the fomites that may induce bruxing during sleep. Dust is a common allergen. Antiallergy bedding such as mattress and pillow covers may be purchased. Down harbors dust mites; down

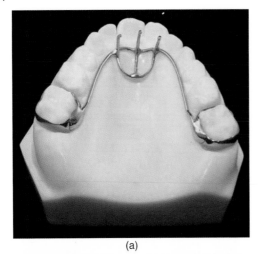

(a)

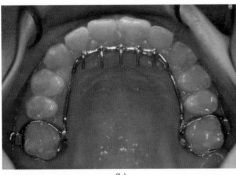

(b)

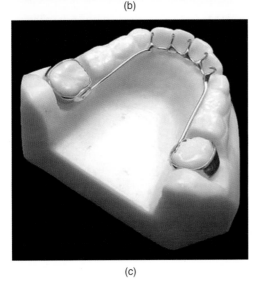

(c)

Figure 22.12 (a) Upper hay-rake for tongue thrust on laboratory model. (b) Intraoral photograph of crib with points on rake. (c) Lower tongue thrust appliance on laboratory model. Source: Image (a) and (c) Courtesy of QC Orthodontics Lab, Inc.

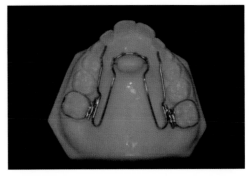

Figure 22.13 Combination appliance on laboratory model. Source: Courtesy of QC Orthodontics Lab, Inc.

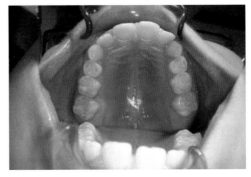

Figure 22.14 Mild attrition of maxillary primary molars.

pillows and comforters should be replaced with cotton. Damp dusting and removal of carpet, stuffed animals, and pets from the bedroom may be advised. In general, childhood bruxing is considered to be a harmless habit that is self-limiting and does not evolve to adult bruxism (AAPD, 2019–2020).

Mild attrition requires no intervention. Significant attrition, with pending pulp exposure, may be restored with high-viscosity glass ionomer cement, placed out of occlusion (Figures 22.14 and 22.15a, b). Primary molars may be restored with stainless-steel crowns, but continued bruxing may create a hole in the occlusal surface of the crown, trapping food under the crown. Preveneered crowns (stainless-steel crowns with a composite facing) are contraindicated, because bruxing

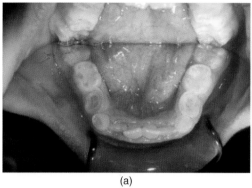
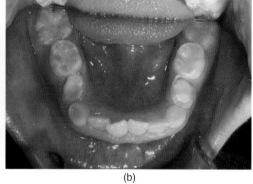

(a)   (b)

Figure 22.15 (a) Severe attrition of mandibular primary molars. (b) Glass ionomer restoration in mandibular first primary molars.

would fracture the facings. A zirconia crown would be the better choice for severe bruxing

with risk of pulp exposure if glass ionomer is not retained.

References

Adair, S. (2003) Pacifier use in children: a review of recent literature. *Pediatric Dentistry*, 25, 449–458.

Amer, A., Abusamaan, M., Li, X., & Fischer, H. (2017) Does pacifier use in infancy decrease the risk of obesity? *Clinical Pediatrics*, 56, 1018–1022.

American Academy of Pediatric Dentistry. (2019–2020) Management of the developing dentition and occlusion in pediatric dentistry. *The Reference Manual of Pediatric Dentistry*. Chicago, IL: American Academy of Pediatric Dentistry; 362–386.

Bauss, O., Freitag, S., Rohling, J., & Rahman, A. (2008) Influence of overjet and lip coverage on the prevalence and severity of incisor trauma. *Journal of Orofacial Orthopedics*, 69, 402–410.

Fricker, J., Kharbanda, O.P., & Dando, J. (2008) Orthodontic diagnosis and treatment in the mixed dentition. In: Cameron, A.C. & Widmer, R.P. (eds.), *Handbook of Pediatric Dentistry*, 3rd edn. London: Mosby; 341–377.

Greenleaf, S. & Mink, J. (2003) A retrospective study of the use of the bluegrass appliance in the cessation of thumb habits. *Pediatric Dentistry*, 25, 587–590.

Insana, S.P., Gozal, D., McNeil, D.W., & Montgomery-Downs, H.E. (2013) Community based study of sleep bruxism during early childhood. *Sleep Medicine*, 14, 183–188.

Kulkarni, G.V. & Lau, D. (2010) A single appliance for the correction of digit-sucking, tongue-thrust, *and posterior crossbite. Pediatric Dentistry*, 32, 61–63.

Marks, M.B. (1980) Bruxing in allergic children. *American Journal of Orthodontics*, 77, 48–59.

Schatz, J.-P., Hakeberg, M., Ostini, E., & Kiliaridis, S. (2013) Prevalence of traumatic injuries to permanent dentition and its association with overjet in a Swiss child population. *Dental Traumatology*, 29, 110–114.

Soxman, J.A. (2007) Non-nutritive sucking with a pacifier: pros and cons. *General Dentistry*, 55, 59–62.

Soxman, J.A. (2013) Upper airway obstruction in the pediatric patient. *General Dentistry*, 61, 13.

Taslan, S., Biren, S., & Ceylanoglu, C. (2010) Tongue pressure changes before, during and after crib appliance therapy. *Angle Orthodontics*, 80, 533–539.

Thakkar, K., Boatright, R.O., Gilger, M.A., & El-Serag, H.B. (2010) Gastroesophageal reflux and asthma in children: a systemic review. *Pediatrics*, 125, e925–e930.

Warren, J.J., Bishara, S.E., Steinbock, K.L., Yonezu, T., & Nowak, A.J. (2001) Effects of oral habits' duration on dental characteristics in the primary dentition. *Journal of the American Dental Association*, 132, 1685–1693.

Warren, J.J., Slayton, R.L., Yonezu, T., Levy, S.M., Yonezu, T., & Kanellis, M.J. (2005) Effects of nonnutritive sucking habits on occlusal characteristics in the mixed dentition. *Pediatric Dentistry*, 27, 445–450.

Zardetto, C.G., Rodrigues, C.R.M.D., & Stefani, F.M. (2002) Effects of different pacifiers on the primary dentition and oral myofunctional structures of preschool children. *Pediatric Dentistry*, 24, 552–560.

23

Behavior Guidance
Jane A. Soxman and Janice A. Townsend

The various forms of behavior that present when treating the pediatric patient can be daunting. Classifying the child's behavior into categories such as fearful, strong avoidance, combative, stubborn, defiant, and hysterical can facilitate behavior guidance treatment planning decisions that permit safe and high-quality treatment. Individual temperament is an individual's characteristic physiologic and emotional state that tends to condition their responses to the various situations of life and significantly influences our ability or inability to modify behavior with basic techniques (Klingberg, 2007). Salem *et al.* (2012) found that dental fear and anxiety were more influenced by temperament than parental influence. Parents/guardians should be informed regarding limitations imposed by a child's behavior on the practitioner's ability to provide quality care. Societal and parental influences are also increasingly influential in our ability to guide behavior (Juntgen *et al.*, 2013). Diverse ethnic communities and various cultural influences increasingly impact our behavior guidance and the compliance of parents/guardians (Goleman, 2014). Nonpharmalogic techniques using tell–show–do, desensitization, modeling, and distraction have proven to be successful, especially for a child who is purely fearful or mildly apprehensive.

Nonpharmacologic Guidance Techniques

Distraction

Distraction is a communicative technique. There is strong evidence supporting the efficacy of distraction for needle-related pain and distress in children and adolescents (Uman *et al.*, 2013). Offering the child a hand mirror to watch the procedure while it is being performed, watching a minute timer, having the child rub his or her palms together, and squeezing a rubber ball may provide distraction for a mildly anxious, but cooperative child (Figures 23.1, 23.2, 23.3, and 23.4). Inhaling lavender oil for 3 minutes prior to a procedure may also be effective to reduce anxiety (Arslan *et al.*, 2020). Telling a story and asking about a family pet (guessing the pet's name, color, etc.) are methods to engage and relax the school-age child during a restorative procedure. He or she can answer with one finger for "yes" and two fingers for "no." Counting backward slowly from 20 or 30, while interjecting comments to increase the amount of time to get to 1, and talking about a movie, song, or anything that might be of interest to the child also engage the child. Audiovisual glasses to watch a movie, watching a ceiling-mounted television ,or listening to patient-chosen music are further

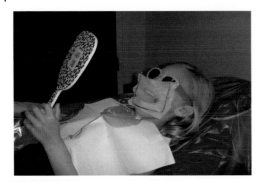

Figure 23.1 Mirror for distraction.

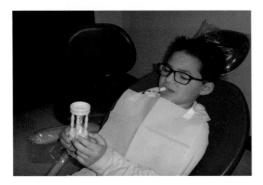

Figure 23.2 Minute timer for distraction.

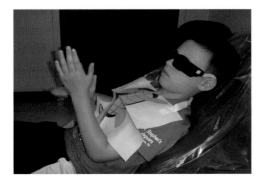

Figure 23.3 Rubbing palms together to reduce anxiety.

very effective distractions for a mildly anxious child (Al-Khotani *et al.*, 2016; Zhang *et al.*, 2019; Custodio *et al.*, 2020) (Figure 23.5a, b). (Distraction is also discussed in Chapter 3 on local anesthesia.)

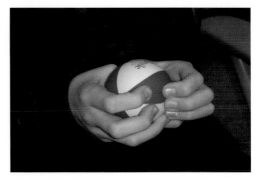

Figure 23.4 Squeezing a soft rubber ball for mild anxiety.

Gagging is fairly common, presents a barrier to care, occurs more often in males, is a manifestation of dental fear, and decreases with age (Katsouda *et al.*, 2020). Gagging is a physiologic manifestation of fear and anxiety that parents/guardians and children feel cannot be modified (Katsouda *et al.*, 2019). A gag reflex may be altered by putting pressure with the eraser end of a pencil into the palm of the hand at the point where the long axis of the middle finger and thumb meet (Scarborough *et al.*, 2008) (Figure 23.6). Another acupressure technique, which may reduce mild anxiety, is squeezing the fleshy area of the hand between the index finger and thumb (Figure 23.7). Bending the leg on the opposite side of the tooth being treated and pressing the foot into the chair are also effective methods to deter a gag reflex (Figure 23.8).

Permitting the child to request a break or communicate can give him or her a sense of control. Escape is a guidance technique in which brief, intermittent breaks may be taken. Permitting a child to leave the operatory chair for a drink of water after the local anesthesia is administered is a good method for reframing to change mindset and an example of escape (Baghdadi, 2001) (Figure 23.9). However, asking a child to tell you anything that is troubling them will focus their attention on potential pain and lead to distress. For example, if you ask a child to raise his or her hand if something is wrong, the hand may be

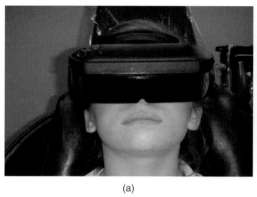
(a)

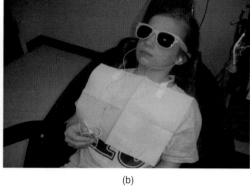
(b)

Figure 23.5 (a) Audiovisual distraction with audiovisual glasses to watch a movie. (b) Auditory distraction with earphones and music.

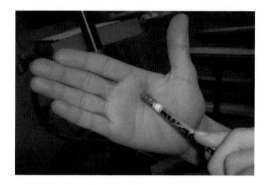

Figure 23.6 Palm pressure to reduce anxiety and decrease gage reflex.

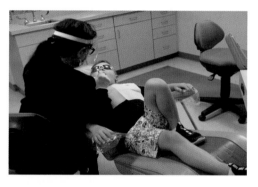

Figure 23.8 Bending leg and pressing foot into the chair to decrease gag reflex.

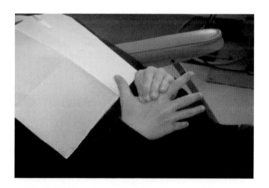

Figure 23.7 Squeezing fleshy area between index finger and thumb to reduce anxiety and gagging.

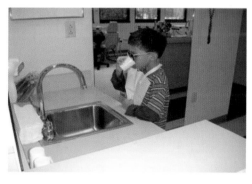

Figure 23.9 Reframing to change mindset.

constantly raised throughout the procedure (Figure 23.10). Asking a child to report discomfort can prompt him or her to focus on possible pain and provoke negative behavior.

Instead, the dentist should constantly evaluate the child for discomfort. Dilated pupils may indicate fear and the need for more empathy and verbal support.

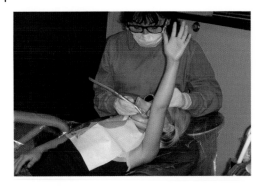

Figure 23.10 Child raising hand during operative procedure in response to anything troubling.

Watching television or playing computer games before a dental visit may relax a child (Campbell *et al.*, 2005). Sitting quietly beside a parent/guardian who is reading a story before treatment may be helpful for an apprehensive child. Systematic desensitization is also useful to reduce anxiety. An effort is made to begin treatment with a procedure that would evoke minimal fear and progress toward more fear-provoking stimuli (Widmer *et al.*, 2008). Think about desensitizing when determining the sequence of a treatment plan, considering local anesthesia and the length of the procedures. Davidovich *et al.* (2013) determined that treatment duration was the main factor influencing behavior for younger and older children. Treatment time should not exceed 30 minutes.

Tell–Show–Do

Tell–show–do, to explain what to expect, is a good tool for guidance at any age, but may begin with the toddler. The procedure is described in as few words as possible, the materials to be used are shown to the child, and the procedure begins (AAPD, 2019–2020) (Figure 23.11a,b). Start with the maxillary incisors, desensitizing the child, before examining or performing prophylaxis on molars.

Direct Observation

Direct observation is an effective method to familiarize a child and/or parent/guardian with a procedure, also providing the opportunity for them to ask questions prior to the procedure. Direct observation may also be helpful for a parent/guardian, who believes a procedure may be too difficult for his or her child to cooperate, by viewing a cooperative child of similar or younger age undergoing the planned treatment. A term for this type of observation is "modeling." Incorporating a video or modeling offer additional types of communicative management technique, in an innocuous environment, prior to actual treatment (AAPD, 2019–2020). Modeling is typically not beneficial until the age of 4 years. Unless the modeling is with a sibling, the parents/guardians of both children should give

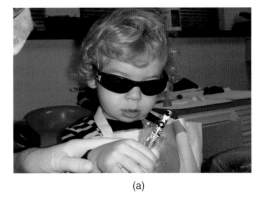

(a)

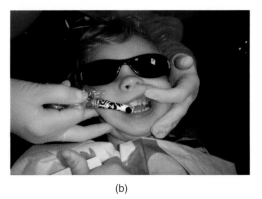

(b)

Figure 23.11 (a) Telling the child about the procedure and showing the prophy angle. (b) Doing the procedure.

Figure 23.12 Direct observation or modeling.

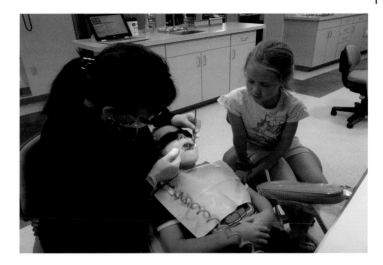

consent for this method of behavior guidance (Figure 23.12).

Voice Control

Voice control is a form of behavior guidance that uses the tone of voice, loudness, or pace to gain cooperation or attention. Parents/guardians should be advised of this technique before use, as some may deem voice control unacceptable (AAPD, 2019–2020). School-age or older children would be preferable for this form of guidance.

Memory Restructuring

Memory restructuring may be used after difficult experiences to focus on the positive aspects of the visit and to extinguish memories of negative aspects. There are four components to restructuring. First, a positive visual reminder, such as a photograph of the child smiling at the time of the initial visit, is shown to the child. Second, the child is reminded of the good job he or she did during a negative experience, and/or of what he or she said to the parent/guardian regarding some positive aspect of the last appointment. Third, the child is praised for anything he or she did to cooperate, such as keeping his or her hands on the lap or opening the mouth wide. Last, the

child demonstrates those behaviors, leading to a sense of accomplishment. The objective of restructuring is to modify behavior with the hope of improvement of behavior for future treatment (AAPD, 2019–2020).

Ask–Tell–Ask

Ask–tell–ask is a technique that involves asking the patient about any concerns for planned procedures, teaching the patient about the procedure with photographs or demonstrations, and finally asking once again about any concerns. This approach explains the procedure, insures the patient's comfort with the procedure, and may curtail uncooperative behavior during treatment prior to proceeding. Consideration of the patient's age and cognitive level is required for this technique (AAPD, 2019–2020).

Parent/Guardian Presence

Contemporary parents/guardians overwhelmingly prefer to be present for treatment (Schroff *et al.*, 2015). A latent, but normal, sense of protection is an emotional need for them. Parents' involvement, along with their questions and concerns, should be welcomed (AAPD,

2019–2020). Kim *et al.* (2012) found that parents who are permitted to choose to be present or absent for the dental visit were more satisfied with the visit, had a more positive attitude toward the dentist, and had a more positive perception of their child's response to the visit. The parent/guardian should be present for treatment for children younger than 4 years and for those with special healthcare needs. Parents/guardians of autistic children will be especially helpful with their knowledge of stress cues and tolerance level.

The parent/guardian who is present is termed the dentist's "silent partner," stressing that his or her mere presence is support for the child. Explain the dentist's need to give the child his or her undivided attention and that the dentist and staff want the child's undivided attention in return (Soxman, 2013). Jain *et al.* (2013) found that 82% of parents comply with these instructions. Instructions to the parent/guardian to remain a passive observer should not adversely impact their satisfaction (Rodriguez *et al.*, 2018). Historical and contemporary studies show that behavior is no different or is improved by parental presence (Vasiliki *et al.*, 2016; Pani *et al.*, 2016).

If the child is doing well and the attending parent/guardian is calm and quiet, he or she may be encouraged to continue to accompany the child for each visit. Changing the attending parent/guardian may negatively impact the child's behavior. However, if the parent/guardian who is present is constantly interjecting comments, repeating the dentist's requests, appears to be very anxious, or has a dental phobia, another parent/guardian or a close relative should be invited to accompany the child. Well- intentioned reassurance such as "Don't worry, everything will be okay" or empathy such as "I know it hurts" by parent/guardians or team members is distress promoting and will negatively impact the child's behavior (Townsend & Wells, 2018).

After a few visits, most parents/guardians do not feel the need to be present for treatment. Separating sends two messages to the child: that the parent/guardian believes the child is capable of undergoing treatment without his or her presence; and also that he or she trusts the dentist. A trusting parent/guardian typically has a trusting child. If a parent/guardian remains in the reception room and the child begins to cry or becomes hysterical, the parent/guardian should be brought to the operatory. In some instances, this may be helpful to complete the procedure. Often, the crying begins with the simple act of placing topical anesthetic. If a parent/guardian perceives improper behavioral guidance by the dentist or staff, ensuing complaints or other problems are likely. Parents/guardians who hear the child crying need to see what is provoking this reaction and receive reassurance of the child's wellbeing. Once the parent/guardian is by the child's side, the door to the operatory may be closed for privacy and to avoid distress for other patients.

Age-Appropriate Expectations

An age-appropriate approach insures that expectations of the dentist, staff, and parent/guardian are realistic regarding the child's ability to cooperate. Toddlers are developing a sense of independence, but a strong attachment to the parent is appropriately present until the age of 2 years. Once a high level of distress is reached, calming the toddler is difficult. If the child is crying or exhibiting avoidance behavior, examine the child as quickly as possible to determine the existence of caries or pathology. The knee-to-knee examination for children 0–2 years of age provides safe, adequate immobilization and ideal visualization for the examination with a positive parental response (Figure 23.13) (Fux-Noy *et al.*, 2020). Apprehensive 2- or 3-year-old children may sit on the parent/guardian's lap for examination or a preventive care visit

Figure 23.13
Knee-to-knee
examination.

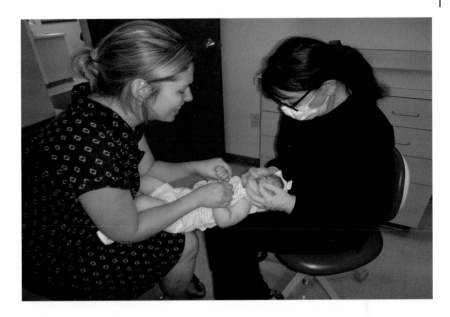

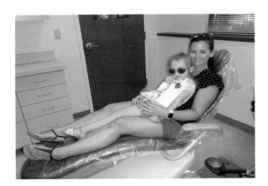

Figure 23.14 Apprehensive young child on parent's lap.

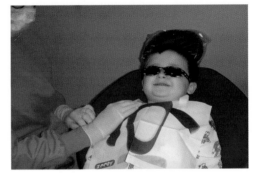

Figure 23.15 Placing hand on child's shoulder before reclining chair.

(Figure 23.14). A neck pillow may be offered for neck support for the parent/guardian. To avoid startling a child, place your hand on his or her shoulder before reclining the chair, while explaining that the chair is going to move backward (Figure 23.15).

Suggest ideas for preparing the preschooler for the first visit, such as the parent/guardian reading a story about going to the dentist, using a reclining chair at home for the child to experience the sensation of the chair moving backward, and using a battery-powered spin brush. Showing positive previsit imagery immediately before the visit can remind families what to expect and facilitate communication (AAPD, 2019–2020). Preschool-age children are in the midst of multiple inoculations; fear of a "shot" may be the predominant concern (Salem *et al.*, 2012). Most preschool children are learning the ABCs and most children can count to 10 by the age of 3 years. Saying the ABCs or counting the teeth during the examination provides distraction and familiarity. Explaining that each baby tooth has a letter and spelling the child's name, touching each tooth with a letter of his or her name, is very engaging. Introduce the mouth mirror by touching the inside of his or her cheek while describing the softness of the mirror. Explain that because you are touching baby teeth, you must be gentle, just as you would be with a baby. Pretending is common play for the preschool child.

The school-age child should be able to sit still and focus. He or she now understands consequences. Competence is gaining value in his or her life, and so accomplishing treatment goals is important not only for the dentist, but also for the child. Positive reinforcement and descriptive praise can help build this sense of accomplishment while shaping desired behaviors (AAPD, 2019–2020). If fearful behavior prohibits completion of the planned procedure, make an effort to accomplish something so the child does not leave the office with a sense of failure. In the same manner, do not permit combative or avoidance behavior to postpone treatment, possibly guaranteeing the same behavior in a manipulative child at the next appointment. Placing sealants is a good procedure to use modeling for behavior guidance.

Advanced Behavior Guidance

Advanced behavior guidance techniques, including protective stabilization, should be considered if behavior does not permit provision of care and lack of treatment would result in pain and/or poor results (McWhorter & Townsend, 2014). Protective stabilization may be performed by the parent/guardian, dentist, or staff, minimizing risks of injury to the child, the parent/guardian, dentist, or staff, and/or enabling the completion of treatment (AAPD, 2019–2020). A parent/guardian may be willing to assist with gently stabilizing a young child for an examination or restorative treatment (Figure 23.16). A parent/guardian straddling the chair is particularly good for this type of assistance for a very young child (Figure 23.17). If the child exhibits extreme fear or hysterical

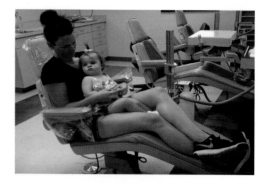

Figure 23.16 Parent stabilizing an apprehensive child.

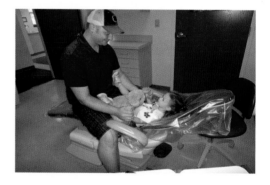

Figure 23.17 Father straddling the chair and assisting with stabilization.

behavior, the stabilization should be released, and the procedure stopped as quickly as possible. Parents/guardians are increasingly concerned about behavior guidance techniques that they perceive as adverse, such as protective stabilization, so written informed consent prior to use and appropriate documentation are advised (AAPD, 2019–2020).

Mouth Props

The Parkell dry-field posterior mouth prop (Parkell, Edgewood, NY, USA) is made of clear, autoclavable plastic, providing a dry field, throat partition, and retraction of the cheek and tongue (Figure 23.18a). An anterior version, to restore an incisor, is also available (Figure 23.18b). The Open Wide® Disposable

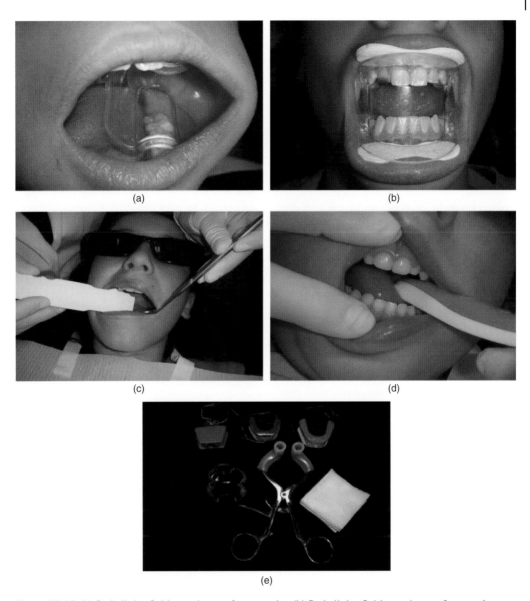

Figure 23.18 (a) Parkell dry-field mouth prop for posterior. (b) Parkell dry-field mouth prop for anterior. (c) Open Wide disposable mouth rest. (d) Toothbrush with rubber handle for mouth prop. (e) Mckesson mouth props, Molt mouth prop, posterior Parkell dry-field mouth prop.

Mouth Rest (Specialized Care Company, Hampton, NH, USA) can be used with any age of child who is unwilling to open his or her mouth or who is unable to reliably maintain an open mouth. This mouth prop is especially useful for children with special needs (Figure 23.18c). The rubber handle of a pediatric toothbrush may also be used (Figure 23.18d). Rubber McKesson mouth props (McKesson, Irving, TX, USA) come in various sizes and are available from many dental supply companies. Molt mouth props work well during sedation or general anesthesia. A few pieces of 2 × 2 gauze should be placed between the cheek and the mouth prop to avoid pressure/injury to the cheek; take care that the lip is not trapped under the mouth prop (Figure 23.18e). The use of a mouth prop in a cooperative child is not considered protective stabilization (AAPD, 2019–2020).

Isolation for Restorative Procedures

Isolation may be challenging in the pediatric population. The floor of the mouth is higher, protective reflexes are diminished, and the tongue is disproportionately large. The rubber dam often incites a strong negative response. Although it provides a reliable throat partition, moisture control, and tongue retraction, an open mouth narrows the oropharyngeal area, significantly reducing the volume of upper airway patency and decreasing tidal volume (Iwatani *et al.*, 2013). If the rubber dam is covering the child's nose, that portion may be cut away with scissors, providing more ventilation and/or less intimidating isolation (Figure 23.19). The term "rubber mustache" is an amusing description for the piece of rubber that is cut from the rubber dam. The use of a Breathe-Right® Nasal Strip (Foundation Consumer Brands, Pittsburgh, PA, USA) can also be very effective to improve airflow through the nose. Isolite® and Isodry® (Zyris, Goleta, CA, USA) provide

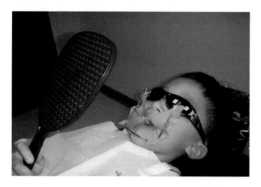

Figure 23.19 Rubber dam with a portion under nose cut away.

a generally well-excepted alternative with a single-use, latex-free unit in various sizes, cheek retractor, throat partition, suction, and an optional light source (Figure 23.20a). This offers easy access and isolation for a partially erupted permanent second molar and the ability to restore the ipsilateral maxillary and mandibular quadrants without removal. The continuous suction also appears to provide a source of distraction and decreases splatter and aerosol. If necessary, the Isolite and Isodry can easily be trimmed with scissors for more custom sizing. Mr. Thirsty® (Zirc, Buffalo, MN, USA) and DryShield® (DryShield, Fountain Valley, CA, USA) have similar features, but DryShield is autoclavable (Figure 23.20b, c). The rubber dam may be preferable for a strong gag reflex and for children younger than 4 years.

Radiographs

When taking radiographs, position the cone head before placing the film, sensor, or plate in the child's mouth. If using conventional radiography with a size 0 film that is too uncomfortable, the film may be bent or positioned vertically (Figure 23.21). Digital sensors cannot be bent. Phosphor plates are smaller, thinner, and more flexible, but bending may damage them. Permit the child to place the film in his or her mouth using a Snap-A-Ray (Dentsply Sirona, York, PA, USA) or similar device, if he or she is reluctant to permit placement by staff or the dentist. Telling the child to open his or her eyes as wide as possible and using a mirror to watch film placement or to lift a foot off the chair are good distraction techniques (Figure 23.22). For a gag reflex, have the child bend his or her knee and press his or her foot into the chair. Placing a small amount of child-flavored toothpaste on the film packet can also decrease gagging. If unable to obtain a traditional anterior periapical radiograph, a size 4 film bent in the middle is an option (Figure 23.23a–b).

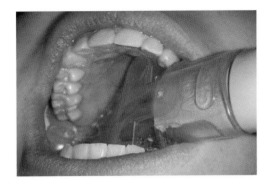

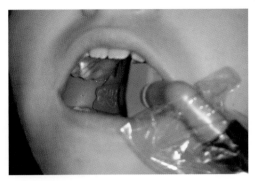

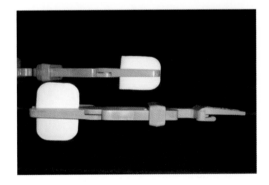

Figure 23.20 (a) Isolite. (b) Mr. Thirsty. (c) DryShield.

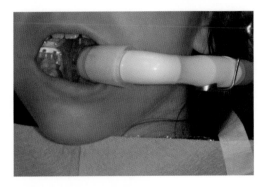

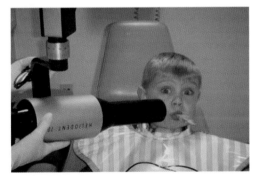

Figure 23.21 Size 0 film bent or placed vertically in a Snap-A-Ray film holder.

Figure 23.22 Eyes wide open for distraction.

Eye Protection

Sunglasses or "fun glasses" shield sensitive young eyes from the bright chair light. They also provide eye protection from splatter and protection from injury with an instrument because of unanticipated movement or accidental dropping. Multicolored sunglasses with various designs can be inexpensively purchased in bulk. Permitting the child to select his or her glasses before the procedure provides a good start, offering a choice. Other options for disposable eye protection are wrap-around glasses (manufactured by Rollens, Centennial, CO, USA) or glasses with adjustable temples, typically used after eye dilation, in adult and child sizes (Practicon, Greenville, NC,

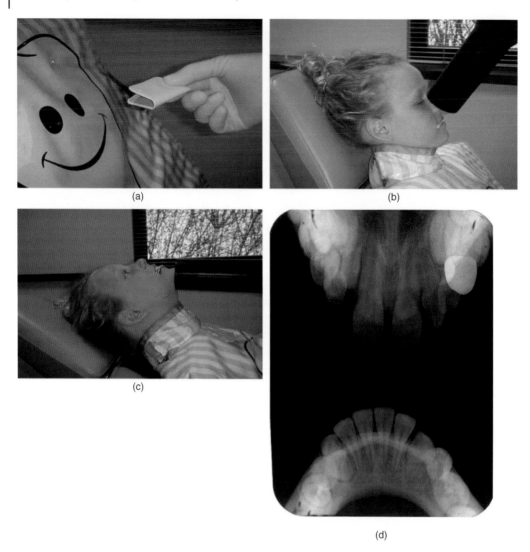

Figure 23.23 (a) Size 4 film bent in the middle to obtain upper/lower occlusal radiograph. (b) Obtaining upper occlusal view with size 4 film. (c) Obtaining lower occlusal view with size 4 film. (d) Upper/lower occlusal radiographic views with size 4 film.

USA) (Figure 23.24a, b). Parents/guardians appreciate the thoughtfulness of reducing the brightness of the light in the child's eyes and providing eye protection.

Frankl Behavioral Rating Scale

This scale uses numbers from 1 to 4 to describe specific behaviors. A rating of 4 is a positive rating given to a cooperative, engaging child.

A rating of 3 is used for mild apprehension or reluctance, and a need for some additional behavior guidance to obtain full cooperation. A rating of 2 describes an uncooperative child, and a rating of 1 indicates fearfulness and/or strong avoidance or combative behavior (AAPD, 2019–2020).

Behavior guidance may be the most challenging aspect of treating pediatric patients. Strong avoidance and combative, hysterical, and/or defiant behaviors prevent our ability

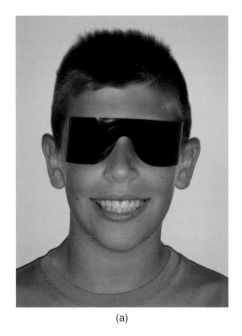

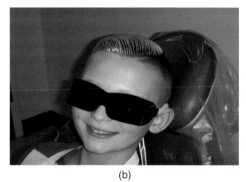

(a)   (b)

Figure 23.24 (a) Disposable wrap-around glasses. (b) Disposable glasses with adjustable temples.

to safely perform restorative treatment and reduce the quality of care we provide. Whenever possible, active surveillance to await more maturity or improved coping skills may be recommended for early lesions. Alternatives to conventional restorations with noninvasive or minimally invasive treatment are discussed in Chapter 1. Restorative appointments should be scheduled during the morning for young children. If sedation or general anesthesia is deemed necessary for treatment, rationale may include young age, acute stress reaction, extent of caries, and medical or emotional circumstances.

References

Al-Khotani, A., Bello, L.A., & Christidis, N. (2016) Effects of audiovisual distraction on children's behaviour during dental treatment: a randomized controlled clinical trial. *Acta Odontologica Scandinavica*, 74, 494–501.

American Academy of Pediatric Dentistry. (2019–2020) Behavior guidance for the pediatric dental patient. *The Reference Manual of Pediatric Dentistry*. Chicago, IL: American Academy of Pediatric Dentistry; 266–279.

Arslan, I., Aydinoglu, S., & Karan, N.B. (2020) Can lavender oil inhalation help to overcome dental anxiety and pain in children? A randomized clinical trial. *European Journal of Pediatrics*, 179, 985–992.

Baghdadi, Z.D. (2001) Principles and application of learning theory in child patient management. *Quintessence International*, 32, 135–141.

Campbell, C., Hosey, M.-T., & McHugh, S. (2005) Coping behavior in children prior to dental general anesthesia: a randomized controlled trail. *Pediatric Anesthesia*, 15, 831–838.

Custodio, N.B., Dos Santos Costa, F., Cademartori, M.G., Pereira da Costa, V.P., & Goettems, M.L. (2020) Effectiveness of virtual reality glasses as a distraction for children during dental care. *Pediatric Dentistry*, 42, 93–100.

Davidovich, E., Wated, A., Shapira, J., & Ram, D. (2013) The influence of location of local anesthesia and complexity/duration of restorative treatment on children's behavior during dental treatment. *Pediatric Dentistry*, 35, 333–336.

Fux-Noy, A., Shmueli, A., Herzog, K., Halperson, E., Moskovitz, M., & Ram, D. (2020) Attitudes of EAPD members toward using the "knee-to-knee" position. *European Archives of Paediatric Dentistry*, 21, 687–691. doi:10.1007/s40368-020-00514-0.

Goleman, J. (2014) Cultural factors affecting behavior guidance and family compliance. *Pediatric Dentistry*, 36, 121–127.

Iwatani, K., Matsuo, K., Kawase, S., Wakimoto, N., Taguchi, A., & Ogasawara, T. (2013) Effects of open mouth and rubber dam on upper airway patency and breathing. *Clinical Oral Investigation*, 17, 1295–1299.

Jain, C., Mathu-Muju, K.R., Nash, D.A., Bush, H.M., Li, H.-F., & Nash, P.P. (2013) Randomized controlled trial: parental compliance with instructions to remain silent in the dental operatory. *Pediatric Dentistry*, 35, 47–51.

Juntgen, L.M., Sanders, B.J., Walker, L.A., Jones, J.E., Weddell, J.A., *et al.* (2013) Factors influencing behavior guidance: a survey of practicing pediatric dentists. *Pediatric Dentistry*, 35, 539–545.

Katsouda, M., Coolidge, T., Simos, G., Kotsanos, N., & Arapostathis, K.N. (2020) Factors associated with gagging during radiographic and intraoral photographic examinations in 4–12-year-old children. *European Archives of Paediatric Dentistry*. doi:10.1007/s40368-020-00535-9.

Katsouda, M., Tollill, C., Coolidge, T., Simos, G., Kotsanos, N., & Arapostathis, K.N. (2019) Gagging prevalence and its association with dental fear in 4–12-year-old children in a dental setting. *International Journal of Paediatric Dentistry*, 29 (2), 169–176. doi:10.1111/ipd.12445.

Kim, J.S., Boynton, J.R., & Inglehart, M.R. (2012) Parents' presence in the operatory during their child's dental visit: a person-environmental fit analysis of parents' perception. *Pediatric Dentistry*, 34, 407–413.

McWhorter, A.G. & Townsend, J.A. (2014) Behavior symposium workshop a report – current guidelines revision. *Pediatric Dentistry*, 36, 152–153.

Pani, S.C., AlAnazi, G.S., AlBaragash, A., & AlMosaihel, M. (2016) Objective assessment of the influence of the parental presence on the fear and behavior of anxious children during their first restorative dental visit. *Journal of International Society of Preventive and Community Dentistry*, 6 (suppl 2), S148–S152.

Rodriguez, H.K., Webman, M.S., Arvealo, O., Roldan, R., & Saman, D.M. (2018) Passive observer instruction on parental satisfaction in a dental setting. *Journal of Clinical Pediatric Dentistry*, 42, 339–343.

Salem, K., Kousha, M., Anissian, A., & Shahabi, A. (2012) Dental fear and concomitant factors in 3–6-year-old children. *Journal of Dental Research, Dental Clinics, Dental Prospects*, 6, 70–74.

Scarborough, D., Bailey-Van Kuren, M., & Hughes, M. (2008) Altering the gag reflex via a palm pressure point. *Journal of the American Dental Association*, 139, 1365–1372.

Shroff S., Hughes C., & Mobley C. (2015) Attitudes and preferences of parents about being present in the dental operatory. *Pediatric Dentistry*, 37, 51–55.

Soxman, J. (2013) Parental presence. *General Dentistry*, 61, 2–3.

Townsend J.A. & Wells M. (2018) Behavior guidance of the pediatric dental patient, In: Nowak, A., Christensen, J., Mabry, T., Townsend, J., & Wells, M. (eds.), *Pediatric Dentistry*, 6th edn. Philadelphia, PA: Elsevier; 352–370.

Uman, L.S., Birnie, K.A., Noel, M., Parker, J.A., Chambers, C.T., *et al.* (2013) Psychological interventions for needle-related procedural pain and distress in children and adolescents. *Cochrane Database of Systematic Reviews*, 10,

CD005179. doi:10.1002/14651858.CD005179. pub3.

Vasiliki, B., Konstantinos, A., Vassilis, K., Nikolaos, K., van Loveren, C., & Jaap, V. (2016) The effect of parental presence on the child's perception and co-operation during dental treatment. *European Archives of Paediatric Dentistry*, 17, 381–386.

Widmer, R., McNeil, D.W., McNeil, C.B., McDonald, J., Alcaino, E.A., & Cooper, M.G. (2008) Child management. In: Cameron, A.C. & Widmer, R.P. (eds.), *Handbook of Pediatric Dentistry*, 3rd edn. London: Mosby; 9–37.

Zhang, C., Qin, D., Shen, L., Ji, P., & Wang, J. (2019) Does audiovisual distraction reduce dental anxiety in children under local anesthesia? A systematic review and meta-analysis. *Oral Disease*, 25, 416–424.

24

Caries Risk Assessment
Christel M. Haberland

Dental caries is a multifactorial and chronic disease process that extends from infection to demineralization and eventually to cavitation. In 2001, the National Institutes of Health (NIH) Consensus Statement officially recognized the paradigm shift in caries management toward the more conservative treatment of caries (National Institutes of Health, 2001). This change consisted of replacement of the surgical management of dental caries with improved prevention, diagnosis, and early treatment of noncavitated lesions. Historically, caries was considered a disease that eventually destroyed the tooth unless the dentist intervened surgically. We now understand that while dental restorations can repair tooth structure, they have a limited life span and are susceptible to the caries disease process. More importantly, they do not stop the process. Therefore, it is crucial to identify and arrest the caries disease process at an early stage. To that end, the American Dental Association (ADA) currently recommends using systematic methods of caries detection, classification, risk assessment, and prevention/risk management strategies (ADA, 2018).

Caries risk assessment (CRA) is the determination of the probability of a patient developing new carious lesions over a specific period and/or the likelihood that there will be changes in the severity or activity of any currently present lesions (Fontana & González-Cabezas, 2019; Riley *et al.*, 2011). To assess the risk for caries development or progression, clinicians need to identify clinical and nonclinical indicators of future caries development (Chaffee *et al.*, 2017).

Many variables may directly or indirectly influence caries risk and include clinical/biologic factors (e.g., previous caries experience of child and caregiver, plaque/microbiology, gingivitis, saliva, developmental tooth defects, health history, genetics); environmental factors (e.g., exposure to fluoride, antibiotic usage); and behavioral/psychosocial/sociodemographic factors (e.g., diet, oral hygiene habits, age, parenting styles, child temperament, beliefs, caregiver's education level, socioeconomic status, insurance status, access to dental care) (Fontana, 2015).

Furthermore, the variables involved in the caries disease process can be classified as either protective or pathologic. This phenomenon is explained using the caries balance and imbalance model. This model was created to emphasize the importance of the balance between pathologic and protective factors involved in the carious disease process (Fontana & González-Cabezas, 2000; Featherstone, 2006; Featherstone *et al.*, 2007) (Figure 24.1).

If the pathologic factors prevail over the protective factors, the caries disease process progresses. Accordingly, a CRA tool should determine the balance between protective factors and pathologic factors and also include the disease indicators, which are either the

Handbook of Clinical Techniques in Pediatric Dentistry, Second Edition. Edited by Jane A. Soxman.

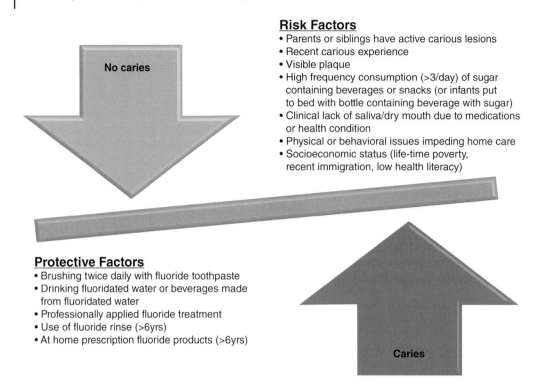

Risk Factors
- Parents or siblings have active carious lesions
- Recent carious experience
- Visible plaque
- High frequency consumption (>3/day) of sugar containing beverages or snacks (or infants put to bed with bottle containing beverage with sugar)
- Clinical lack of saliva/dry mouth due to medications or health condition
- Physical or behavioral issues impeding home care
- Socioeconomic status (life-time poverty, recent immigration, low health literacy)

No caries

Protective Factors
- Brushing twice daily with fluoride toothpaste
- Drinking fluoridated water or beverages made from fluoridated water
- Professionally applied fluoride treatment
- Use of fluoride rinse (>6yrs)
- At home prescription fluoride products (>6yrs)

Caries

Figure 24.1 Caries imbalance: risk factors vs. protective factors for caries. Source: Modified from Featherstone (2006).

presence of current active initial lesions (i.e., enamel lesions or white spots) or existing active lesions (cavitations). Based on these findings, it establishes a category of risk: low, medium, or high. It primarily seeks to identify patients at the highest risk of disease, to guide treatment decisions, and to determine appropriate recalls (Christian *et al.*, 2018).

There are several CRA tools in use today, including tools from the ADA and the American Academy of Pediatric Dentistry (AAPD), and tools based on the Caries Management by Risk Assessment (CAMBRA) philosophy, as well as software-based prediction tools such as Cariogram (Halasa-Rappel *et al.*, 2019). The ADA CRA tools were designed for children 0 through 6 years of age (ADA, 2011a) and patients older than 6 years (ADA, 2011b). For this tool, the absence of moderate- or high-risk factors places a patient in a low-risk category, and high risk exists when

at least one high-risk factor is identified or if the overall score exceeds 9. The AAPD tools were designed for children 0 through 5 years of age and patients who are 6 years and older (AAPD, 2019–2020). A patient is considered at low risk in the absence of moderate- or high-risk factors and high risk when the presence of at least one high-risk factor is identified. The CAMBRA tool was designed for children ages 0 through 5 years and for patients 6 years and older (Featherstone & Chaffee, 2018). A patient is classified as at low, moderate, high, or extremely high risk based on clinical judgment, addressing the balance among disease indicators and pathologic and preventive factors. The CARIOGRAM tool is a computer program that graphically represents the patient's risk for developing new caries in the future, which is expressed as a percentage "chance to avoid new caries" (Bratthall & Hänsel Petersson, 2005). This tool consists of

Table 24.1 Links for available CRA tools.

ADA CRA TOOL 0–6 yrs	https://www.ada.org/en/~/media/ADA/Member%20Center/FIles/topics_caries_under6
ADA CRA TOOL >6 yrs	http://www.ada.org/~/media/ADA/Science%20and%20Research/Files/topic_caries_over6.ashx
AAPD CRA TOOL 0–5 yrs	https://www.aapd.org/media/Policies_Guidelines/BP_CariesRiskAssessment.pdf
AAPD CRA TOOL ≥6 yrs	https://www.aapd.org/media/Policies_Guidelines/BP_CariesRiskAssessment.pdf
CAMBRA 0–5 yrs	https://www.cdafoundation.org/Portals/0/pdfs/cambra_handbook.pdf
CAMBRA ≥6 yrs	https://www.cdafoundation.org/Portals/0/pdfs/cambra_handbook.pdf
CARIOGRAM	https://www.mah.se/upload/FAKULTETER/OD/cariogram%20program%20caries/cariogmanual201net.pdf

nine items and the risk level is generated based on a predetermined "weighted" algorithm. Links for accessing these CRA tools are given in Table 24.1.

The CRA tools listed collect similar information on the protective and pathologic factors involved in the caries disease process, just with slight variations. To compare them, Table 24.2 lists the different factors and disease indicators collected for each CRA tool for patients under 6 years of age, and Table 24.3 lists those for patients over 6 years of age.

In 2018 the ADA convened an expert panel discussion on guidance for CRA in children (ADA, 2018). They reviewed the current literature on CRA in children and developed a comprehensive guide on the categorization of risk to educate, treatment plan, and improve care for dental caries. They focused on the individual factors that were predictive of caries risk to include them in the CRA tool, and considered the strength of those associations and how to weigh them in determining the overall caries risk status. Their literature review and discussion lead to the identification of 15 factors that were predictive of caries risk (Table 24.4).

The ADA panel also discussed the impact of socioeconomic status (SES) and caries risk. They found that although there is significant evidence supporting a strong correlation between SES and caries experience (Schwendicke *et al.*, 2015), there was not enough evidence to establish that SES is a risk factor apart from the other disease indicators/risk factors identified in Table 24.4. The panel concluded that SES can be included in establishing a patient's caries risk status, but that it should be based on individual determinants such as lifetime poverty, recent immigration, and low health literacy, and not by more generalized determinants such as "belonging to a government plan" (e.g., Medicaid, CHIP, Head Start).

The CRA tools analyzed by the panel used the 15 factors identified in the table and addressed risk based on combinations of different factors rather than single risk factors. However, to date, there is limited evidence to determine the combination or weighting of risk factors to define distinct risk categories (Twetman, 2016). A risk factor's predictive ability and, therefore, the validity of any CRA tool will vary with the baseline prevalence of the disease in the defined population in which it is being used. Thus, the ADA panel advised practitioners that it is essential to assess caries risk by educating patients/caregivers and managing modifiable risk factors based on the best available evidence, despite the limited evidence on whether assessing caries risk by itself results in improved oral health (Tinanoff *et al.*, 2019). They concluded that current or

Table 24.2 Comparison of CRA tools for 0–5-year-old patients.

	ADA*	AAPD	CAMBRA	CARIOGRAM
Risk factors/ contributing conditions	Sugary foods or drinks (including juice, carbonated or noncarbonated soft drinks, energy drinks, medicinal syrups)	Child has frequent exposure (>3 times/day) to between-meal sugar-containing snacks or beverages per day	Frequent snacking (>3 times daily)	Dietary sugar content (fermentable carbohydrates) (very low, low, moderate, or high content)
	Eligible for government programs (WIC, Head Start, Medicaid or SCHIP)	Child uses bottle or nonspill cup containing natural or added sugar frequently, between meals, and/or at bedtime	Uses bottle/nonspill cup containing other than water or milk	Frequency of daily meals and snacks (very low, low, high, very high)
	Caries experience of mother, caregiver, and/or other siblings	Mother/primary caregiver has active dental caries	Mother/primary caregiver or sibling has current decay or a recent history of decay	
		Parent/caregiver has a lifetime of poverty and low health literacy	Family has low socioeconomic/health literacy status	
		Child is a recent immigrant		
Protective factors	Fluoride exposure (through drinking water, supplements, professional applications, toothpaste)	Child receives optimally fluoridated drinking water or fluoride supplements	Lives in a fluoridated drinking water area	Fluoride exposure assessment (fluoride toothpaste and constant use of additional fluoride measures; fluoride toothpaste plus occasional use of additional measures; fluoride toothpaste only; fluoride not used in any form)
	Dental home: established patient of record in a dental office	Child has teeth brushed daily with fluoridated toothpaste	Drinks fluoridated water	
		Child receives topical fluoride from health professional	Uses fluoride-containing toothpaste at least two times daily (a smear for ages 0–2 years and pea size for ages 3–6 years)	
		Child has dental home/ regular dental care	Has had fluoride varnish applied in the last 6 months	

Table 24.2 (Continued)

	ADA[a]	AAPD	CAMBRA	CARIOGRAM
Clinical findings/conditions	Visual or radiographically evident restorations/cavitated carious lesions	Child has noncavitated (incipient/white spot) caries or enamel defects	Heavy plaque on the teeth	Caries experience (DMFT, DMFS, new caries experience in the past one year)
	Noncavitated (incipient) carious lesions	Child has visible cavities or fillings or missing teeth due to caries	Evident tooth decay or white spots	Silness-Löe Plaque Index (no plaque, some plaque not visible to the naked eye, moderate plaque visible, abundant plaque)
	Teeth missing due to caries	Child has visible plaque on teeth	Recent restorations in last 2 years (new patient) or the last year (patient of record)	
	Visible plaque			Stimulated saliva secretion rate
	Dental/orthodontic appliances present (fixed or removable)			Saliva buffering capacity (chairside test)
	Salivary flow (low)			Estimation of *Mutans streptococci* in saliva (chairside testing)
General health conditions	Special healthcare needs (developmental, physical, medical, or mental disabilities that prevent or limit the performance of adequate oral healthcare by the child or caregivers)	Child has special healthcare needs	Medications that induce hyposalivation	Related general diseases or conditions associated with caries risk

a) ADA tool is for 0–6-year-olds.

Table 24.3 Comparison of CRA tools for ≥6-year-old patients.

	ADA	AAPD	CAMBRA	CARIOGRAM*
Risk factors/ contributing conditions	Sugary foods or drinks (including juice, carbonated or noncarbonated soft drinks, energy drinks, medicinal syrups)	Child has frequent exposure (>3 times/day) to between-meal sugar-containing snacks or beverages per day	Frequent snacking (more than 3 times daily)	Dietary sugar content estimation (fermentable carbohydrates) (very low, low, moderate, or high content)
	Caries experience of mother, caregiver, and/or other siblings	Parent/caregiver has a lifetime of poverty and low health literacy		Frequency of daily meals and snacks (very low, low, high, very high)
		Child is a recent immigrant		
Protective factors	Fluoride exposure (through drinking water, supplements, professional applications, toothpaste)	Patient receives optimally fluoridated drinking water	Fluoridated water	Fluoride exposure assessment (fluoride toothpaste and constant use of additional fluoride measures; fluoride toothpaste plus occasional use of additional measures; fluoride toothpaste only; fluoride not used in any form)
		Patient brushes daily with fluoridated toothpaste	Fluoride toothpaste once a day	
	Dental home: established patient of record in a dental office, receiving regular dental care in a dental office	Patient receives topical fluoride from health professional	Uses fluoride-containing toothpaste 2 times daily or more	
		Patient has dental home/regular dental care	5000 ppm fluoride toothpaste	
			Has had fluoride varnish applied in the last 6 months	
			0.05% NaF mouth rinse daily	
			0.12% Chlorhexidine gluconate mouth rinse daily for 7 days a month	
			Normal salivary function	

Table 24.3 (Continued)

	ADA	AAPD	CAMBRA	CARIOGRAM[a]
Clinical findings/conditions	Cavitated or noncavitated (incipient) carious lesions or restorations (visually or radiographically evident)	Patient has ≥1 interproximal caries lesions	New cavities or lesion(s) into dentin (radiographically)	Caries experience (DMFT, DMFS, new caries experience in the past 1 year)
	Teeth missing due to caries in the past 36 months	Patient has active noncavitated (white spot) caries lesions or enamel defects	New white spot lesions on smooth surfaces	Silness-Löe Plaque Index (no plaque, some plaque not visible to the naked eye, moderate plaque visible, abundant plaque)
	Unusual tooth morphology that compromises oral hygiene	Patient has low salivary flow	New noncavitated lesion(s) in enamel (radiographically)	Stimulated saliva secretion rate
	Visible plaque	Patient has defective restorations	Existing restorations in last 3 years (new patient) or the last year (patient of record)	Saliva buffering capacity (chairside test)
	Interproximal restorations (1 or more)	Patient wears an intraoral appliance	Heavy plaque on teeth	Estimation of *Mutans streptococci* in saliva (chairside testing)
	Exposed root surfaces present		Reduced salivary function (measured low flow rate)	
	Restorations with overhangs and/or open margins, open contacts with food impaction		Deep pits and fissures	
	Dental/orthodontic appliances present (fixed or removable)		Exposed tooth roots	
	Severe dry mouth (xerostomia)		Orthodontic appliances	
General health conditions	Special healthcare needs	Child has special healthcare needs	Hyposalivatory medications	Related general diseases or conditions associated with caries risk
	Chemo/radiation therapy		Recreational drug use	
	Eating disorder			
	Medications that reduce salivary flow			
	Drug/alcohol abuse			

a) CARIOGRAM tool is the same for patient of all ages.

Table 24.4 The 15 most predictive factors and disease indicators for new caries formation in children, according to an ADA expert panel.

Risk Factors	Protective Factors	Disease Indicators
Consumes more than 3 sugary beverages or snacks between meals each day (or infants put to bed with a bottle containing beverage with sugar)	Brushes twice a day with toothpaste containing fluoride	Current active initial lesion(s) (i.e., enamel lesions, white spots)
Physical or behavioral health issues that impede home care	Predominantly drinks fluoridated water/beverages made from fluoridated water	Current active moderate or advanced lesion(s)
Clinically, little saliva or dry mouth due to medical condition or medication	Receives professionally applied fluoride	
Recent caries experience (past moderate or advanced lesion(s) since last assessment or in the last 3 years)	Uses over-the-counter fluoride mouth rinse (over age 6 years)	
Parents or siblings have cavitated lesion(s) in the last year (consider for children under age 14 years)	Uses at-home prescription fluoride products (over age 6 years)	
Visible plaque		
Uncoalesced and unsealed pits and fissures		

Source: ADA (2018); Schwendicke et al. (2015).

recent history of carious lesions is the most valid predictor of elevated caries risk, and in infants (<3 years old), the presence of one or more carious lesions indicates increased risk. The final recommendation from the panel was that the CRA tool should be used to measure the effectiveness of an intervention to reduce future caries risk and predict the occurrence of new carious lesions.

Overall, the CRA tool has great potential to enhance patient care by allowing the oral healthcare practitioner and the patient to understand the specific reasons for their caries activity and to tailor their care plans and recall intervals accordingly (Domejean *et al.*, 2017). Risk-based, patient-centered decision-making, supported by best available evidence, is an essential component for the correct prevention and management of dental caries, especially for infants (< 3 years old) (Ramos-Gomez *et al.*, 2007). Healthcare professionals (especially pediatric dentists) should perform a CRA evaluation for children by age 1 year (or as soon as their first tooth erupts), and this evaluation should be reassessed periodically over time.

In conclusion, assessing caries risk is an essential element in the planning of preventive and therapeutic strategies. Caries risk assessment has excellent potential to enhance patient care, as it is a critical component in a minimally invasive care plan, allowing determination of the appropriate noninvasive and invasive interventions and recall strategies (Cagetti *et al.*, 2018; Rechmann *et al.*, 2019).

References

American Association of Pediatric Dentistry. (2019–2020) Caries-risk assessment and management for infants, children and adolescents. *The Reference Manual of Pediatric Dentistry*. Chicago, IL: American Association of Pediatric Dentistry; 209–219.

American Dental Association (ADA). (2011a) Caries Risk Assessment Form (Age 0–6). Retrieved from https://www.ada.org/en/~/media/ADA/Member%20Center/FIles/topics_caries_under6. Accessed December 2, 2020.

American Dental Association (ADA). (2011) Caries Risk Assessment Form (Age >6yrs). Retrieved from http://www.ada.org/~/media/ADA/Science%20and%20Research/Files/topic_caries_over6.ashx. Accessed December 2, 2020.

American Dental Association. (2018) *Guidance on caries risk assessment in children. Retrieved from* Retrieved from https://www.ada.org/~/media/ADA/DQA/CRA_Report.pdf?la=en. Accessed December 2, 2020.

Bratthall, D. & Hänsel Petersson, G. (2005) Cariogram—a multifactorial risk assessment model for a multifactorial disease. *Community Dentistry and Oral Epidemiology*, 33 (4), 256–264. doi:10.1111/j.1600-0528.2005.00233.x.

Cagetti, M.G., Bonta, G., Cocco, F., Lingstrom, P., Strohmenger, L., & Campus, G. (2018). Are standardized caries risk assessment models effective in assessing actual caries status and future caries increment? *A systematic review. BMC Oral Health*, 18 (1), 123. doi:10.1186/s12903-018-0585-4.

Chaffee, B.W., Featherstone, J.D.B., & Zhan, L. (2017). Pediatric caries risk assessment as a predictor of caries outcomes. *Pediatric Dentistry*, 39 (3), 219–232.

Christian, B., Armstrong, R., Calache, H., Carpenter, L., Gibbs, L., & Gussy, M. (2018). A systematic review to assess the methodological quality of studies on measurement properties for caries risk assessment tools for young children. *International Journal of Paediatric Dentistry*, doi:10.1111/ipd.12446.

Domejean, S., Banerjee, A., & Featherstone, J.D.B. (2017). Caries risk/susceptibility assessment: its value in minimum intervention oral healthcare. *British Dental Journal*, 223 (3), 191–197. doi:10.1038/sj.bdj.2017.665.

Featherstone, J.D. (2006). Caries prevention and reversal based on the caries balance. *Pediatric Dentistry*, 28 (2), 128–132; discussion 192-198.

Featherstone, J.D., Domejean-Orliaguet, S., Jenson, L., Wolff, M., & Young, D.A. (2007). Caries risk assessment in practice for age 6 through adult. *Journal of the California Dental Association*, 35 (10), 703–707, 710–713.

Featherstone, J.D.B. & Chaffee, B.W. (2018). The evidence for Caries Management by Risk Assessment (CAMBRA(R)). *Advances in Dental Research*, 29 (1), 9–14. doi:10.1177/0022034517736500.

Fontana, M. (2015). The clinical, environmental, and behavioral factors that foster early childhood caries: evidence for caries risk assessment. *Pediatric Dentistry*, 37 (3), 217–225.

Fontana, M. & González-Cabezas, C. (2019). Evidence-based dentistry caries risk assessment and disease management. *Dental Clinics of North America*, 63 (1), 119–128. doi:10.1016/j.cden.2018.08.007.

Fontana, M. & González-Cabezas, C. (2000). Secondary caries and restoration replacement: an unresolved problem. *Compendium of Continuing Education in Dentistry*, **21** (1), 15–18, 21–14, 26 passim; quiz 30.

Halasa-Rappel, Y. A., Ng, M. W., Gaumer, G., & Banks, D. A. (2019, Feb). How useful are current caries risk assessment tools in informing the oral health care decision-making process? *J Am Dent Assoc, 150*(2), 91-102.e102. https://doi.org/10.1016/j.adaj.2018.11.011

National Institutes of Health. (2001) National Institutes of Health Consensus Development Conference statement. Diagnosis and management of dental caries throughout life. *Journal of the American Dental Association*, 132 (8), 1153–1161. doi:10.14219/jada .archive.2001.0343.

Ramos-Gomez, F.J., Crall, J., Gansky, S.A., Slayton, R.L., & Featherstone, J.D. (2007). Caries risk assessment appropriate for the age 1 visit (infants and toddlers). *Journal of the California Dental Association*, 35 (10), 687–702.

Rechmann, P., Chaffee, B.W., Rechmann, B.M.T., & Featherstone, J.D.B. (2019). Caries management by risk assessment: results from a practice-based research network study. *Journal of the California Dental Association*, 47 (1), 15–24.

Riley, J.L., 3rd, Gordan, V.V., Ajmo, C.T., Bockman, H., Jackson, M.B., *et al.* (2011). Dentists' use of caries risk assessment and individualized caries prevention for their adult patients: findings from the Dental Practice-Based Research Network. *Community Dentistry and Oral Epidemiology*, **39** (6), 564–573. doi:10.1111/j.1600-0528.2011.00626.x.

Schwendicke, F., Dorfer, C.E., Schlattmann, P., Foster Page, L., Thomson, W.M., & Paris, S. (2015). Socioeconomic inequality and caries: a systematic review and meta-analysis. *Journal of Dental Research*, 94 (1), 10–18. doi:10.1177/0022034514557546.

Tinanoff, N., Baez, R.J., Diaz Guillory, C., Donly, K.J., Feldens, C.A., et al. (2019). Early childhood caries epidemiology, aetiology, risk assessment, societal burden, management, education, and policy: global perspective. *International Journal of Paediatric Dentistry*, 29 (3), 238–248. doi:10.1111/ipd.12484.

Twetman, S. (2016). Caries risk assessment in children: how accurate are we? *European Archives of Paediatric Dentistry*, 17 (1), 27–32. doi:10.1007/s40368-015-0195-7.

25

Clinical Examination of the Infant
Jane A. Soxman and S. Thikkurissy

Infant Oral Health Exam

Children are not born with the bacteria that cause caries. This is acquired through either horizontal (peer groups/nonfamily members) or vertical (primary caregiver) transmission of bacteria. It should be noted that while the American Academy of Pediatric Dentistry states that for all children "Parents should be encouraged establish a dental home for infants by 12 months of age," it should be noted that an addendum to that statement reads "(or within six months of eruption of the first tooth)" (AAPD, 2019–2020). Establishment of the dental home is an individualized process that is dependent on the child in question. Some sources describe infancy as the first 12 months of life, while others define infancy as the first 2 years of life (Quinonez *et al.*, 2018; Elkind, 1994, p. 4). This chapter will discuss considerations for the 12–24 month-old child. (See Chapter 23 for the infant examination with knee-to-knee exam position.)

During the infant oral health visit, as with a medical well child visit, there is a myriad of items to address. Among these are (AAPD, 2019–2020):

- Infant's risk for developing caries based on protective factors (such as fluoride exposure) and pathologic factors (such as sugar-sweetened beverage use).
- Counseling regarding non-nutritive sucking habits and sequelae.
- Injury prevention associated with developing mobility or play.
- Assessment and evaluation of frenal attachments.
- Counseling regarding teething.
- Review of how medical condition, medications, or allergies may impact delivery of oral healthcare.

Evidence proves that education alone is not effective for reducing early childhood caries. The shortfall seems to be related to educators' inattention to the parent/caregiver's readiness to modify or change existing behaviors. Motivational interviewing (MI) is an approach used for counseling with suggestions regarding open-ended questioning, nonjudgmental affirmation, and reflective listening. MI raises parent/caregiver's awareness of the infant's oral health and his or her ability and readiness to incorporate the counseling is determined. MI has been reported to be a successful method to change health behaviors (Quinonez *et al.*, 2018; AAPD, 2019–2020; Faghihian *et al.*, 2020). Other considerations during the exam are the following:

- The use of a fluoridated dentifrice at 1 year of age is included in discussion regarding protective factors. The amount of fluoridated toothpaste to be dispensed is described as the size of a grain of rice. The vertical route of bacteria transmission from parent/caregiver to the child is discussed, with information regarding transmission via sharing utensils with the infant, for instance tasting food to check temperature. Biofilm and its role in contributing to early childhood caries are mentioned. Parents/caregivers are advised to wipe the entire oral cavity with a clean, wet cloth or paper towel each time the diaper is changed in order to disrupt the biofilm. Fluoride varnish should be applied to infants' teeth with high caries risk (AAPD, 2019–2020). (See Chapter 24 for caries risk assessment.) Sippy cup use and content should be included in the counseling (Quinonez *et al.*, 2018). Use of sippy cups should be avoided in general. Sippy cups containing juice promote repeated exposure of sugar and acid to the teeth, resulting in early childhood caries. Juice should be consumed only at meals. If a sippy cup is used, the cup may contain only water. By 12 months of age, babies can push the tongue tip upward, lifting it to swallow. A sippy cup with a long spout can hold the tongue down, promoting tongue thrust and interfering with the development of a "mature" swallowing pattern. A spill-proof straw cup is a better choice.

- Counseling regarding non-nutritive sucking, and in particular the pros and cons of pacifier habits, is an integral part of this first visit. Prolonged use of a pacifier for more than 6 hours a day and higher intensity of sucking may result in functional crossbite, posterior crossbite, increased overjet, and open bite. If recurrent bouts of otitis media are reported in the medical history, advice regarding restricted use of the pacifier is prudent. Ingression of oral bacteria via saliva into the Eustachian tube may occur with sucking while in a supine position. Pacifiers during sleep may reduce the risk of sudden infant death syndrome. Pacifier sucking during sleep lowers the auditory threshold, which positively affects arousal during a deep sleep and diminishes episodes of apnea (Soxman, 2007; see Chapter 22 on non-nutritive sucking and parafunctional habits).

- Injury prevention should be discussed, including electric cord safety and anticipatory guidance for avulsion or tooth fracture with excessive overjet. Avulsed primary incisors are not replanted. Intruded incisors will typically re-erupt. With complete intrusion, the incisor may appear to be avulsed. Between 12 months and 2 years of age, damage to the permanent successor with avulsion or intrusion should not be a concern. Parents/caregivers are reminded of the value of the "dental home," because children who experience trauma are more likely to have another incident. A photograph of the injury can be texted or emailed to determine the need for immediate treatment and counseling for the injury. In the event of palatal displacement of a maxillary primary incisor, the displacement may cause an inability to occlude the teeth due to interference or pain. Immediate repositioning is necessary. (See Chapter 14 on traumatic injury to the primary incisors.)

- Low, thick maxillary frenulum attachments often result in lacerations as children progress though crawling, walking, and running. This injury frequently causes profuse bleeding. Sutures are not necessary. Anticipatory guidance is given with instruction to offer a wet washcloth or a popsicle to hasten hemostasis with the coldness of the popsicle, lip pressure on the frenulum, and a calming effect. Parents/caregivers are informed that one drop of blood, mixed with a lot of saliva, gives the appearance of much more blood.

- Teething usually occurs from birth to 36 months of age, although this can greatly vary depending on parental tooth eruption history. In some cases, the first tooth may not appear until 14 months of age. In the absence of a syndrome, this is not considered to be of any concern. Systemic illness such as fever, tugging, diarrhea, or any sign of infection should not be attributed to teething, as this assumption may delay necessary medical intervention. Because maternal antibodies are diminishing by 6 months of age, the infant may be more susceptible to illness. Normal responses to teething may be drooling; sucking on a blanket, fingers, or hands; some interruption in sleep or feeding habits; and/or some irritability. Onset of salivary gland activity is at its maximum just before tooth eruption, and the infant may not yet be able to swallow all the saliva being produced, with the consequence of drooling. Topical anesthetics, including over-the-counter teething gels, should never be used. Plastic teething rings may break. Better choices are a clean, cold, damp washcloth or a cooled (not frozen) rubber teething ring. Massaging the gingiva with a clean finger is soothing. The eruption hematoma should be described, with assurance that this painless purple elevation on the gingiva sometimes appears just before a primary tooth erupts and is of no concern. The usual ages and sequence of primary tooth eruption may be provided with a chart (Soxman, 2002; AAPD, 2019–2020). The parent/caregiver should be informed that the sequence of eruption may not occur exactly as described in the chart and that this is typically of no consequence.

- Enamel defects increase caries risk and may be the result of premature birth or signal questions or follow-up for celiac disease. Baby bottle tooth decay may be a hallmark for anemia due to overconsumption of milk and decreased appetite for food (Quinonez *et al.*, 2018). Liquid oral medications taken routinely increase bacterial counts and biofilm. Medications to treat asthma decrease salivary flow and may cause gastroesophageal reflux due to relaxation of the esophageal sphincter, increasing caries risk. Counseling should be provided regarding the need to rinse the mouth and offer water after asthma medication. The need to brush the teeth, as well as wiping cheeks and tongue after the bedtime dose of liquid medications with their high sugar content, is included.

The first visit during infancy provides an opportunity to impact the dental and general health of a child for a lifetime. In addition to the intraoral examination, gathering information and parental/caregiver education are essential goals. The first visit during infancy provides the opportunity for active surveillance to monitor caries progression, interim therapeutic restoration, and application of silver diamine fluoride prior to advanced carious involvement requiring sedation or general anesthesia. Both the parent and the infant benefit, with the parent/caregiver's peace of mind at the establishment of a dental home, and the comfort level that comes from the infant's familiarity with the dental experience beginning at a young age.

References

American Academy of Pediatric Dentistry (AAPD). (2019–2020) Perinatal and infant oral health care. *The Reference Manual of Pediatric Dentistry*. Chicago, IL: American Academy of Pediatric Dentistry; 228–232.

Elkind, D. (1994) *A Sympathetic Understanding of the Child*, 3rd edn. Needham Heights, MA: Allyn and Bacon.

Faghihian, R., Faghihian, E., Kazemi, A., Tarrahi, M.J., & Zakizade, M. (2020) Impact of motivational interviewing on early childhood caries. A systematic review and meta-analysis. *Journal of the American Dental Association*, 151, 650–659.

Quinonez, R., Lou, J., Amini, H., & Chuang, A. (2018) Prenatal, perinatal and early childhood oral health (ECOH). In: Nowak, A.J. & Casamassimo, P.S. (eds.). *The Handbook of Pediatric Dentistry*, 5th edn. Chicago, IL: American Academy of Pediatric Dentistry; 1–15.

Soxman, J.A. (2002) The first dental visit. *General Dentistry*, 50, 148–155.

Soxman, J.A. (2007) Non-nutritive sucking with a pacifier: pros and cons. *General Dentistry*, 55, 59–62.

26

Clinical Examination of the Patient with Special Healthcare Needs

S. Thikkurissy, Giulia M. Castrigano, and AnnMarie Matusak

The patient with special healthcare needs represents a particularly vulnerable population. This population, as with infants, is often dependent on a caregiver for general and oral hygiene. The Centers for Disease Control note that approximately one-third of children have dental caries by the time they reach kindergarten (US Department of Health and Human Services, 2000). Additionally, all caries risk assessment tools recognize that special healthcare needs elevate a person's risk. This can be due to the nature of the special need, medication, or delayed global development (AAPD, 2019–2020).

Communication with Parents of Children with Special Healthcare Needs: Setting Expectations

Estimates are that 13–19% of children in the United States have special healthcare needs (SHCN), defined as "Children who have or are at an increased risk for a chronic physical, developmental, behavioral or emotional condition and who also require health and health related services of a type or amount beyond that required by children in general."

It is also significant to note that approximately 10% of children with SHCN have some impact or limitation on their functional mobility. Establishing a dental home is a critical part of overall healthcare delivery for all children, but particularly those with SHCN. It is estimated that the healthcare expenses of children with SHCN may be three or four times that of their nonaffected peers. It is not uncommon to see oral health de-prioritized in the light of other systemic medical issues. It is therefore critical to establish a common ground of expectations for the family with regard to oral health maintenance. This common ground should contain reasonable oral hygiene practice recommendations that are mindful of and consistent with physician-based recommendations (Denboba *et al.*, 2006). An example of this would be that if a child is diagnosed as failure to thrive, they may be placed on caloric supplementation through liquids such as Pediasure®, which contains 18 g of sugar per 8 oz (Abbott Nutrition, n.d.). The challenge for the dentist is to work a suitable oral cleansing regimen into the daily habit of a child needing this high-carbohydrate drink for weight gain.

Common ground on expectations can often be found in term of establishing what oral findings may be related to the special need, versus what oral findings are related to poor oral hygiene. It is not uncommon for caregivers to associate all oral findings with the special need, and assume a fatalistic approach that decay is "inevitable." The dentist plays a role early on to empower caregivers to establish healthy routines, while still being mindful of medical/medication requirements.

Kratz *et al.* (2009) noted that parents of children with SHCN often play multiple roles, which can include healthcare coordinator, medical expert, and advocate. In addition to these there is the seminal role of parent, which may become secondary based on the medical complexity of the child's condition. These parents, while often hypervigilant, may be prone to emotional exhaustion. This can make them less likely to comply with overzealous oral hygiene recommendations.

The oral healthcare team must be aware of the home care regimens that families follow and incorporate oral hygiene recommendations so that they are a relatively seamless addition.

Patient Positioning: Wheelchair Transfer

Statistics out of Canada reveal that approximately 50% of all wheelchair users do so due to a special need (McManus *et al.*, 2016). While the Americans with Disabilities Act recommends use of wheelchair ramps and spacing of dental chairs and restrooms to accommodate wheelchairs, this is only required if the dental practice takes federal/state money for providing dental care. Rashid-Kandvani *et al.* (2015) identified seven specific challenges faced by wheelchair users within the dental care pathway. Among these challenges were "transferring into the dental chair" and "overcoming discomfort on the dental chair." Most study participants preferred to stay in their wheelchair during the dental examination, specifically related to discomfort and pain associated with extended periods in the dental chair. This was at odds with most practitioners, who preferred the patient in the dental chair. The process of transfer and remaining in the dental chair was particularly difficult for patients who suffered from any type of partial or complete paralysis.

While treatment in the wheelchair is in many cases ideal for the patient and preferred,

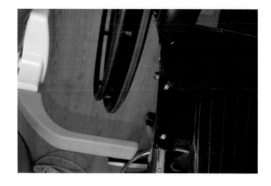

Figure 26.1 Insure lights, dental chair armrests, etc. are clear of the path of transfer. Dental chair armrest with the path of the wheelchair.

it is not always feasible due to the nature of the dental work being completed. The dental team should ensure that transfer is required for treatment rather than assuming it needs to be done. In light of this possibility, it is critical to understand the elements of the wheelchair transfer (Shields, 2004). The US Department of Health and Human Services through the NIH/NIDCR has published documents with five steps for successful wheelchair transfer (National Institutes of Health, 2009).

Determining the patient's needs, including the preferred transfer method, the ability to help, and the potential for spasms during transfer, is illustrated in Figures 26.1, 26.2, 26.3, and 26.4. Finally, position the patient carefully in the dental chair after transfer, including centering the patient, insuring comfort, and,

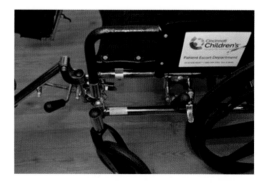

Figure 26.2 Prepare the wheelchair, including removing footrests.

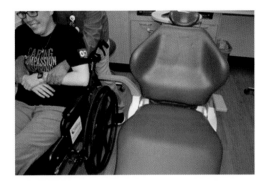

Figure 26.3 Place wheelchair parallel to dental chair and lock wheelchair wheels.

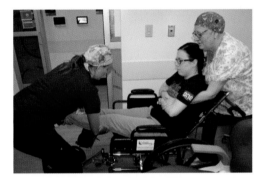

Figure 26.4 For a two-person transfer: first staff member behind patient with arms across patient's chest, second staff member with both hands under patient's lower thighs.

if a urine collecting device is used, position it above the level of the bladder.

Adjuncts to Keep the Mouth Open

A patient who does not progress from infantile reflexes (such as a startle reflex) to adult reflex patterns has what are known as "over-retained reflexes." In light of this, it is not uncommon to require adjuncts to keep the mouth open during dental work/examination of patients with SHCN. Various adjuncts to keep the mouth open have advantages and disadvantages. These adjuncts fall into three general categories:

- Latex-free intraoral bite block. These come in various sizes and are selected to optimize patient comfort while still keeping the mouth open. They can be spit out, which may be an issue with those patients who have developmental delay. Additionally, if the patient opens the mouth wider than the bite block, the bite block can be dislodged, interfering with the dental work being conducted.
- Molt mouth prop. This adjunct is controlled more by the dental team as, once it is placed, a member of the dental team can press it gently against the patient's face. There is a caveat, in that it is not unheard of for the patient's cheek to get caught in the gears of the mouth prop if the dental team is not careful. Additionally, if the dental team is overzealous in placement of the prop against resistance (the patient biting down), it can lead to luxation and, in severe cases, avulsion of teeth.
- Foam bite blocks are seen as a less invasive alternative for quick procedures, or for examinations/dental prophylaxis. While they tend to be softer than rigid mouth props, they are still somewhat stiff and patients who are initially resistant may need to be coaxed to open their mouth.

References

1 Abbott Nutrition. (n.d.) Pediasure® Grow & Gain shake. https://abbottnutrition.com/pediasure-grow-and-gain. Accessed July 20, 2020.

2 American Academy of Pediatric Dentistry. (2019–2020) Caries-risk assessment and management for infants, children, and adolescents. *The Reference Manual of Pediatric Dentistry*. Chicago, IL: American Academy of Pediatric Dentistry; 220–224.

3 Denboba, D., McPherson, M.G., Kenney, M.K., Strickland, B., & Newacheck, P.W.

(2006) Achieving family and provider partnerships for children with special health care needs. *Pediatrics*, 118 (4), 1607–1615.

4 Kratz, L., Uding, N., Trahms, C.M., Villareale, N., & Kieckhefer, G.M. (2009) Managing childhood chronic illness: parent perspectives and implications for parent-provider relationships. *Families, Systems & Health*, 27, 303–313.

5 McManus, B.M., Prosser, L.A., & Gannotti, M.E. (2016) Which children are not getting their needs for therapy or mobility aids met? Data from the 2009-2010 National Survey of Children with Special Health Care Needs. *Physical Therapy*, 96 (2), 222–231. doi:10.2522/ptj.20150055.

6 National Institutes of Health. (2009) Wheechair Transfer: A health care provider's guide. NIH 09-5195. https://www.nidcr.nih.gov/sites/default/files/2020-10/wheelchair-transfer-provider-guide.pdf. Accessed December 1, 2020.

7 Rashid-Kandvani, F., Nicolau, B., & Bedos, C. (2015) Access to dental services for people using a wheelchair. *American Journal of Public Health*, **105**, 2311–2317.

8 Shields, M. (2004) *Use of wheelchairs and other mobility support devices. Health Reports*, **15**, 37–41.

9 U.S. Department of Health and Human Services. (2000) *Oral Health in America: A Report of the Surgeon General.* Rockville, MD.: U.S. Department of Health and Human Services, National Institute of Dental and Craniofacial Research, National Institutes of Health.

27

Sleep Disordered Breathing in Children
Cristina V. Perez

Sleep disordered breathing (SDB) refers to a continuum of conditions in which a patient is not able to intake the ideal amount of air during sleep. There are different levels of severity of SDB; however, in any of its presentations it may produce important consequences that include cardiovascular, metabolic, growth and development, and cognitive impairments. The dentist's area of expertise may present with SDB characteristics that they should be aware of to provide a timely referral and avoid these consequences. Dentists also play an important role in the multidisciplinary approach to treating these conditions in children and adolescents.

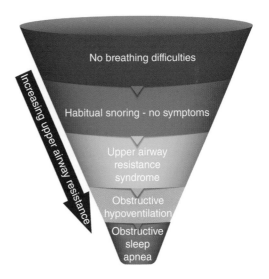

Figure 27.1 Sleep disordered breathing is a continuum spanning from primary snoring to obstructive sleep apnea. Source: Modified from Carroll (2003).

Sleep Disordered Breathing

SBD is a term that comprises a continuum of all air intake anomalies in a child during sleep. It spans from primary snoring with no associated hypoxia or sleep disruption, to obstructive sleep apnea (OSA) with complete obstruction of the airway and cessation of air intake during sleep (Figure 27.1) (Carroll, 2003). SDB can manifest with symptoms such as snoring, gasping, apneas, and restless sleep (Chinnadurai *et al.*, 2017). SBD is highly prevalent in the child population, with 5–25% of the population affected under the age of 12, and is now considered a public health concern due to the increasing number of children affected (Bixler *et al.*, 2009). Although only complete

obstruction of air intake during sleep was considered harmful in the past, today any form of SDB in a child should be concerning, since it has been shown that even the least severe of these conditions may have important consequences in the quality of life and overall health of a child.

Sleep in Children

Children spend more than half their lives sleeping. Any activity practiced for this long a

Handbook of Clinical Techniques in Pediatric Dentistry, Second Edition. Edited by Jane A. Soxman.
© 2022 John Wiley & Sons, Inc. Published 2022 by John Wiley & Sons, Inc.

period must have a great importance. Sleep is fundamental for a child's attention, behavior, cognitive functioning, emotional regulation, and physical health. More importantly, lack of sleep is related to increased risk for cardiovascular disease, psychologic dysfunction, growth impairment, obesity, poor academic achievement, depression, and reduced quality of life/wellbeing (Chan *et al.*, 2004; Dutil & Chaput, 2017).

Based on physiologic measures and a polysomnograph, sleep can be divided into rapid eye movement sleep (REM) and non-rapid eye movement sleep (NON-REM). Both REM and NON-REM sleep are very important for a child to recuperate from a day's activity and to develop both physically and neurologically. During REM sleep most muscles are completely inactive, except for the eye muscles and diaphragm. During this time brain activity is at its highest; an electroencephalogram taken during REM sleep looks very much like the child is awake, but the child is completely unresponsive. REM sleep is essential for the brain to recover from a long day's intellectual activities and is thought to play a role in maintaining and establishing new neuronal connections during development (Bathory & Tomopoulos, 2017). During REM sleep, short reductions in airflow are prevalent and considered normal due to low muscle tone and lack of neurologic response; however, in most patients these do not cause side effects. During NON-REM sleep, the brain is very quiet and muscle tone returns; it functions as a restorative phase. NON-REM sleep is essential for the body to recover from a day's physical activity.

Newborns spend up to 16 hours each day sleeping, and much of this sleep is in REM sleep. As a child reaches 6 months, longevity of sleep should decrease and most sleep should occur during the night. At 6 years of age a child's sleep pattern should be much like an adult's, although they require more time sleeping; for example, a 6-year-old requires 11 hours of sleep a day. A child's sleep should follow a predictable cyclic pattern, from shallow NON-REM sleep to deep NON-REM sleep and finally to REM sleep. Children should have 4–6 of these cycles per night.

Sleep is essential for life. Lack of reparative sleep can cause impaired attention and concentration, impaired quality of life, reduced productivity, as well as accidents, coronary artery disease, heart failure, high blood pressure, obesity, type II diabetes, stroke memory impairments, and depression (Chokroverty, 2010).

In today's society children are exposed to multiple sources of electronic media, many of which are used during a child's induction to sleep, therefore displacing it. This may put at risk a child's sleep duration, appropriate timing, quality, and regularity (Paruthi *et al.*, 2016).

Obstructive apneas, the most severe form of SDB, occur mostly during REM sleep. Therefore, a child with OSA may be physically well rested, but his or her brain does not get a chance to "reset" during sleep. This is manifested in children who demonstrate lack of neurologic rest by hyperactivity, not necessarily sleepiness like adults.

Obstructive Sleep Apnea: Definition, Diagnostic Criteria, and Prevalence

SDB encompasses all air intake insufficiencies during sleep. The most severe on this continuum is OSA. OSA in children is defined by the American Academy of Pediatrics as a "disorder of breathing during sleep characterized by prolonged partial upper airway obstruction (hypopnea) and/or intermittent complete obstruction (apnea) that disrupt normal ventilation during sleep and normal sleep patterns" (Marcus *et al.*, 2012). OSA is found in approximately 2–5% of the child population and is an important health concern, due to its consequences that impact the child's physical and mental development.

To be able to effectively diagnose OSA, an overnight sleep study (polysomnography or PSG) must be performed. A PSG can give the practitioner information on the number and duration of partial or complete obstructions of the airway. A partial obstruction or hypopnea is determined when a 50% or greater reduction in air intake is observed' this is accompanied by at least a 4% decrease in blood oxygen saturation or is associated to an arousal. A complete obstruction or apnea is determined when there is complete cessation of air flow into the lungs for 5 seconds or more (American Thoracic Society, 1996).

The PSG provides a numeric value called an apnea hypopnea index or AHI. An AHI of 1 indicates that a child suffered either one partial or complete obstruction of the airway using the criteria given previously. Due to the consequences OSA can have on a child, the diagnostic criteria are more stringent than cutoffs in adults. While in an adult an AHI of 1–5 is considered normal, in a child OSA is diagnosed if a child has an AHI of 1 or above (American Society of Anesthesiologists Task Force, 2014). OSA can be divided into mild (AHI 1–5), moderate (AHI 6–10), or severe (AHI 10 and above).

Prevalence

SBD is quite prevalent in children (5–25%) and on many occasions goes undiagnosed. OSA, the most severe form of SDB, is also prevalent in children, although to a lesser degree. Studies find that OSA occurs in 1.2–5% of the child population, many cases of which also remain undiagnosed (Abad & Guilleminault, 2009; Bixler *et al.*, 2009). The most prevalent age for OSA is between 2 and 8 years, due to the increased size of the tonsils and adenoids in an airway that still has much growing to do. However, hypertrophic tonsils and adenoids are not the only factor affecting the prevalence of this

condition: recent studies show an increase in OSA related to child obesity.

The typical patient with OSA has changed in recent years. A thin child with an elongated face and large tonsils and adenoids has been replaced with an overweight child that has a similar presentation to an adult with OSA, with an increased BMI and waist circumference. Although the first phenotype is still present, dentists must be alert to this new presentation (Bixler *et al.*, 2009).

Risk Factors

Certain physical and physiologic characteristics place a child at risk for having or developing SDB. These risk factors can be related to gender: before puberty both sexes show similar risk, but after puberty males are more affected than females; this responds to longer pharyngeal length, therefore more possibility of collapse.

Within races, African Americans, Hispanics, and Asians are more at risk due to their craniofacial form. Caucasian children with increased levels of obesity are also at increased risk.

BMI and higher waist circumference are strong predictors for OSA in children, with almost 50% of obese children presenting with OSA; if we add snoring to obesity, the risk increases to 90%. Adipose tissue within the airway may be one of the factors associated with this increased risk, which may help explain why an increasing number of obese children with OSA are not cured by adenotonsillectomy (Ye, 2009).

Adenotonsillar hypertrophy has been proven to increase the risk for OSA, as large adenoids and tonsils can occupy almost an entire airway once the neuromuscular control that holds the airway open is decreased during sleep.

Chronic respiratory ailments (allergic rhinitis and asthma) are related to SDB due to respiratory tract inflammation, decreasing the airway diameter.

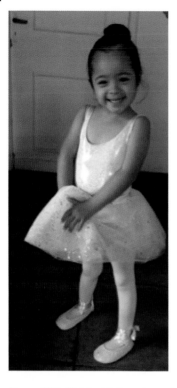

Figure 27.2 Child with Down's syndrome. All children with Down's syndrome should be evaluated for obstructure sleep apnea before age 4 years.

Children with craniofacial anomalies such as craniofacial synostosis (Apert, Crouzon, and Pfeiffer syndromes), hypoplastic mandibles (Treacher Collins or Pierre Robin sequence), hypoplastic maxilla (achondroplasia), or cleft lip and palate have small and narrow airways or altered airway dynamics that can influence the amount of air that passes through to the lungs at night.

Down's syndrome children are especially prone to OSA (Figure 27.2), with 31–100% suffering from it. They present with relative macroglossia, mandibular hypoplasia, midface hypoplasia, hypotonia, and glossoptosis, characteristics that increase the risk for these children. Due to these statistics, all children with Down's syndrome should be evaluated for OSA by age 4 (Horne *et al.*, 2018b).

Pathophysiology

SDB can be attributed to a discrepancy between the three-dimensional size of the airway and the neuromuscular control designed to keep it open. The diameter of airway is proportionally related to the resistance of airflow. Resistance increases exponentially with a small decrease in diameter. The volume of the airway can be decreased by anatomic variables such as abundant adenotonsillar and other lymphoid tissue (Waldeyer's tonsillar ring; Figure 27.3), macroglossia or retro-positioned tongue, micrognathia or retro-positioned mandible, maxillary constriction, shortened lower dental arch, altered nasal anatomy, and increased adipose tissue distribution.

The airway is a long, collapsible tube made of soft tissues and must be continuously kept open by upper airway dilator muscles. This neuromuscular control can be affected by chronic inflammation, altered reflexes, neuromuscular disease, and hypotonia. It has been shown that children with OSA have to work twice as hard to keep their airway open during the day, so these children cannot continue with this effort during the night, leading to decreased muscle activity in keeping the airway open. Additionally, REM sleep produces a further decrease in muscle tone and complete lack of voluntary control, increasing collapsibility. Furthermore, in obese children adipose tissue releases proinflammatory molecules that reduce muscle and diaphragm contractibility (Tan *et al.*, 2013).

Consequences

SDB and more so OSA cause a disruption of normal ventilation, intermittent lack of oxygenation, increased CO_2 in the blood, and sleep arousals that lead to sleep fragmentation. In a growing child these have been found to have a significant effect on the cardiovascular,

Figure 27.3 Waldeyer's tonsillar ring, lymphatic tissue surrounding the airway. Source: Reproduced with permission from Suvilehto (2009).

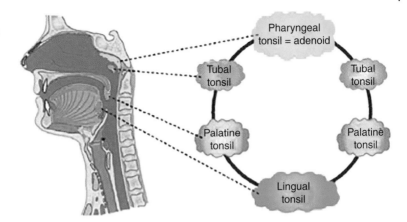

metabolic, and central nervous systems and somatic growth, therefore decreasing their quality of life. Although overall sleep duration is important for a child's growth and development, the disruption of the sleep process, where a child does not reach the deep, reparative stages of sleep, or does not have enough REM sleep, seems to be responsible for many of the consequences described below (Capdevila *et al.*, 2008). Fortunately, the severity of most of the complications seen in childhood can be halted and recovered from, if treated early.

Neurologic

Sleep plays an important role in attentional capacity, memory, intelligence, and learning. NON-REM sleep is involved in consolidation and integration of memory and REM sleep helps in accommodation of new memories into an association network. If sleep is disrupted, the learning process may be altered. Studies demonstrate that children with OSA present impaired learning and school performance, and reduced attentional capacity; if the severity of OSA is increased, then children may show reduced memory and overall intelligence. Authors believe that these deficits are due to prefrontal cortex (PFC) dysfunction as a consequence of sleep disruption, hypoxemia, and hypercarbia. The PFC is important in the development of cognitive flexibility, reasoning,

and memory. PFC dysfunction may eventually lead to a disruption of executive functions, a domain that includes processes governing the ability to focus, plan, remember instructions, and successfully juggle multiple tasks. The prefrontal cortex shows decreased activity during all sleep stages, demonstrating its ability to recalibrate. Hypoxemia and sleep fragmentation may affect this area disproportionately due to its late maturity (Kennedy *et al.*, 2004). Many authors have proven that treating OSA leads to improvements in memory and learning substrates.

Behavioral

Children with SDB exhibit a number of behavioral symptoms, including aggressiveness, impulsivity, hyperactivity, and decreased attention. Additionally, SDB is associated with the diagnosis in children and adolescents of attention-deficit/hyperactivity disorder (ADHD), depression, oppositional defiant disorder, and abnormal social behavior. Repeated arousals or micro awakenings from sleep are common in children with SDB as a way for the child to overcome an obstructive event and receive the necessary oxygen required; multiple awakenings during the night are common and are the cause of sleep fragmentation. This is thought to be the major causative factor for behavioral problems in children with SDB. Sleep deprivation studies found behavioral effects even after one night of sleep deprivation; if this deprivation continues for a week, the behavioral changes are more severe. Treating children with behavioral issues like ADHD for SDB shows an important decrease in ADHD symptoms. Studies suggest that all children diagnosed with ADHD should be evaluated for SDB before a medication regimen is initiated (Sedky *et al.*, 2014).

Cardiovascular

Current literature demonstrates that children with SDB have early signs of cardiovascular dysfunction. The mechanisms of this dysfunction are related to chronic intermittent hypoxia, hypercapnia, and changes in intrathoracic pressures produced during SDB events. They cause a dramatic change in blood pressure, vascular remodeling, endothelial dysfunction, and elevated pulmonary artery pressure. These autonomic changes may leave a child with important cardiovascular consequences, including systemic hypertension, increased heart rate, nocturnal cardiac strain, and left ventricle remodeling. These consequences are related to the severity of SDB; however, they are concerning since they may be accumulative, leading to a lifetime of cardiovascular problems as an adult (Bhattacharjee *et al.*, 2009).

Growth

SDB is a risk factor for growth failure. Growth hormone is preferably secreted during the deep stages of NON-REM sleep. If sleep is disrupted by continuous arousals during the night, this stage of sleep may not be reached. Additionally, children with SDB have shown increased caloric consumption during the night due to continuous awakenings to open their obstructed airway. Furthermore, these children have also been shown to have hyperactivity during the day. Both are related to increased caloric expenditure and lack of

growth. Fortunately, when children with SBD are treated effectively and in a timely manner, their growth seems to be able to "catch up" to normal patterns (Bonuck *et al.*, 2009).

Screening in a Dental Setting

Dentists can initiate a diagnosis of SDB through patient history-taking and examination. A through medical history questionnaire should include questions on craniofacial anomalies, neuromuscular disorders, syndromes including Down's syndrome, premature birth (35 weeks or less), cardiovascular disease, ADHD, and systemic growth anomalies. During the patient interview information can be gained by asking parents about frequent snoring (3 nights a week or more), labored breathing during sleep, gasps, snorting noises, observed episodes of apnea (especially in the early-morning hours), sleep enuresis (bed wetting, especially 6 months or more after bladder control is obtained), sleeping in a seated position or with the neck hyperextended (Figure 27.4), headaches on awakening, daytime sleepiness, mood alterations, and learning problems.

Dentists treating children should consider calculating all patients' BMI due to the proven correlation between increased BMI and SDB. It has been shown that for every 1 kg/m^2 increase in BMI, above the mean for age and sex, there is a 12% increased risk of developing OSA (Horne *et al.*, 2018a). Due to a child's continuous change in height and weight, BMI is best expressed as a percentile; many BMI percentile calculating tools are available online. Concern should be expressed to a parent whose child is in the 95th percentile or greater, especially if the child has other symptoms related to SDB. Sleep questionnaires such as I'M SLEEPY, STOP-BNG, Sleep Health Habit Questionnaire, and Pediatric Sleep Questionnaire are available to assess sleep habits and to screen for SDB; however, they are not a diagnostic tool.

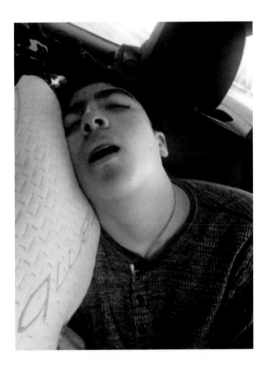

Figure 27.4 Sleeping in an open mouth position with a hyperextended neck.

The clinical examination is an important moment to assess for clinical manifestations related to SDB. Clinical examination should be performed systematically, starting with an exhaustive extraoral exam in which the dentist should observe the child's facial shape and extraoral features. Although the phenotype of a child with SDB is changing, a child with SDB may present with an elongated facial type (dolichocephalic, adenoid facies), and the nasal apertures may be small and atonic, demonstrating lack of nasal breathing. The size of the mandible and its relation to the maxillary bone should also be evaluated, since children with SDB may have micrognathia or retrognathia.

During the intraoral examination the dentist should start by observing the soft tissues. Red and inflamed anterior gingival tissues with lack of abundant plaque may be associated with mouth breathing. Large tongue, long soft palate and uvula, and large pharyngeal tonsil that occupies much of the open airway should

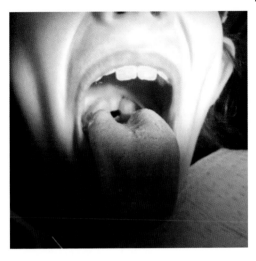

Figure 27.5 Large pharyngeal tonsils on intraoral examination.

be noted (Figure 27.5). A good time to evaluate tonsil size is when examining the tongue with gauze (Figure 27.6). A high-arched palate with maxillary constriction may imply the mouth is open for a prolonged period of time, therefore implying the tongue does not rest on the palate (Figure 27.7) (Capua *et al.*, 2009).

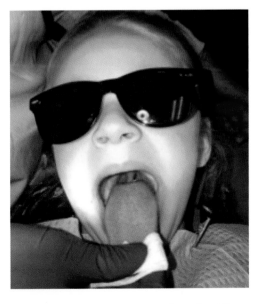

Figure 27.6 Evaluating pharyngeal tonsils while examining tongue.

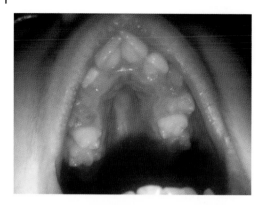

Figure 27.7 High-arched, constricted palate.

Radiographic studies may provide additional information for a patient who may be at risk for SDB. Lateral cephalometric radiographs and panoramic radiographs are useful in diagnosing airway narrowing and lymphatic tissue overgrowth. Although magnification of up to 25% exists, the correlation between structures remains (Figure 27.8). Radiographs may be a good instrument to attach when referring a patient to a physician to be evaluated for SDB.

During treatment a dentist should be aware of certain signs related to obstructive airways. If a child is unable to breathe through his/her nose during the administration of N₂O and no respiratory ailments are reported, dentists should be alert to possible adenoidal hypertrophy. If a child receives sedation medications and the monitors indicate the intake of air has decreased significantly, it is possible that the sedation medications are causing a decrease in muscle tone, reproducing an obstructive event that the child may experience during sleep (Stark *et al.*, 2018).

If the history, clinical exam, radiographic exam, or signs during treatment lead the dentist to believe the patient is likely to have SDB, a referral to a specialist should be made. This professional can make a final diagnosis after requesting an overnight sleep study (Trosman, 2013).

Management

Due to the nature of SDB and its many levels of obstruction, its management usually responds to the severity of the SDB or to the patient's symptoms. It was assumed for many years that adenotonsillectomy (AT) was the only treatment for OSA; however, many patients with OSA do not improve after this procedure, therefore other options have been evaluated.

Surgery

Hypertrophic adenoid tissue (pharyngeal tonsils and adenoids) is one of the most well-documented causes of SDB, specifically in its most severe form OSA, therefore the removal of tonsils and adenoids (AT) is the first-line treatment for OSA. While AT is effective in completely eliminating obstructive events in only 60–80% of cases, other parameters, including behavioral and quality of life, seem to have improved outcomes. The children prone to be refractory to AT are those with craniofacial anomalies, neuromuscular disease, Down's syndrome, obesity, those with high preoperative AHI (AHI > 20/h), as well as those older than 7 years of age (Lee *et al.*, 2016). AT is not without risks, which include dehydration, primary and secondary hemorrhage, velopharyngeal insufficiency, nasopharyngeal stenosis, and atlantoaxial subluxation, therefore all options for treatment should be evaluated (Capdevila *et al.*, 2008; Tan *et al.*, 2013).

Continuous Positive Airway Pressure

Continuous positive airway pressure (CPAP) is a device that forces air into the airway providing a mechanical stent, therefore preventing its collapse. It is the gold standard therapy for OSA in adults and is effective in eliminating OSA. In children, however, this therapy is indicated when AT is ineffective or

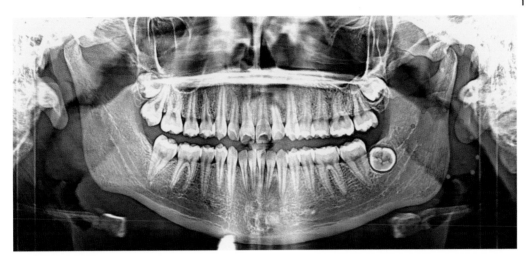

Figure 27.8 Panoramic radiograph showing shadow of pharyngeal tonsils (surrounded by blue dots).

contraindicated. Additionally, this therapy is not US Food and Drug Administration (FDA) approved for children <30 kg and may cause maxillary growth restriction due to the pressure of the mask on the maxilla. Furthermore, if used on a child with orthodontic therapy, it may irritate the soft tissues on the inside of the upper lip. Although reports indicate that CPAP can be well tolerated by children, long-term adherence to treatment is low; on average, the device is only used for 5 months and in many cases for no more than 3 hours per night (Marcus *et al.*, 2006).

Medications

Medications are a good alternative for those children with mild to moderate OSA but for whom AT is not a good option, or for parents looking for an alternative to surgery. The medications most used are corticosteroid nasal sprays, leukotriene antagonists, and daily antihistamines. The mechanism of action is systemic or local. Systemically, leukotriene antagonists like montelukast show a reduction in adenotonsillar proliferation and reduction in the concentrations of tumor necrosis factor α. Locally, nasal fluticasone and budesonide

target the glucocorticoid receptors in the adenoid tissue, reducing its size. These treatments have been shown to decrease the AHI; however, their use must be prolonged to observe significant improvements (Baldassari & Choi, 2018).

Dental Treatment

Mandibular Advancement Devices

Mandibular advancement devices (MAD) are removable oral appliances worn simultaneously on the mandible and maxilla that protrude the mandible, and thereby also the tongue (Figure 27.9a, b). Since the tongue is inserted along the inner border of the mandible, this appliance lifts the tongue off the posterior wall of the pharynx, opening the airway. Appliances have been proven to increase the airway volume and resting tone of the pharyngeal musculature, helping keep the airway open during sleep (Idris *et al.*, 2018). MAD have been proven effective in reducing the AHI of patients with mild to moderate OSA, although not as effectively as CPAP. Caution should be applied in young children, since long-term use may alter growth, producing dentoalveolar, skeletal, and soft tissue

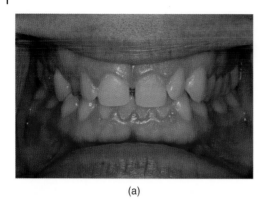
(a)

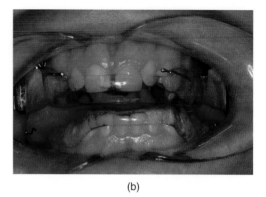
(b)

Figure 27.9 (a) Initial bite of patient needing mandibular advancement device therapy. (b) Mandibular advancement device (dorsal fin) advancing the mandible to treat obstructive sleep apnea.

effects, including proclination of mandibular incisors, retroclination of maxillary incisors, reduction of overjet and overbite, distal movement of maxillary molars, mesial movement of mandibular molars, increase in mandibular length, and forward posturing of the mandible. A good candidate for MAD is young adult or adolescent who has finished growth and is not able to use CPAP or who was refractory to AT (Nazarali *et al.*, 2015).

Rapid Maxillary Expansion

Many patients with SDB present with a constricted maxilla and posterior crossbite. These characteristics are associated with a mouth-breathing patient with an elongated facial form (Figure 27.10).

Rapid maxillary expansion (RME) is an orthodontic therapy used to expand the maxilla's transverse dimension and therefore correct the maxillary constriction and aberrant tooth relation. RME is achieved by a fixed maxillary appliance that, through distraction osteogenesis, widens the transversal dimensions of the maxillary bone. Changes are seen soon after the appliance is activated by observing a midline diastema. The mechanism of action of RME for the treatment of OSA is to increase the volume of the nasal and oral cavity, therefore allowing more room for the structures occupying these areas. RME also

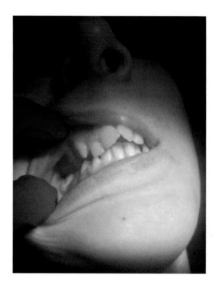

Figure 27.10 Posterior crossbite with maxillary constriction.

works by repositioning the tongue, providing a wide horizontal palate for its resting position, lifting it off the oropharynx. Additionally, the newly positioned tongue adopts an improved swallowing pattern, increasing its muscle tone and helping avoid its collapse during sleep.

RME has shown to be favorable in reducing OSA in children with a high-arched palate and maxillary constriction (Camacho *et al.*, 2017; Villa *et al.*, 2007).

Conclusion

SDB is a prevalent and underdiagnosed condition affecting the child and adolescent population. Studies show that the phenotypical characteristics of patients with SDB are changing and that adenotonsillar hypertrophy may not be the only factor influencing its appearance. Dentists play an important role in the diagnosis, referral, and treatment of this condition. Becoming familiarized with SDB characteristics found during medical history, interview, and examination will prepare the dentist to help their child patients with this life-altering condition in a timely manner, avoiding long-term consequences.

References

Abad, V.C., & Guilleminault, C. (2009) Treatment options for obstructive sleep apnea. *Current Treatment Options in Neurology*, 11 (5), 358–367.

American Society of Anesthesiologists Task Force on Perioperative Management of patients with obstructive sleep apnea. (2014) Practice guidelines for the perioperative management of patients with obstructive sleep apnea: an updated report by the American Society of Anesthesiologists Task Force on Perioperative Management of patients with obstructive sleep apnea. *Anesthesiology*, 120 (2), 268–286.

American Thoracic Society. (1996) Standards and indications for cardiopulmonary sleep studies in children. American Thoracic Society. *American Journal of Respiratory and Critical Care Medicine*, 153 (2), 866–878.

Baldassari, C.M. & Choi, S. (2018) Mild obstructive sleep apnea in children: what is the best management option? *Laryngoscope*, 128 (12), 2671–2672.

Bathory, E. & Tomopoulos, S. (2017) Sleep regulation, physiology and development, sleep duration and patterns, and sleep hygiene in infants, toddlers, and preschool-age children. *Current Problems in Pediatric and Adolescent Health Care*, 47 (2), 29–42.

Bhattacharjee, R., Kheirandish-Gozal, L., Pillar, G., & Gozal, D. (2009) Cardiovascular complications of obstructive sleep apnea syndrome: evidence from children. *Progress in Cardiovascular Diseases*, 51 (5), 416–433.

Bixler, E.O., Vgontzas, A.N., Lin, H., Liao, D., Calhoun, S., *et al.* (2009) Sleep disordered breathing in children in a general population sample: prevalence and risk factors. *Sleep*, 32 (6), 731–736.

Bonuck, K.A., Freeman, K., & Henderson, J. (2009) Growth and growth biomarker changes after adenotonsillectomy: systematic review and meta-analysis. *Archives of Disease in Childhood*, 94 (2), 83–91.

Camacho, M., Chang, E.T., Song, S.A., Abdullatif, J., Zaghi, S., *et al.* (2017) Rapid maxillary expansion for pediatric obstructive sleep apnea: a systematic review and meta-analysis. *Laryngoscope*, 127 (7), 1712–1719.

Capdevila, O.S., Kheirandish-Gozal, L., Dayyat, E., & Gozal, D. (2008) Pediatric obstructive sleep apnea: complications, management, and long-term outcomes. *Proceedings of the American Thoracic Society*, 5 (2), 274–282.

Capua, M., Ahmadi, N., & Shapiro, C. (2009). Overview of obstructive sleep apnea in children: exploring the role of dentists in diagnosis and treatment. *Journal of the Canadian Dental Association*, 75 (4), 285–289.

Carroll, J.L. (2003). Obstructive sleep-disordered breathing in children: new controversies, new directions. *Clinical Chest Medicine*, 24 (2), 261–282.

Chan, J., Edman, J.C., & Koltai, P.J. (2004) Obstructive sleep apnea in children. *American Family Physician*, 69 (5), 1147–1154.

Chinnadurai, S., Jordan, A.K., Sathe, N.A., Fonnesbeck, C., McPheeters, M.L., & Francis,

D.O. (2017) Tonsillectomy for obstructive sleep-disordered breathing: a meta-analysis. *Pediatrics*, 139 (2), e20163491.

Chokroverty, S. (2010) Overview of sleep & sleep disorders. *Indian Journal of Medical Research*, 131, 126–140.

Dutil, C. & Chaput, J.P. (2017) Inadequate sleep as a contributor to type 2 diabetes in children and adolescents. *Nutrition & Diabetes*, 7 (5), e266.

Horne, R.S.C., Shandler, G., Tamanyan, K., Weichard, A., Odoi, A., *et al.* (2018a). The impact of sleep disordered breathing on cardiovascular health in overweight children. *Sleep Medicine*, 41, 58–68.

Horne, R.S., Wijayaratne, P., Nixon, G.M., & Walter, L.M. (2018b) Sleep and sleep disordered breathing in children with Down syndrome: effects on behaviour, *neurocognition and the cardiovascular system*. *Sleep Medicine Reviews*, 44, 1–11.

Idris, G., Galland, B., Robertson, C.J., Gray, A., & Farella, M. (2018) Mandibular advancement appliances for sleep-disordered breathing in children: a randomized crossover clinical trial. *Journal of Dentistry*, 71, 9–17.

Kennedy, J.D., Blunden, S., Hirte, C., Parsons, D.W., Martin, A.J., *et al.*(2004) Reduced neurocognition in children who snore. *Pediatric Pulmonology*, 37 (4), 330–337.

Lee, C.H., Hsu, W.C., Chang, W.H., *et al.* (2016) Polysomnographic findings after adenotonsillectomy for obstructive sleep apnoea in obese and non-obese children: a systematic review and meta-analysis. *Clinical Otolaryngology*, 41 (5), 498–510.

Marcus, C.L., Brooks, L.J., Draper, K.A., Gozal, D., Halbower, A.C., *et al.* (2012) Diagnosis and management of childhood obstructive sleep apnea syndrome. *Pediatrics*, 130 (3), e714–e755.

Marcus, C.L., Rosen, G., Ward, S.L., Halbower, A.C., Sterni, L., *et al.* (2006) Adherence to and effectiveness of positive airway pressure therapy in children with obstructive sleep apnea. *Pediatrics*, 117 (3), e442–e451.

Nazarali, N., Altalibi, M., Nazarali, S., Major, M.P., Flores-Mir, C., & Major, P.W. (2015) Mandibular advancement appliances for the treatment of paediatric obstructive sleep apnea: a systematic review. *European Journal of Orthodontistry*, 37 (6), 618–626.

Paruthi, S., Brooks, L.J., D'Ambrosio, C., Hall, W.A., Kotagai, S., *et al.* (2016). Consensus statement of the American Academy of Sleep Medicine on the recommended amount of sleep for healthy children: methodology and discussion. *Journal of Clinical Sleep Medicine*, 12 (11), 1549–1561.

Sedky, K., Bennett, D.S., & Carvalho, K.S. (2014). Attention deficit hyperactivity disorder and sleep disordered breathing in pediatric populations: a meta-analysis. *Sleep Medicine Reviews*, 18 (4), 349–356.

Stark, T.R., Pozo-Alonso, M., Daniels, R., & Camacho, M. (2018) Pediatric considerations for dental sleep medicine. *Sleep Medicine Clinics*, 13 (4), 531–548.

Suvilehto, J. (2009) Immunodeficiencies, pathogens and sex in upper respiratory diseases. Dissertation, University of Helsinki. Retrieved from https://helda.helsinki.fi/bitstream/handle/10138/20506/immunode.pdf?sequence=2&isAllowed=y. Accessed December 2, 2020.

Tan, H.L., Gozal, D., & Kheirandish-Gozal, L. (2013) Obstructive sleep apnea in children: a critical update. *Nature and Science of Sleep*, 5, 109–123.

Trosman, I. (2013) Childhood obstructive sleep apnea syndrome: a review of the 2012 American Academy of Pediatrics guidelines. *Pediatric Annals*, 42 (10), 195–199.

Villa, M.P., Malagola, C., Pagani, J., Montesano, M., Rizzoli, A., *et al.* (2007) Rapid maxillary expansion in children with obstructive sleep apnea syndrome: 12-month follow-up. *Sleep Medicine*, 8 (2), 128–134.

Ye, J. (2009) Emerging role of adipose tissue hypoxia in obesity and insulin resistance. *International Journal of Obesity*, 33 (1), 54–66.

28

Pediatric Oral Medicine

Christel M. Haberland

The oral mucosa of children can present with various infections and benign pathologies that require either definitive or palliative treatment. However, due to a lack of clinical trials, many medications used for oral medicine conditions are often prescribed "off-label" (Frattarelli *et al.*, 2014). Additionally, the safety, efficacy, effectiveness, and adverse reactions of medications used in adults may vary in children, especially those under the age of 2 years. Therefore, practitioners must be careful when prescribing medications for children, even if they have been found beneficial in adults.

In general, benign conditions are more commonly seen in children, and of these, fungal and viral are the most prevalent (Pinto *et al.*, 2014). Other benign lesions that are frequently seen in children are oral ulcerations, which can result from immune-mediated conditions, trauma, or systemic diseases. These oral ulcerations are often painful and require treatment (Flaitz & Baker, 2000). Clinicians should be familiar with the oral presentations of these conditions and be able to prescribe the appropriate medications for treatment or palliative care.

Oral Candidiasis

Oral candidiasis is the most common fungal infection in children. The causative organism is usually *Candida albicans*, but other species like *C. glabrata*, *C. tropicalis*, and *C. guilliermondii*

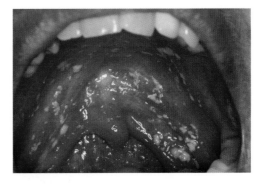

Figure 28.1 Pseudomembranous candidiasis ("thrush") in palate secondary to topical corticosteroid use.

can also be responsible. Approximately 30–50% of the population are asymptomatic *C. albicans* carriers, which means that the yeast is part of the oral flora and is present in the oral mucosa, but does not cause disease. However, changes in the host microenvironment can favor its proliferation, allowing candida to invade the mucosa (Vila *et al.*, 2020). Therefore, candidiasis is an indicator of immune dysfunction and an opportunistic infection frequently seen in immunocompromised patients, secondary to cellular immune deficiencies, immunosuppressive treatment, or antineoplastic therapy (Flaitz & Hicks, 1999). Various other conditions have been associated with predisposition to oral candidiasis (Table 28.1). Occasionally, candidiasis can also be seen in healthy patients without any associated conditions.

Handbook of Clinical Techniques in Pediatric Dentistry, Second Edition. Edited by Jane A. Soxman.
© 2022 John Wiley & Sons, Inc. Published 2022 by John Wiley & Sons, Inc.

Table 28.1 Predisposing factors for oral candidiasis in children and adolescents.

Local Factors	Systemic Factors
Xerostomia	Primary immunodeficiency
Smoking	Immunosuppressive therapy
Use of topical corticosteroids	Chemotherapy treatment
Use of corticosteroid inhaler	Malnutrition
Poor oral hygiene	Blood dyscrasias or malignancies (e.g., leukemia)
Intraoral appliance	Broad-spectrum antibiotic use
Dysbiosis (altered or immature oral flora)	Congenital conditions (e.g., familial candidiasis)
Impaired local defense mechanisms	Acquired immunodeficiency (e.g., HIV-related)
Loss of vertical dimension	Vitamin deficiencies (e.g., vitamin B_{12})
Altered oral mucosa (atrophic, decreased blood supply secondary to radiotherapy)	Endocrine disease (e.g., diabetes mellitus, hypothyroidism, hypoparathyroidism)
Chronic lip licking, thumb sucking, or use of petroleum-based lip products	

Samaranayake *et al.* (2009).

Oral candidiasis can present clinically in many different forms (Holmstrup & Axéll, 1990). A combination of host factors and microbial factors is most likely responsible for determining the occurrence of a particular clinical presentation. Oral candidiasis can be classified into three general forms: (i) acute infections; (ii) chronic infections; and (iii) chronic mucocutaneous candidiasis syndromes (Vila *et al.*, 2020). The most common acute infections in children are pseudomembranous candidiasis, known colloquially as "thrush," and acute erythematous candidiasis, or "antibiotic sore mouth." The other clinical forms that can be seen in children include central papillary atrophy (previously known as median rhomboid glossitis), chronic erythematous candidiasis (denture stomatitis), and angular cheilitis. Hyperplastic candidiasis, familial candidiasis, and endocrine-candidiasis syndrome are much less commonly seen. Table 28.2 describes the clinical presentations of oral fungal infections in children.

Oral candidiasis is most frequently treated with topical antifungal medications (Groll & Tragiannidis, 2010; Williams *et al.*, 2011). Of these, the most commonly used is nystatin. However, in chronic candidiasis associated with immunosuppression, topical agents may not be effective and may require the use of systemic medications (Singh *et al.*, 2014). Additionally, for the management of candidiasis, the underlying associated factors have to be addressed. Table 28.3 presents the most commonly used medications for the treatment of oral candidiasis.

Oral and Perioral Viral Infections

The clinical manifestations of viral infection in children are different than those seen in adults. These differences can be attributed to a child's immature immune system, rendering some infections more severe (Fenton & Unkel, 1997). Additionally, children are also highly effective incubators for viral replication and are promoters of the spread of viral infections, especially when they become mobile and tend to exchange infected fluids more effectively than adults because of a lack of hygiene.

Viral infections of the oral cavity usually manifest as either vesicles or ulcerations. They typically present with an abrupt onset and are associated with concomitant systemic symptoms such as fever, malaise, and

Table 28.2 Clinical manifestations of oral candidiasis

	Condition	Clinical Presentation	Associated Factors
Acute candida infections	Pseudomembranous candidiasis ("thrush")	Acute infection presenting with multiple white "cottage cheese-like" plaques that are wipeable, leaving an erythematous base. Commonly located on buccal mucosa, hard and soft palate, and tongue. They may be painful, or patients may complain of a "cottony" feeling or roughness in the mouth. Additionally, there may be a loss of taste or pain on swallowing (Figure 28.1).	• Associated with immunosuppression (especially HIV-related) or steroid use (systemic, topical, or inhaled). • Patients using a steroid inhaler should rinse their mouth with water following its use. • Seen in newborns or neonates attributed to an immature immune system. • In order to prevent reinfection, items placed in infants' mouth (e.g., bottle nipples, pacifiers) need to be sterilized or disinfected.
	Acute erythematous candidiasis ("antibiotic sore mouth")	Sudden onset of multiple red macules located on dorsal tongue, secondary to loss or atrophy of the filiform papillae. Patients can have a painful, burning sensation.	• Associated with antibiotic use (proliferation of candida secondary to reduction of oral bacterial microflora). • Has also been associated with the use of a steroid inhaler.
Chronic candida infections	Central papillary atrophy	Well-demarcated area of localized erythema on the midline posterior dorsal tongue. Results from the loss/atrophy of filiform papillae. This condition is usually asymptomatic. Used to be known as "median rhomboid glossitis," but this term is no longer applicable (Baughman, 1971) (Figure 28.2).	• Associated with antibiotic use, steroid inhaler use, tobacco smoking, or immunosuppression, or it may be idiopathic.
	Chronic erythematous candidiasis/candida-associated denture stomatitis	Erythema confined to the palatal denture-bearing mucosa. In children, it can be seen in patients with intraoral appliances with acrylic palatal coverage (e.g., Hawley retainer) (Hibino *et al.*, 2009). It is usually asymptomatic (Figure 28.3).	• Associated with the use of a palatal-bearing appliance, especially if it is kept in at night, is ill-fitting, or not cleaned properly (the area beneath the denture provides an ideal environment for candida to grow). • Candida is also present on the acrylic surface of appliance, so that needs to be treated as well in order to eradicate the colonization.

(continued)

Table 28.2 (Continued)

Condition	Clinical Presentation	Associated Factors
Angular cheilitis (Park et al., 2011)	Erythema and fissuring on the labial commissures. Lesions are most often bilateral. It may cause pain and can wax and wane. It commonly occurs in patients with another form of intraoral candidiasis through direct spread and colonization of candida in the angles of the mouth.	• Infection caused by excessive moisture and maceration of tissue from saliva resulting in a secondary infection with *Candida albicans* and in 20% of cases a bacterial co-infection with *Staphylococcus aureus*. • Associated with immunosuppression (especially HIV-related). • Related to a loss of vertical dimension and secondary saliva pooling in the area. • Other causes include nutritional deficiencies, such as B_9 (folic acid), zinc, B_6 (pyridoxine), B_2 (riboflavin), or B_3 (niacin) deficiency.
Cheilocandidosis	Erythema, crusting and ulceration of lips.	• Secondary to overuse of petroleum-based lip products, chronic lip licking, or thumb sucking.
Chronic multifocal candidiasis	Areas of localized erythema on the dorsal surface of the tongue, plus associated erythematous lesions on the junction of the hard and soft palate and in some cases angular cheilitis too.	• Associated with xerostomia, immunosuppression, or it can be idiopathic.
Hyperplastic candidiasis	Chronic thickened nonwipeable white plaque located on the tongue (lateral or dorsal surface) or anterior buccal mucosa (retrocommisural area).	• Any remaining white lesion that persists after antifungal treatment must be biopsied, since it may represent a premalignancy.
Chronic mucocutaneous candidiasis (CMC) syndromes	Familial candidiasis (Campois et al., 2015)	This includes a group of rare disorders characterized by altered immune responses, selective against *Candida* species, and resulting in persistent and/or recurrent infections of the skin, nails, and mucous membranes (including oral mucosa). Commonly presents with pseudomembranous candidiasis in the oral mucosa.	• Inherited autosomal dominant or autosomal recessive.
	Autoimmune polyendocrinopathy-candidiasis-ectodermal dystrophy (APECED) (Capalbo et al., 2013)	Characterized by (i) chronic mucocutaneous candidiasis; (ii) hypoparathyroidism; and (iii) adrenal gland insufficiency. Commonly presents with pseudomembranous candidiasis in oral mucosa. The ectodermal dystrophy present affects mainly nails and the tooth enamel, resulting in enamel defects.	• Rare condition, with incidence of 1 in 90,000–200,000. • Inherited autosomal recessive or autosomal dominant.

Table 28.3 Commonly prescribed medications for oral candidiasis.

Medication	Prescription	Indications	Side Effects	Special Considerations
Clotrimazole troches	**Rx:** Clotrimazole (Mycelex®) oral troches 10 mg **Disp:** 50–70 troches **Sig:** Slowly dissolve in mouth 5 times daily for 10–14 days (*avoid chewing the troches*)	Pseudomembranous candidiasis, erythematous candidiasis	Choking hazard for infants <4 years Medication has 60% sucrose, insure good oral hygiene to avoid increase in dental caries	• FDA approval in infants 3 years or older
Clotrimazole cream	**Rx:** Clotrimazole cream 1% (prescription) or Lotrimin AF®, Mycelex®, Trivagizole® (OTC) **Disp:** 15 g tube (prescription) or 12 g or 2 4g (OTC) **Sig:** Apply a thin layer on affected area 4 times a day, after meals and before bedtime	Angular cheilitis, cheilocandidosis		• Available as prescription or OTC
Fluconazole suspension/ tablets	**Rx:** Fluconazole (Diflucan®) oral suspension 10 mg/mL, 40 mg/mL Fluconazole (Diflucan®) 100 mg tablets (also available in 50 mg, 150 mg, or 200 mg)		Adverse effects include nausea, vomiting, headaches, rash, abdominal pain, and diarrhea Hepatic toxicity, including fatalities, has been reported rarely	• Efficacy has not been established in infants younger than 6 months • The drug requires acidic pH in the stomach to disintegrate and dissolve for oral absorption; therefore, absorption is decreased by medications that increase gastric pH • Contraindicated use with drugs metabolized by CYP3A4 and known to prolong QT interval, such as cisapride, astemizole, erythromycin, pimozide, and quinidine

(continued)

Table 28.3 (Continued)

Medication	Prescription	Indications	Side Effects	Special Considerations
	Disp: 35 mL bottle or 15 tabs **Sig:**	Pseudomembranous or erythematous candidiasis that is refractory to topical treatment in immunocompetent patients		• For recalcitrant lesions, it is recommended to perform fungal culture and susceptibility testing
	6 mg/kg orally once on the first day, followed by 3 mg/kg once per day for a total of 7–14 days (for neonates >14 days old)	Moderate or severe pseudomembranous candidiasis in immunocompetent infants/children		
	200mg orally initial loading dose and 100 mg daily thereafter for 7–14 days	Pseudomembranous or erythematous candidiasis in immunosuppressed patients (initial dose maximum 200 mg for non-HIV-exposed/positive children and 400 mg for HIV-exposed/positive; followed by maximum dose 100 mg for non-HIV-exposed/positive children, 400 mg for HIV-exposed/positive children)		
Gentian violet	**Rx:** Gentian violet 0.5% solution (OTC) **Disp:** 1 bottle **Sig:** apply 1.5 mL twice daily until lesions resolve	Pseudomembranous candidiasis in infants	Has been associated with increased risk in cancer; stains lips, clothes Prolonged use can cause ulceration of oral mucosa (Leung, 1988)	• Given the availability of other effective agents, use of gentian violet is not suggested
Miconazole mucoadhesive buccal tablet	**Rx:** Miconazole (Oravig®) buccal tablet 50 mg	Pseudomembranous candidiasis, erythematous candidiasis	Diarrhea, nausea, altered taste	• Safety and effectiveness have *not* been established for pediatric <16 years of age

Table 28.3 (Continued)

Medication	Prescription	Indications	Side Effects	Special Considerations
	Disp: 14 tabs **Sig:** Apply tablet to the mucosal surface over the canine fossa once daily for 7–14 days (patients >16 years of age)			
Miconazole ointment	**Rx:** Miconazole 2% ointment, available as prescription (Monistat Derm®) or OTC (Micatin®) **Disp:** 15 g tube (prescription), 15 g or 30 g (OTC) **Sig:** Apply a thin layer to affected area 3-4 times a day after meals and before bedtime	Angular cheilitis, cheilocandidosis		• FDA approved in ages ≥2 years and adults • Available in prescription and OTC preparations
Nystatin suspension	**Rx:** Nystatin (Mycostatin®, Nilstat®) oral suspension 100,000 U/mL **Disp:** 120 mL infants <12 months; 300 mL child/adult **Sig:** Swab oral tissues with 2 mL 4 times a day. Use for 14 days and reevaluate. Encourage swallowing and avoid feeding 30 minutes after use	Pseudomembranous candidiasis immunocompetent infants/children	Has a high glucose content, which can increase risk for dental caries, must maintain good oral hygiene	• Treatment should be extended 1–2 days after lesions disappear in order to lower rate or risk of recurrence of candidiasis • Bottle nipples and pacifiers should be sterilized or disinfected to avoid reinfection

(continued)

Table 28.3 (Continued)

Medication	Prescription	Indications	Side Effects	Special Considerations
	Swish and swallow 5 mL 3–4 times a day (child/adult). Use for 14 days and reevaluate. For older children, swish and hold in the mouth as long as possible before swallowing			
Nystatin lozenges	**Rx:** Nystatin lozenges 200,000 U **Disp:** 56 (112) tablets **Sig:** Dissolve 1 or 2 lozenges in mouth 4 times a day for 7–14 days		Choking hazard for infants <4 years Medication has high glucose content, must ensure good oral hygiene to avoid increase risk of dental caries	• Lozenges no longer marketed in the USA
Nystatin ointment	**Rx:** Nystatin ointment 100,000 U/g **Disp:** 15 g tube **Sig:** Apply 3–4 times daily on affected area (can be applied inside removable oral appliance)	Angular cheilitis, cheilocandidosis, denture stomatitis		• FDA approval for infants >2 months

Table 28.3 (Continued)

Medication	Prescription	Indications	Side Effects	Special Considerations
Nystatin and triamcinolone ointment	**Rx:** Nystatin 100,000 U and triamcinolone acetonide 0.1% (Mycolog-II®) **Disp:** 15 g tube **Sig:** Apply a thin layer to affected area 3 times a day after meals and before bedtime for 5 days	Angular cheilitis, cheilocandidosis		• FDA approval for infants >2 months • Best choice for chronic cases of angular cheilitis because it combines anti-inflammatory and antifungal properties
Iodoquinolol and hydrocortisone cream	**Rx:** Iodoquinolol and hydrocortisone cream (Vytone®) **Disp:** 1 oz tube **Sig:** Apply a thin layer to the affected area 3 times a day after meals and before bedtime for 5 days	Angular cheilitis, cheilocandidosis		• Safety and effectiveness in pediatric patients <12 years have not been established • Best for chronic cases since it combines anti-inflammatory and antifungal properties
Chlorhexidine gluconate	**Rx:** Chlorhexidine gluconate 0.12% (Peridex®) **Disp:** 16 oz bottle **Sig:** Soak oral appliance in solution overnight for 15 minutes twice daily or overnight	Denture stomatitis (chronic erythematous candidiasis)		Chlorhexidine not only has activity against gram-positive and gram-negative organisms, facultative anaerobes, and aerobes, but also yeast

FDA, Food and Drug Administration; OTC, over the counter.
Pappas *et al.* (2016).

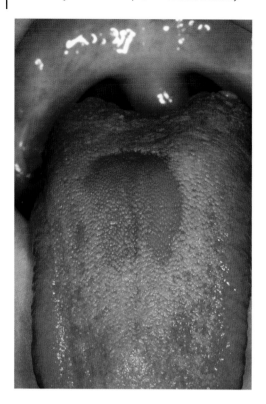

Figure 28.2 Central papillary atrophy in dorsal tongue.

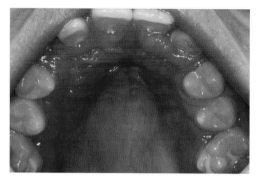

Figure 28.3 Chronic erythematous candidiasis ("denture stomatitis") associated with use of a Hawley appliance.

lymphadenopathy (Sällberg, 2009; Santosh & Muddana, 2020). The most common viral infections in children are primary herpetic gingivostomatitis, herpangina, and hand foot and mouth disease.

Human papillomavirus (HPV) infections are also common in children (Summersgill *et al.*, 2001). HPV is an epidermotropic DNA virus and there are more than 200 HPV types identified; of these more than 30 types are known to infect the oral mucosa. The HPV virus can cause benign or malignant tumors of the mucosa or skin, depending on the HPV subtype involved. The low-risk types are 6, 11,

13, 32, 40, 42, 44, 54, 55, 61, 62, 64, 67, 69, 70, 71, 72, and 81, and the high-risk types are 16, 18, 31, 33, 35, 39, 45, 51, 52, 56, 58, 59, 66, 68, and 73 (Mammas *et al.*, 2009, 2019).

Oral viral infections are frequently seen in the pediatric dental practice. Table 28.4 describes the viruses that are associated with oral and perioral infections in children. Many of these viruses either produce symptoms in the oral cavity or can be effectively spread during dental treatment.

Oral viral infections in children are treated with a combination of palliative care and antivirals. Milder, symptomatic patients can receive supportive care, which includes maintenance of fluids, antipyretics, and use of topical anesthetics or coating agents for topical pain relief. More severe infections require systemic antiviral treatment. Most perioral lesions are treated with topical antivirals. HPV-related oral lesions in children are treated by excision or in some cases topical agents. Table 28.5 lists the medications commonly used for oral viral infections.

Table 28.4 Oral and perioral viral infections in children.

Viral Infection	Clinical Condition	Epidemiology	Clinical Description
Herpes simplex virus (HSV) Type 1 or 2 or human herpesvirus (HHV) Type 1 or 2	Primary herpetic gingivostomatitis	• Typically occurs in children younger than the age of 5, but can also occur in adolescents and young adults • HSV-1 responsible for 90% of infections • Lower socioeconomic status correlates with earlier exposure to the virus • Virus is acquired through direct contact with oral lesions or saliva of an infected person, or through saliva of an asymptomatic person shedding the virus in the absence of clinical disease • HSV-1 or -2 can be present in genital mucosa and can be transmitted by oral–genital contact as well • Many infections are asymptomatic and subclinical • After the primary infection, HSV migrates to the trigeminal ganglion, where it remains latent and can be reactivated	• Oral lesions start off as 1–3 mm vesicles that later ulcerate and coalesce • Typically affects marginal gingiva as edema, inflammation, and bleeding and punched-out ulcers • Other oral sites include tongue, hard and soft palate, floor of mouth, and buccal mucosa • Lips and perioral skin are affected in two-thirds of cases and can show crusting • Associated systemic signs and symptoms include fever, irritability, malaise, sleeplessness, cervical lymphadenopathy, and headaches • Lesion are painful and patients complain of pain on eating, drinking, and swallowing. • In young adults and adults, primary infection can present as pharyngotonsillitis, with lesion in soft palate and tonsillar pillars and associated sore throat and fever (Figure 28.4)

(continued)

Table 28.4 (Continued)

Viral Infection	Clinical Condition	Epidemiology	Clinical Description
	Recurrent herpes labialis ("cold sore" or "fever blister")	• Occurs less frequently, only 15–40% of seropositive patients ever experience symptomatic reactivation of HSV-1 or -2 located in trigeminal ganglion • Reactivation may be secondary to exposure to sunlight, cold, trauma (e.g., after dental procedure), stress, increased age, or immunosuppression • Autoinoculation of virus can occur when vesicles rupture and the viral-filled fluid is released	• The prodrome presents with tingling, burning sensation, erythema, or pain in the area • Lesions start off as vesicles that later rupture and ulcerate and crust over • Lesions are usually located on vermillion of lips/perioral skin (Figure 28.5)
	Recurrent intraoral herpes	• Occurs less frequently than herpes labialis • Reactivation may be secondary to traumatic dental procedure (local anesthesia or extraction)	• In immunocompetent patient, lesions located only on keratinized mucosa (attached gingiva and palate) • Lesions start off as 1–3 mm vesicles that rupture, forming erosions that coalesce and later ulcerate • Lesions are usually asymptomatic, patients can complain of "rough feeling" in mouth • In immunocompromised patients, nonkeratinized mucosa (tongue and buccal mucosa) can be affected. Lesions also last longer, are more painful and do not respond to therapy
Varicella zoster virus (VZV) or HHV-3	Varicella (chickenpox)	• Primary infection with VZV in nonimmune hosts • Acquired by direct contact with infected person or airborne transmission of infected droplets (highly contagious). • Incidence is low due to vaccination (introduced in 1995)	• Prodrome with aching muscles, nausea, decreased appetite, and headache • Skin lesions develop and present as a rash, then vesicles develop, usually on skin of face and trunk. Skin lesions occur in crops and are typically at different stages of evolution • Oral lesions may precede skin lesions, begin as small vesicles that eventually rupture to form small ulcers on the palate and buccal mucosa (similar to primary herpetic gingivostomatitis, but less painful)

Table 28.4 (Continued)

Viral Infection	Clinical Condition	Epidemiology	Clinical Description
	Herpes zoster ("shingles") (Katakam *et al.*, 2016)	• Reactivation of VZV that remains latent in the sensory ganglia of the cranial nerve or dorsal root ganglia • Most commonly occurs in people with depressed immune systems or those over the age of 50 • Rarely occurs in children, but children with depressed immune systems have a greater risk and may experience more severe symptoms. This includes patients with immunosuppression secondary to malignancy; undergoing immunosuppressive treatment for malignancy, organ transplantation, or for chronic diseases, such as rheumatoid arthritis; and children with HIV infection • Children who had chickenpox during the first year of life, or whose mothers had chickenpox very late in pregnancy, are also at risk	• Prodrome with intense pain (burning sensation, prickling, tingling) in affected area (innervated by sensory nerve). May also have fever, malaise, and headaches • Acute phase shows 1–4 mm vesicles on an erythematous base, which ulcerate and crust over, located on both keratinized and nonkeratinized mucosa • In the oral cavity, lesions are secondary to trigeminal nerve involvement and extend to the midline but do not cross it. Overlying skin can also be involved • Teeth in affected area may show pulpitis, necrosis, or root resorption • Chronic phase consists of neuralgia (postherpetic neuralgia), with pain persisting after lesions resolve
Epstein–Barr virus or HHV-4	Infectious mononucleosis ("kissing disease")	• Infection occurs through contact with infected saliva via fingers, toys, other objects, or kissing • In the USA it is more commonly seen in adolescents and young adults	• Most children are asymptomatic, less than 10% develop any signs/symptoms • Classic presentation is fever, lymphadenopathy, pharyngitis, and atypical lymphocytosis • Intraoral lesions typically consist of tonsillar enlargement with surface exudate and secondary abscesses. Patients can also present with petechiae in the hard and soft palate • Occasionally patients can develop necrotizing ulcerative gingivitis (NUG), especially NUG-like pericoronitis. • Children <4 years can present with hepatosplenomegaly • Complications include ruptured spleen, thrombocytopenia, hemolytic anemia, aplastic anemia, myocarditis

(continued)

Table 28.4 (Continued)

Viral Infection	Clinical Condition	Epidemiology	Clinical Description
Cytomegalovirus (CMV) or HHV-5	CMV infection	• CMV is an ubiquitous virus that infects people of all ages • Transmission occurs by contact with maternal cervicovaginal secretions during delivery, from breast milk, or from blood transfusions	• CMV infection ranges from asymptomatic or mild disease in immunologically normal infants and children, to severe and potentially life-threatening disease in immunocompromised children • In 10% of cases there may be symptoms, including a mononucleosis–like syndrome • Most common manifestations are fever, fatigue, pharyngitis, adenopathy (especially cervical adenopathy), and hepatitis • CMV disease in immunocompromised children is often linked to the underlying disease process responsible for the immunosuppression:graft loss in renal transplant patients; hepatitis and colitis in liver transplant patients; pneumonitis in lung and bone marrow transplant patients; myocarditis followed by late atherosclerosis in heart transplant patients
Coxsackievirus infections	Hand–foot–mouth disease	• Coxsackieviruses A16 and A6 are most commonly involved (also enterovirus A71) • Most cases occur in infants and children, particularly those less than 5–7 years old • Typically occurs during the summer and early autumn • Transmission is by person to person, via fecal–oral route	• No prodrome • Presents as fever (<101°F), oral or pharyngeal pain (in verbal children), or refusal to eat (in nonverbal children) • Oral lesions are multiple (2–30) 2–7 mm vesicles that ulcerate, located on buccal mucosa, labial mucosa, and tongue, but can affect any site. Oral lesions precede the skin lesions • Skin lesions are a macular, maculopapular, or vesicular rash, which is nonpruritic and nonpainful, involving the hands (dorsum of the fingers, interdigital area, palms), feet (dorsum of the toes, lateral border of the feet, soles, heels), buttocks, legs (upper thighs), and arms

Table 28.4 (Continued)

Viral Infection	Clinical Condition	Epidemiology	Clinical Description
	Herpangina	• Coxsackieviruses A1–6, 8, 10, and 22 most commonly involved • Occurs most frequently in summer and early autumn • Transmission is through direct contact via fecal–oral route	• Symptoms start with high fevers (>101 °F) • Some patients may experience malaise, headache, sore throat, dysphagia, and abdominal pain • A small number of lesions (2–6) develop in the soft palate/tonsillar pillar area. Lesions are 2–4 mm red macules initially, then form vesicles, which later ulcerate
Paramyxovirus	Measles (rubeola)	• Infection caused by measles (rubeola) virus, a paramyxovirus • Transmission is through direct contact • In the USA, there has been an increase in measles cases, rising from 371 cases in 2018 to 1261 cases in 2019, as reported by the Centers for Disease Control	• Prodrome consists of fever, malaise, conjunctivitis, and cough • Koplik spots found in the prodrome in over 70% of cases. These are 1–3 mm white macules surrounded by erythema, usually located on the buccal mucosa. They are thought to represent foci of epithelial necrosis and typically last for 12–72 hours before sloughing off • Skin lesions consists of an erythematous, maculopapular, blanching rash, which classically begins on the face and spreads from head to toe and from the trunk to the extremities • Enamel pitting on permanent teeth has been reported in children who develop measles in early childhood
	Mumps	• Highly contagious viral infection caused by Rubulavirus, a paramyxovirus • It is transmitted by respiratory droplets, direct contact, or through fomites • Outbreaks occur in unvaccinated regions	• Prodrome with fever, headache, myalgia, fatigue, and anorexia • This is followed by the development of parotid gland swelling within 48 hours (most often bilateral, but can be unilateral), lasting up to 10 days • Stenson's duct (parotid duct) is often erythematous and swollen, and there can also be swelling of the sublingual and submandibular glands • Orchitis is the second most common manifestation

(continued)

Table 28.4 (Continued)

Viral Infection	Clinical Condition	Epidemiology	Clinical Description
Rubella virus	Rubella ("German measles")	• Rubella virus is a member of the Togavirus family • If acquired in pregnancy it can cause birth defects in the developing fetus • Transmission is through respiratory droplets • In 2015, rubella was officially declared eliminated from the Americas • Currently cases continue to be reported in African and Southeast Asian countries	• In children it presents with the acute onset of a maculopapular rash with minimal systemic symptoms • The rash consists of pinpoint, pink maculopapules, which first appear on the face and then spread to trunk and extremities • Oral lesions are known as Forchheimer sign and consist of small, dark red papules (petechiae) that develop in soft palate (and can extend to the hard palate)
Human immunodeficiency virus (HIV-1) (Lauritano et al., 2020)	HIV disease and acquired immunodeficiency syndrome (AIDS)	• Most HIV infections in children are acquired via mother-to-child transmission during pregnancy, labor, delivery, or breastfeeding • In developed countries incidence is low; the highest number of cases are reported in Sub-Saharan Africa	• The most common lesions associated with pediatric HIV infection are angular cheilitis, erythematous candidiasis, pseudomembranous candidiasis, HSV infections, linear gingival erythema, parotid enlargement, and recurrent aphthous ulcers
Human papillomavirus (HPV) (Summersgill et al., 2001)	Verruca vulgaris ("warts")	Common benign skin lesion in children Caused by HPV subtype 2 In oral and perioral mucosa lesions occur due to autoinoculation from skin lesions	• Presents as <5 mm white papule, which can be pedunculated or sessile and has papillary projections or pebbly surface • Commonly located on vermillion border of lip, labial mucosa, anterior dorsum of tongue
	Squamous papilloma ("papilloma")	HPV subtypes 6, 11	• Presents as 5–10 mm papule, can have white color or normal mucosal color, and is usually pedunculated • Common locations include labial mucosa • tongue and soft palate (Figure 28.6)

Table 28.4 (Continued)

Viral Infection	Clinical Condition	Epidemiology	Clinical Description
	Condyloma accuminatum ("genital wart")	HPV subtypes 6, 11, 16, 18	• Typically presents as a larger pink papule, 10–15 mm, with a sessile base and blunt papillary projections • Located on labial mucosa, lingual frenum, or soft palate
	Multifocal epithelial hyperplasia ("Heck's disease") (Carlos & Sedano, 1994)	HPV subtypes 13 and 32	• Presents as multiple papules more frequently seen in children • Papulonodular variant: multiple smooth-surfaced pink papules that vary in size (between 1 mm and 10 mm) • Papillomatous variant: multiple white or pink papules of varying sizes between 1 mm and 10 mm with pebbly surface (Figure 28.7)

Source: Sällberg (2009).

Table 28.5 Commonly prescribed treatments for oral and perioral viral infections.

Condition	Management Recommendations	Side Effects	Special Considerations
Primary herpetic gingivostomatitis/ acute herpetic gingivostomatitis (Arduino & Porter, 2008)	*Hydration* • Adequate fluid intake should be encouraged to avoid dehydration. Children who are unable to drink sufficiently to maintain hydration should be hospitalized for parenteral fluid therapy *Pain/fever management* **Rx**: Acetaminophen (Tylenol®), oral solution 60 mg/5 mL, 500 mg/5 mL, 500 mg/15 mL or chewable tabs 80 mg or 160 mg **Disp**: mL varies by weight or 20–40 tabs **Sig**:: Take 10/15 mg/kg (for patients <12 years) orally every 4–6 hours as required for pain/fever or Take 325, 650, or 1000 mg (for patients >12 years) orally every 4–6 hours as required for pain/fever **Rx**: Ibuprofen (oral suspension 100 mg/5 mL or 200, 400, 600 mg tabs) **Disp**: mL varies by weight or 20–40 tabs **Sig**: Take 10 mg/kg (for patients <12 years) every 4–6 hours as required for pain or fever or Take 400–600 mg for patients >12 years orally every 4–6 hours as required for pain/fever	Acetaminophen has been associated with cases of acute liver failure, at times resulting in liver transplant and death	To lower the risk for hepatotoxicity, limit daily dose to ≤75 mg/kg/day (maximum of 5 daily doses), not to exceed 4000 mg/day Maximum daily dose is 40 mg/kg/day or 2400 mg/day

Table 28.5 (Continued)

Condition	Management Recommendations	Side Effects	Special Considerations
	Rx: Hydrocodone/acetaminophen (Lortab elixir® 10 mg hydrocodone/300 mg acetaminophen/15mL), Hycet® oral solution (7.5 mg hydrocodone and 325 mg acetaminophen/15 mL) or Lorcet®, Lortab® (5 mg hydrocodone and 325 mg acetaminophen, 7.5mg hydrocodone and 325 mg acetaminophen, 10 mg hydrocodone and 325 mg acetaminophen tabs) **Disp.:** mL varies by weight or 9–24 tabs **Sig:** 0.1–0.2 mg/kg hydrocodone (for patients <50 kg) every 4–8 hours or 5–10 mg hydrocodone (for patients >50 kg) every 4–8 hours *Pain/palliative*	Opiates should be used with caution, because potential adverse effects include respiratory depression, central nervous system depression, hypotension, and constipation	For severe cases (e.g., patients who cannot sleep or eat), the use of oral opiates such as hydrocodone may be required

(continued)

Table 28.5 (Continued)

Condition	Management Recommendations	Side Effects	Special Considerations
	Rx: *Diphenhydramine HCL (Children's Benadryl®) 12.5 mg/5 mL and **Maalox® mix in a 1 : 1 ratio **Disp.:** 200 mL **Sig:** Rinse with 1–2 teaspoons (5–10 mL) every 4 hours for 2 minutes and spit out. If unable to rinse, swab inside of mouth with a cleansing sponge (Toothette®) or a cotton-tipped applicator every 4 hours		*Alcohol-free diphenhydramine HCL (Benadryl®) should be used if possible **Kaopectate® or other magnesium aluminum hydroxide solution can be substituted for Maalox®
	Rx: Diphenhydramine HCL (Children's Benadryl®) 12.5 mg/5 mL/**Maalox®/viscous lidocaine 2%; mix in a 1 : 1 : 1 ratio **Disp.:** 200 mL **Sig:** Rinse with 1–2 teaspoons (5–10 mL) every 4 hours for 2 minutes and spit out ●Topical benzocaine should not be used in children because of reports of methemoglobinemia	Seizures, cardiopulmonary arrest, and death in patients <3 years have been reported.	The use of lidocaine in patients < 3 years of age should be limited to those situations where safer alternatives are not available or have been tried but failed
	Rx: Dyclonine HCL 0.1% spray (OTC) (Cepacol® Sore Throat) can be used for pain relive in children >4 years of age *Adjunctive management* **Rx:** Chlorhexidine gluconate 0.12% (Peridex®) can be helpful in managing residual gingivitis after the gingival ulcers have healed. There is also some evidence that it may have antiviral properties	It can also predispose to self-injury if the child chews on anesthetized oral mucosa or chokes on secretions secondary to pharyngeal anesthesia	Chlorhexidine gluconate 0.12% alcohol-free (Paroex®) can be substituted and may be better tolerated by some patients

Table 28.5 (Continued)

Condition	Management Recommendations	Side Effects	Special Considerations
	• Patients/parents should be instructed to restrict contact with active lesions and to avoid fingers in mouth in order to prevent autoinoculation or spread to others.		
	Antivirals		
	For immunocompetent children:		
	Rx: Oral acyclovir (Zovirax®) suspension (200 mg/5mL) or 400 mg, 800 mg tablets	Maximum dose of acyclovir is 80 mg/kg/day	Recommend for immunocompetent infants/children who present within 3–4 days of disease onset and/or those in great pain or who are unable to eat or drink.
	Disp.: mL varies by weight or 35–70 tabs		For children who present ≥4 days after illness, only supportive care is recommended
	Sig: Take 15 mg/kg/dose 5 times per day, swish and swallow for 5–7 days, or 400–800 mg 5 times per day for 7–14 days		
	For immunosuppressed children:		Antivirals are recommended for all immunocompromised children. In severe cases intravenous antivirals may be indicated. This will be dictated by the degree of immunosuppression, suspicion for dissemination, severity, and ability to absorb oral acyclovir from the gastrointestinal tract.
	Rx: Oral acyclovir (Zovirax®) suspension (200 mg/5 mL) or 400 mg, 800 mg tablets		
	Disp.: mL varies by weight		
	Sig.: Take 1000 mg/day divided in 3–5 doses (for children >2 years old) for 10–14 days		
	• Topical antiviral agents are not helpful in the treatment of primary herpes gingivostomatitis in immunocompetent patients and are not recommended		

(continued)

Table 28.5 (Continued)

Condition	Management Recommendations	Side Effects	Special Considerations
Recurrent herpes labialis ("cold sore" or "fever blister") (Raborn *et al.*, 2002)	*Prevention* •Use of PABA-free (OTC) sunscreen for lips is recommended before sun exposure and reapplication every hour •Additionally, use of a wide-brimmed hat or visor plus sunscreen on the face is also recommended for maximum protection when excessive sunlight exposure is the triggering factor *Topical antivirals* **Rx:** Penciclovir (Denavir®) cream 1% **Disp.:** 2 g tube **Sig.:** Apply to affected area every 2 hours for a period of 4 days, beginning as soon as first symptoms occur **Rx:** Acyclovir (Zovirax®) ointment 5% **Disp.:** 15 mg tube **Sig.:** Apply to affected area every hour at the onset of initial signs or symptoms for 7 days or when lesion resolves **Rx:** Docosanol (Abreva®) OTC **Disp.:** 2 g tube **Sig.:** Apply to affected area 5 times a day for up to 10 days		Topical antivirals may act as a protective emollient over the lesion, but they have not been found to have a significant clinical benefit in immunocompetent children For maximum efficacy, they should be applied at the earliest sign or symptom, which can be difficult to establish in young children

Table 28.5 (Continued)

Condition	Management Recommendations	Side Effects	Special Considerations
	Oral antivirals	Maximum dose of acyclovir is 80 mg/kg/day	In placebo-controlled clinical trials, oral antiviral therapy has been shown to accelerate healing of lesions when treatment is started in prodrome
	Rx: Oral acyclovir (Zovirax®) suspension (200 mg/5 mL) or 200 mg, 400 mg tablets	Safety and efficacy in children have not been established	
	Disp.: mL varies by weight or 15–25 tabs	Safety and efficacy in children have not been established	
	Sig: Take 20 mg/kg/dose 5 times per day for 5–7 days		
	or		
	200 mg 5 times a day for 5 days		
	400 mg 3 times a day for 5 days		
	Rx: Valacyclovir (Valtrex®) 500 mg or 1 g tablet		
	Disp.: 4–8 tabs		
	Sig.: 2 g 2 times a day for 2 days (start at first sign or symptom)		
	Rx: Famciclovir (Famvir®) 500 mg tablets		
	Disp.: 3 tabs		
	Sig.: Take 1.5 g (3 tabs) as a single dose at first sign or symptom		

(continued)

Table 28.5 (Continued)

Condition	Management Recommendations	Side Effects	Special Considerations
For immunosuppressed children			
	Rx: *Acyclovir (Zovirax®) 400 mg*	Maximum dose of acyclovir is 400 mg/dose. Maximum dose is 80 mg/kg/day	
	Disp.: 15–30 tabs		
	Sig.: Take 1 tab orally 3 times a day for 5–10 days	Safety and efficacy in children have not been established	
	Rx: Valacyclovir (Valtrex®) 1 g tablet	Safety and efficacy in children have not been established	
	Disp.: 10–20 tabs		
	Sig.: Take 1 tab orally 2 times a day for 5–10 days	Safety and efficacy in children have not been established	
	Rx: Famciclovir (Famvir®) 500 mg	Safety and efficacy in children have not been established	
	Disp.: 10–20 tabs		
	Sig.: Take 1 tab orally 2 times a day for 5–10 days		
	Prophylaxis		
	Rx: Acyclovir (Zovirax®) 400 mg		
	Disp.: 60 tabs		
	Sig.: Take 1 tab orally 2 times a day		

Table 28.5 (Continued)

Condition	Management Recommendations	Side Effects	Special Considerations
	Rx: Valacyclovir (Valtrex®) 500 mg		
	Disp.: 30 tabs		
	Sig.: Take one tab orally daily		
	Rx: Famciclovir (Famvir®) 250 mg		
	Disp.: 60t abs		
	Sig.: Take one tab orally 2 times a day		
	Secondary bacterial infections on skin		
	Rx: Mupirocin ointment 2% (Bactrobam®)		
	Disp.: 22 g tube		
	Sig.: Apply a thin layer to affected area 3 times a day		
Recurrent intraoral herpes	• Most patients do not require treatment because lesions are not painful		
	• In cases where patients complain of pain, chlorhexidine gluconate 0.12% (Peridex®) has shown antiviral properties and can be used. Alternatively, chlorhexidine gluconate 0.12% alcohol-free (Paroex®)		
	Rx: Acyclovir suspension 200 mg/5 mL can also be used alone or in combination with chlorhexidine gluconate 0.12% (Peridex®). Alternatively, chlorhexidine gluconate 0.12% alcohol-free (Paroex®)		

(continued)

Table 28.5 (Continued)

Condition	Management Recommendations	Side Effects	Special Considerations
Herpes zoster "shingles" (Mustafa et al., 2009)	**Rx:** Acyclovir (Zovirax®) 800 mg Disp.: 35–50 tabs Sig.: Take 1 tab orally 5 times a day for 7–10 days **Rx:** Valacyclovir (Valtrex®) 1000 mg Disp.: 21 tabs Sig.: Take 1 tab orally 3 times a day for 7 days **Rx:** Famciclovir (Famvir®) 500 mg Disp.: 21 tabs Sig.: Take 1 tab orally 3 times a day for 7 days *Analgesia for Neuritis* Mild pain: **Rx:** Acetaminophen or ibuprofen Moderate to severe pain: **Rx:** Opioid analgesics (oxycodone or oral morphine)	Although the doses for treatment of herpes zoster are higher than those used for herpes simplex, adverse events are uncommon, but can include nausea, diarrhea, or headache	Treatment should start within 48–72 hours after onset of symptoms/signs to be most effective and maximize potential benefits of the therapy Immunocompromised patients should receive therapy, even if they present after >72 hours of onset of symptoms Some randomized double-blind studies have shown that the resolution of neuritis was accelerated with the use of valacyclovir compared to treatment with acyclovir Antiviral therapy reduces pain associated with neuritis, but in some cases pain can be severe
Hand–foot–mouth disease/ herpangina (Ooi et al., 2010)	• Supportive treatment. No antiviral therapy available • Maintain adequate hydration *Pain and fever management* **Rx:** Ibuprofen 10 mg/kg (for patients <12 years) every 4–6 hours, or 400–600 mg (for patients >12 years) orally every 4–6 hours **Rx:** Acetaminophen 10–15 mg/kg (for patients <12 years) orally every 4–6 hours or		

Table 28.5 (Continued)

Condition	Management Recommendations	Side Effects	Special Considerations
	325, 650, or 1000 mg (for patients >12 years) orally every 4–6 hours *Topical medications* **Rx:** Diphenhydramine HCL (Children's Benadryl®) 12.5mg/5 mL and Maalox®/Kaopectate® mix in a 1 : 1 ratio **Rx:** Diphenhydramine hydrochloride (Children's Benadryl®) 12.5 mg/5 mL/Maalox® or Kaopectate®/viscous lidocaine 2%*; mix in a 1 : 1 : 1 ratio (*only for patients who can expectorate) **Rx:** Topical dyclonine HCL 0.1% spray (OTC) (Cepacol® Sore Throat)	Lidocaine should not be used in children who cannot expectorate because of potential risk of aspiration or toxicity	There is limited evidence on the benefit of topical medications in the management of these conditions
Verruca vulgaris	• Surgical excision • Laser • Cryotherapy • Electrosurgery		Low chance of recurrence, no malignant transformation. Lesions may spontaneously resolve
Squamous papilloma	• Surgical excision		No malignant transformation. Rare recurrence

(continued)

Table 28.5 (Continued)

Condition	Management Recommendations	Side Effects	Special Considerations
Condyloma acuminatum (Syrjänen, 2018)	• Surgical excision • Cryotherapy • Laser ablation (may produce infectious HPV plume) **Rx:** Topical agents: Imiquimod 5% cream Podophyllotoxin 0.15% cream Sinecatechins 15% ointment		Sexually transmitted lesion, in children suspected sexual abuse should be reported No malignant transformation has been reported Topical agents are used in anogenital lesions, but not used routinely for oral lesions
Multifocal epithelial hyperplasia "Heck's disease" (Said et al., 2013)	• Conservative surgical excision • Cryotherapy • Laser • Electrosurgery removal to confirm diagnosis or improve esthetics. **Rx:** Topical agents (limited case reports): Topical interferon beta Intralesional interferon-alpha Topical imiquimod cream 5%		May resolve spontaneously after months or years. Rarely seen in adults. No malignant transformation reported

OTC, over the counter; PABA, para-aminobenzoic acid.

Table 28.6 Oral ulcers in children and their management.

		Etiology	Clinical Description	Management
Acute Ulcers				
Single	**Traumatic ulcer**	These can occur secondary to:		
		• Sources of irritation to oral mucosa: brackets, wires, rough tooth surfaces, broken-down restorations	Ulcers with ragged borders, occasionally raised white (hyperkeratotic) borders	• Remove source of irritation if applicable Palliative care **Rx:** Diphenhydramine HCL 12.5 mg/5 mL and Maalox®/Kaopectate® 1 : 1 ratio
		• Thermal burns from eating foods or drinking liquids that are too hot	Ulcers or erosions on the anterior palate, ill-defined borders	**Rx:** Diphenhydramine HCL 12.5 mg/5 mL, Maalox®/Kaopectate® plus lidocaine suspension 2%* ratio 1 : 1 : 1 (*only for patients who can expectorate) **Rx:** Viscous lidocaine 2% suspension (only for patients who can expectorate)
		• Lip biting or cheek biting: related to unfamiliar sensation after local anesthesia mandibular nerve block	Ulceration on lower labial mucosa or buccal mucosa with ragged borders	• Provide clear postoperative instructions, parents/caregivers to monitor patient closely • Avoid eating or drinking for at least 3–4 hours postoperatively • Placement of barrier (long cotton roll, tongue depressor) between teeth and soft tissue • Use of phentolamine mesylate (OraVerse®) to reverse local anesthesia for children >15 kg (dose is 0.5–1 cartridge, 0.2–0.4 mg) • For severe pain, palliative care: **Rx:** Diphenhydramine HCL 12.5 mg/5 mL and Maalox® ± lidocaine 2%* (*only for patients who can expectorate) • Follow-up and assurance to parents that it is not an infection

(continued)

Table 28.6 (Continued)

	Etiology	Clinical Description	Management
	• Riga–Fede disease: appears between 1 week and 1 year old, caused by repetitive trauma of tongue by natal/neonatal teeth on protrusive and retrusive movements (Padmanabhan et al., 2010)	Ulcer located on anterior ventral tongue (area in contact with tooth), usually has ragged borders	• If natal/neonatal tooth has +3 mobility, extraction is indicated (high risk of swallowing or aspiration) • If tooth is not mobile: -smoothing incisal surface -covering incisal surface (composite/glass ionomer or creating a shield) • Biopsy is indicated if lesion remains after source of trauma is removed
Iatrogenic ulcer	• Secondary to caustic materials inadvertently applied to the oral soft tissues during dental procedures (e.g., formocresol, sodium hypochlorite)	Ulcer present after dental procedure, usually located on gingiva or labial mucosa with ragged borders	• Prevention of exposure is important • Use of rubber dam/barriers to avoid exposure to mucosa, care while using caustic agents intraorally *Palliative care for pain* **Rx:** Diphenhydramine HCL 12.5 mg/5 mL plus Maalox®/Kaopectate® ± viscous lidocaine 2%* suspension (*only for patients who can expectorate)
Self-induced ulcer (Limeres et al., 2013)	• Ulcerations caused by biting or by using fingernail or other object to cause harm to mucosa • May be seen in patients with certain syndromes with known self-injurious behaviors (Lesh–Nyhan syndrome, familial dysautonomia (Riley–Day syndrome), congenital indifference to pain, Gaucher disease, cerebral palsy, or Tourette syndrome)	If associated with biting, will be located in accessible areas such as lower labial mucosa, buccal mucosa, or tongue. Injuries caused by fingernails or other objects are usually located on gingiva	*Palliative care* **Rx:** Viscous lidocaine 2%* suspension or topical anesthetics) (*only for patients who can expectorate) • Fabrication of oral appliances (bite guards or lip bumpers) to serve as barriers • In severe cases prophylactic dental extractions may be needed

Table 28.6 (Continued)

	Etiology	Clinical Description	Management
Recurrent aphthous ulcers (RAU) "canker sores" (Scully & Porter, 2008)	• The exact cause is unknown, but most researchers support the concept of immune dysregulation involving the oral mucosa leading to an exaggerated inflammatory process. There is also a genetic predisposition and most patients have a family history • Onset of ulcers can be exacerbated by trauma of the mucosa, such as biting or undergoing a dental procedure • Most patients start developing lesion between 10 and 30 years and these can continue until middle age, but their frequency diminishes • If patients have associated systemic symptoms, other causes have to be investigated (see below). For patients with more severe disease or patients who develop lesions later in life, an underlying cause should be investigated *Laboratory studies* Complete blood count (CBC), erythrocyte sedimentation rate (ESR), and assessment of nutritional deficiencies (vitamin B_{12}, folate, iron) should be done. Correction of these could potentially lead to resolution or improvement of the ulcers	Ulcers have a characteristic clinical course: -Well-defined ulcers round to oval in shape surrounded by an erythematous halo -Located on nonattached (nonkeratinized) mucosa. Most commonly sites are the buccal and labial mucosa, followed by ventral tongue, floor of the mouth, and soft palate (Figure 28.8) -Involvement of the keratinized mucosa is extremely rare and represents extension -Can be single or multiple (1–5 ulcers) -Size can vary, but usually between 1 mm and 3 mm (rarely >10 mm) • Morphological classification: --Minor (80%; Mikulicz aphthae): 3–10 mm in size, common in labial or buccal mucosa, heal in 7–14 days without scarring (Figure 28.9) --Major (10%; Sutton disease, periadenitis mucosa necrotica recurrens): 1–3 cm in size, deeper, can occur in posterior soft palate, tonsillar pillar, or pharynx, and can take weeks or months to heal and may scar	• Avoid trauma to mucosa • Avoid toothpaste containing sodium laurel sulfate (SLS), since it has been found to exacerbate RAU in some patients *Pain control/palliative care* **Rx:** Viscous lidocaine 2%* (*only for patients who can expectorate) **Rx:** Diphenhydramine HCL liquid 12.5 mg/5 mL (alcohol free) **Rx:** Diphenhydramine liquid 12.5 mg/5 mL and Maalox®/Kaopectate® 1 : 1 ratio **Rx:** Diphenhydramine 12.5 mg/5 mL, Maalox®/Kaopectate® and lidocaine* 2% suspension, ratio 1 : 1 : 1 (*only for patients who can expectorate) **Rx:** Sucralfate oral suspension 1 g/10 mL **Disp.:** 200 mL **Sig:** Rinse with 1–2 teaspoons (5–10 mL) 4 times a day and spit out *Topical therapies* Topical corticosteroids are used for patients with mild to moderate RAU. Not indicated for patients <2 years old. They are more effective if initiated early in the course of the episode and if used in small amounts multiple times a day. They should not be used for >7 days, to reduce the risk of adrenal suppression. Elixirs are preferred if multiple lesions present or if located in soft palate or areas not accessible for gel placement. Gels are more easily used intraorally than ointments. Topical corticosteroids are classified according to their potency: ultra-high, high, moderate, and low

(continued)

Table 28.6 (Continued)

Etiology	Clinical Description	Management
• Additional laboratory assessment should be considered in patients with signs or symptoms suggesting an underlying or associated systemic disease	--Herpetiform (10%): multiple small 1–3 mm ulcers, clustered or grouped together, most common in nonkeratinized mucosa but can affect keratinized mucosa, female predilection, and occur more common in adulthood. These ulcers heal within 7–10 days without scarring	*Low potency* **Rx:** Dexamethasone elixir 0.5 mg/5 mL **Disp.:** 237 mL **Sig.:** Swish with 5 mL and spit out, 3–4 times a day. Try to keep medication in mouth for 5 minutes. Do not rinse mouth afterward and avoid eating or drinking for 30 minutes
• Therefore, for the initial diagnosis it is important to ask about systemic symptoms/signs to rule out these conditions	• Also classified according to clinical course:	*Considerations:* Contains alcohol and may cause slight burning sensation in some patients. Useful in patients with multiple lesion and lesions in soft palate/tonsillar pillars.
	--Simple aphthosis: patients have few lesions that heal in 10–14 days and recur infrequently	*Moderate potency* **Rx:** Triamcinolone acetonide 0.1% in Orabase® paste **Disp.:** 5 g tube
	--Complex aphthosis: Patients have >3 ulcers that recur frequently (present almost constantly) and are larger in size and extremely painful. Patients can also have genital or perianal lesions, but no associated systemic disease (Letsinger et al., 2005)	**Sig.:** Apply to affected area 3–4 times a day *Considerations:* Orabase is a thick paste, like adhesive. It may not be appealing to many patients
	-Aphthous ulcers are very painful and the pain correlates with the size of the lesions.	*High potency* **Rx:** Fluocinonide gel 0.05% (Lidex®) **Disp.:** 60 g tube
	-More frequently seen in children and young adults (usually before age 30)	
	-Patients typically have a history of multiple recurrences	

Table 28.6 (Continued)

Etiology	Clinical Description	Management
	-Mucosal barrier is important in prevention. There is an increased frequency of lesions when mucosal barrier decreases: trauma, smoking cessation -Lesions usually resolve in 10–14 days. Usually minor ulcers heal without scarring, while major ulcers may scar	**Sig.:** Apply a small amount with cotton applicator to affected area 3–4 times a day (after meals and before bedtime) **Rx:** Betamethasone dipropionate augmented 0.05% gel (Diprolene®) **Disp.:** 15 g tube **Sig**: Apply a small amount with cotton applicator to affected area 3–4 times a day (after meals and before bedtime) *Ultra-high potency* **Rx:** Clobetasol gel 0.05% (Temovate®) **Disp.:** 15 g tube **Sig:** Apply a small amount with cotton applicator to affected area 3–4 times a day (after meals and before bedtime) *Considerations*: Used for major aphthous ulcers or when other topical steroids are not effective. To be used in patients >12 years old **Rx:** Amlexanox paste 5% **Disp.:** 5 g tube **Sig.:** Apply small amounts to affected area 3–4 times a day *Considerations*: Has been shown to increase healing by 1 day. Also helps with pain relief Intralesional injection of corticosteroids (can be used for major aphthous ulcers): triamcinolone acetonide 40 mg/mL.

(*continued*)

Table 28.6 (Continued)

	Etiology	Clinical Description	Management
			For patients with complex disease and those in which topical therapies are not effective, systemic steroids may be indicated. A short course of oral prednisone may be beneficial (20–40 mg per day for 4–7 days) or prednisolone oral suspension 15 mg/5 mL in a swish-and-swallow application to obtain both topical and systemic therapy. Other treatments include colchicine, dapsone, and thalidomide.
			Other treatments
			-Laser therapy: laser cauterization has been studied and may provide rapid pain relief and reduce healing time
			-Nutritional supplements: supplementation with vitamin B_{12} has been shown to be beneficial in one randomized clinical trial
Aphthous-like ulcers associated with systemic disease (Rogers, 1997)	If patients experience associated signs and symptoms, systemic conditions should be evaluated, including the following		
	• **Behcet's syndrome** Rare disease characterized by recurrent oral aphthous ulcers and any of several systemic manifestations, including genital ulcerations, ocular disease, skin lesions, gastrointestinal disease, neurologic disease, vascular disease, and arthritis. Usually presents in the 3rd-4th decades of life and is most prevalent in Turkey, Japan, Korea, and Middle Eastern and Mediterranean countries	Oral ulcers are the most common and frequent sign. They tend to be more extensive and often multiple. They are present for 1–3 weeks and recur, or they can be present continuously.	Some patients can be treated with potent topical steroids or intralesional steroids.
			-**Rx:** Clobetasol gel 0.05% (Temovate®)
			-**Rx:** Triamcinolone 40 mg/mL injection
			Others may require systemic management
			Rx: Prednisone (15 mg/day),
			Rx: Colchicine (1–2 mg/day in divided doses)
			or
			Rx: Apremilast (Otezla®, 10 mg/day)

Table 28.6 (Continued)

Etiology	Clinical Description	Management
• **MAGIC syndrome** Mouth and genital ulcers with inflamed cartilage. Rare condition with only around 20 cases reported. There is a slight female predilection and is more common in 3rd–4th decades. Inflamed cartilage presents as bilateral auricular chondritis, polyarthritis, or nasal chondritis	Oral ulcers described as "aphthous ulcer-like"	Treatment can include nonsteroidal anti-inflammatory drugs (NSAIDs), dapsone, colchicine, prednisone, immunosuppressants (azathioprine, cyclophosphamide, methotrexate) and biologics (infliximab, tocilizumab).
• **Gluten-sensitive enteropathy (GSE) (celiac disease/celiac sprue)** Immune-mediated inflammatory disease of the small intestine caused by sensitivity to dietary gluten. Patients have gastrointestinal complains (diarrhea, bloating, abdominal pain, constipation, weight loss, vomiting) or known gluten intolerance	There is evidence that patients with GSE may have an increased prevalence of oral ulcers, which may not respond to routine medications. Also, enamel defects (yellow-brown opacities, grooves, or pits) have been described in permanent dentition, symmetric in all four quadrants.	Treated with a gluten-free diet and relapses when gluten is reintroduced
• **Inflammatory bowel disease(IBD)/Crohn's disease (CD)** CD can involve mucosa of any portion of the gastrointestinal tract from the oral cavity to the anus and is characterized by transmural inflammation. Peak incidence at 15–30 years. Gastrointestinal symptoms include abdominal pain, weight loss, lack of appetite, diarrhea	Extraintestinal manifestations include oral ulcers. Seen in 10–40% of children. Many different clinical presentations: oral "aphthous-like" ulcers, vestibular linear ulcerations, cobblestoning of mucosa, mucosal tags, lip swelling, pyostomatitis vegetans	Isolated orofacial inflammation can occur in the absence of bowel disease or may precede the development of bowel disease by several years. In these patients, biopsy of inflamed lips, buccal mucosa is indicated for early diagnosis

(continued)

Table 28.6 (Continued)

Etiology	Clinical Description	Management
•**Cyclic neutropenia** Rare autosomal dominant disorder of bone marrow progenitor cells resulting in recurrent neutropenia (every 21 days). Associated symptoms include fever, malaise, pharyngitis, and aphthous stomatitis. Usually noted during infancy or early childhood	Recurrent oral ulcerations. Gingivitis and periodontal breakdown associated with early tooth loss.	Granulocyte-colony-stimulating-factor (G-CSF) (filgrastim or pegfilgratim). Supportive care includes dental care with regular prophylaxis to decrease gingivitis **Rx:** Chlorhexidine gluconate 0.12% (Peridex®) rinse (twice daily) can be prescribed to help reduce gingivitis. Alternatively chlorhexidine gluconate 0.12% alcohol-free (Paroex®)
•**PFAPA** Periodic **fever** with **aphthous** stomatitis, **pharyngitis**, and **adenitis** has a pattern of recurrence approximately once a month. It is an autoinflammatory diseases characterized by inflammation without any significant levels of either autoantibodies or autoreactive T cells. Seen in patients 1–4 years old	Fever of sudden onset, lasting 2–7 days. Oral ulcers on the labial or buccal mucosa. Pharyngitis with exudates and cervical lymphadenopathy.	*Antipyretics* **Rx:** Acetaminophen **Rx:** Ibuprofen Some patients/caregivers may elect no treatment since it is a self-limited disease *For moderate/severe cases* **Rx:** Prednisone (1–2 mg/kg) *For more severe cases with more frequent occurrence* **Rx:** Cimetidine (20–40 mg/kg/day) **Rx:** Colchicine (0.6–1.2 mg/day) Elective tonsillectomy (severe cases)
•**HIV-Associated Aphthous Ulcers** Less common manifestation of immunosuppression	Herpetiform variant is more commonly seen. As immunosuppression is more severe, major aphthous ulcers are more frequent	•Managed with cART (combination antiretroviral therapy) *Potent topical corticosteroids* **Rx:** Clobetasol gel 0.05% (Temovate®) •Lesions that appear atypical or do not respond to therapy must be biopsied to rule out other infections or neoplasms •Treated with nutritional supplements as needed

Table 28.6 (Continued)

	Etiology	Clinical Description	Management
	•**Nutritional deficiencies— iron, folate, zinc, vitamins B_1, B_2, B_6, and B_{12}** Vitamin and mineral deficiencies have been implicated in the pathogenesis of aphthous ulcers, in particular vitamin B_{12} deficiency.		
Multiple	**Erythema multiforme (EM)** (Samim et al., 2013)		
	•Acute, immune-mediated condition characterized by appearance of distinctive target-like lesions on skin and erosions/ulcers on oral, genital, and/or ocular mucosa •Common in young patients 20–40 years, with slight male predominance •In 90% of cases it is precipitated by infections (HSV is the most common) and only 10% associated with medications (penicillin, NSAIDs, oral antibiotics) (Figure 28.10)	Common lesions, seen in 70% of patients with EM. Affects vermillion lips with crusting and intraorally on buccal, labial mucosa, tongue, and nonattached gingiva (Figure 28.10)	•Self-limited disease. Resolves spontaneously. Usually lasts 2 weeks *Topical steroids* **Rx**: Clobetasol 0.05%) gel *Palliative mouthwash* **Rx**: Diphenhydramine 12.5 mg/5 mL, Maalox® /Kaopectate® and lidocaine 2%* in 1 : 1 :1 ratio (*only for patients who can expectorate) •Severe cases with extensive oral lesions leading to inability to eat, systemic therapy **Rx**: Prednisone (0.5–1 mg/kg or 40–6 0mg per day) tapered over 2–4 weeks •HSV-induced EM should be treated with antiviral therapy *Continuous antiviral therapy* **Rx**: Acyclovir 20 mg/kg/day for 6 months or acyclovir 400 mg twice a day **Rx**: Valacyclovir 500 mg twice a day **Rx**: Famciclovir 500 mg twice a day

(continued)

Table 28.6 (Continued)

	Etiology	Clinical Description	Management
Steven–Johnson syndrome/ toxic epidermal necrolysis	• Acute, immune-mediated condition that is triggered by drug exposure (more than 200 medications identified)	Steven–Johnson is seen more frequently and occurs in young patients. Initially patients have prodrome with fever, malaise, sore throat, and loss of appetite. They have erythematous macules in trunk initially and then sloughing of skin and bullae formation (10% body surface). Patients also have oral mucosal ulcerations and other mucosal sites (genital, ocular) Toxic epidermal necrolysis is more severe (affecting >30% of body surfaces), has lower incidence, and occurs in patients >60 years	Early recognition and diagnosis, and discontinuing triggering medication immediately Hospital admission to burns unit for care and management Mortality rate for Steven–Johnson is 1–5% and for toxic epidermal necrolysis is 25–30%
Necrotizing ulcerative gingivitis	• Acute, rapid-onset gingivitis associated with oral spirochetes (*Borrelia Vincenti*) and fusobacteria (*Prevotella intermedia, Fusobacterium nucleatum*) • Usually associated with stress	Commonly seen in young adults. Inflammation of interdental papillae, edema, and hemorrhage. Papillae are blunted and have "punched-out" areas of necrosis. May have fetid odor. May have lymphadenopathy, fever, and malaise	• Debridement, scaling, curettage *Palliative care* Topical anesthetics **Rx:** Lidocaine 2% suspension (only for patients who can expectorate) *Adjunctive care* **Rx:** Chlorhexidine gluconate 0.12%. Alternatively chlorhexidine gluconate 0.12% alcohol-free (Paroex®) Diluted hydrogen peroxide rinses (OTC) *Antibiotics* (if fever and lymphadenopathy present): **Rx:** Metronidazole 250 or 500 mg 3 times a day for 7–14 days **Rx:** Augmentin 500 or 875 mg 2 times a day for 7–14 days

Table 28.6 (Continued)

	Etiology	Clinical Description	Management
Chronic ulcers			
Single			
Chronic traumatic ulcer/ self-induced	Chronic (>2 weeks) longstanding ulcers associated with source of trauma intraorally or may be self-inflicted. May be associated with neurologic conditions with self-mutilation (see above) or may be related to attention-seeking behavior in teenagers	Common sites include tongue, labial mucosa, buccal mucosa. Also may be seen in gingiva. Ulcers can have a rolled white (hyperkeratotic) border. Ulcers can last months, especially if source of trauma is not removed or patient continues self-harm	• Remove source of trauma • Stop self-harm behavior • Place a barrier (lip bumper or bite guard) *Palliative care* **Rx:** Lidocaine 2% suspension (only for patients who can expectorate) • Biopsy is indicated if source of trauma not identified or patient does not disclose self-harm
Multiple			
Erosive lichen planus	Common dermatologic immunologically mediated disease that can affect oral mucosa	Disease commonly seen in middle-aged adults, but has been reported in teenagers/young adults (Patel *et al.*, 2005) Areas of atrophy, erosion, or ulceration with periphery of white striations (lines). In some cases only affects the gingiva and the term "desquamative gingivitis" is used	• Biopsy indicated for diagnosis, in some cases submission of tissue for immunofluorescence studies is necessary to rule out other conditions (pemphigus, pemphigoid, lupus erythematosus) *Topical corticosteroids* **Rx:** Clobetasol gel 0.05% (Temovate®) **Rx:** Dexamethasone elixir 0.5 mg/5 mL • May see iatrogenic oral candidiasis associated with topical steroid use
Chronic graft vs. host disease (GVHD)	Reaction seen after allogenic bone marrow transplantation. Transplanted stem cells identify host as a foreign body. Chronic GVHD occurs >100 days after transplantation (and in some cases years later) (Rocha *et al.*, 2000)	Oral involvement seen in 30–75% of patients. Presents as white striations (lines), or papules associated with erosion or ulcerations located on buccal mucosa, tongue, or labial mucosa.	• Biopsy needed for diagnosis, correlation with clinical history, and findings *Topical corticosteroids* (used for focal ulcers to improve healing) **Rx:** Clobetasol gel 0.05% (Temovate®) • For recalcitrant ulcers or those not responding to topical steroids: **Rx:** Tacrolimus 0.1% (Protopic®) ointment

OTC, over the counter.

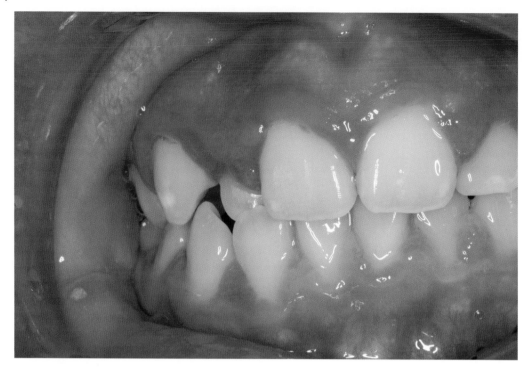

Figure 28.4 Primary herpetic gingivostomatitis with gingival edema, inflammation, and ulcers on buccal mucosa in a teenager.

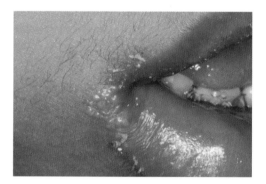

Figure 28.5 Recurrent herpes labialis ("cold sore/fever blister") in a child, presenting as multiple vesicles in right commissure.

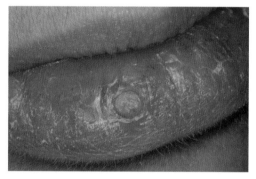

Figure 28.6 Squamous papilloma in the lower lip in a teenager.

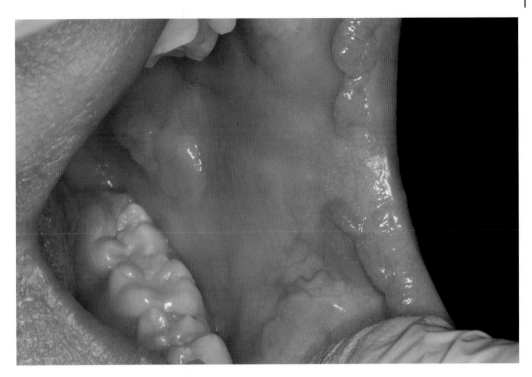

Figure 28.7 Multifocal epithelial hyperplasia ("Heck's disease") in a teenager, with multiple smooth-surfaced papules on buccal mucosa.

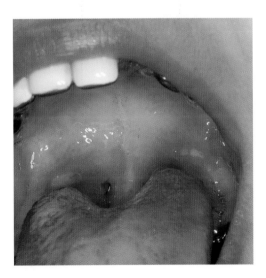

Figure 28.8 Multiple recurrent aphthous ulcers located on the posterior oropharynx in a child one day post intubation for comprehensive dental treatment under general anesthesia.

Oral Mucosal Ulcerations

Oral ulcers are a common clinical condition in children (Stoopler & Al Zamel, 2014). An ulcer is defined as a discontinuity of the surface epithelium, covered by a fibrin clot (pseudomembrane), and thus giving the lesion a yellowish appearance. The borders of ulcers can be either well defined (traceable) or ill defined. Clinically, ulcers can present as a single or multiple, they can present in attached or unattached mucosa, and they can have sudden onset (acute) or be longstanding (chronic) (Bilodeau & Lalla, 2019; Fitzpatrick *et al.*, 2019). Traumatic ulcers are the most common oral ulcers in children. Viral infections can also cause oral ulcerations, and these have been discussed in Table 28.3. A review of oral ulcerations (nonviral) seen in children and their management is offered in Table 28.5.

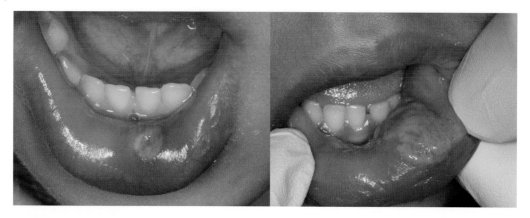

| Recurrent Aphthous Ulcer | Traumatic ulcer post nerve block anesthesia |

Figure 28.9 Comparison of clinical appearance of a recurrent aphthous ulcer and a traumatic ulcer post anesthesia with mandibular block in the lower lip.

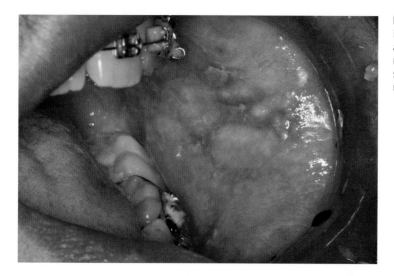

Figure 28.10 Oral lesions in erythema multiforme in a teenager, with multiple ragged-bordered ulcers of sudden onset in the buccal mucosa.

References

Arduino, P.G. & Porter, S.R. (2008) Herpes simplex virus type 1 infection: overview on relevant clinico-pathological features. *Journal of Oral Pathology Medicine*, 37 (2), 107–121. doi:10.1111/j.1600-0714.2007.00586.x.

Baughman, R. (1971) Median rhomboid glossitis: a developmental anomaly? *Oral Surgery, Oral Medicine, Oral Pathology*, 31 (1), 56–65. doi:10.1016/0030-4220(71)90034-x.

Bilodeau, E.A. & Lalla, R.V. (2019) Recurrent oral ulceration: etiology, classification, management, and diagnostic algorithm. *Periodontology 2000*, 80 (1), 49–60. doi:10.1111/prd.12262.

Campois, T.G., Zucoloto, A.Z., de Almeida Araujo, E.J., Svidizinski, T.I.E., Almeida, R.S., *et al.* (2015) Immunological and histopathological characterization of cutaneous candidiasis. *Journal of Medical Microbiology*, 64 (8), 810–817. doi:10.1099/jmm.0.000095.

Capalbo, D., Improda, N., Esposito, A., De Martino, L., Barbieri, F., *et al.* (2013) Autoimmune polyendocrinopathy-candidiasis-ectodermal dystrophy from the pediatric perspective. *Journal of Endocrinological Investigation*, 36 (10), 903–912. doi:10.3275/8999.

Carlos, R. & Sedano, H.O. (1994) Multifocal papilloma virus epithelial hyperplasia. *Oral Surgery, Oral Medicine, Oral Pathology*, 77 (6), 631–635. doi:10.1016/0030-4220(94)90325-5.

Fenton, S.J. & Unkel, J.H. (1997) Viral infections of the oral mucosa in children: a clinical review. *Practical Periodontics and Aesthetic Dentistry*, 9 (6), 683–690; quiz 692.

Fitzpatrick, S.G., Cohen, D.M., & Clark, A.N. (2019) Ulcerated lesions of the oral mucosa: clinical and histologic review. *Head and Neck Pathology*, 13 (1), 91–102. doi:10.1007/s12105-018-0981-8.

Flaitz, C.M. & Baker, K.A. (2000) Treatment approaches to common symptomatic oral lesions in children. *Dental Clinics of North America*, 44 (3), 671–696.

Flaitz, C.M. & Hicks, M.J. (1999) Oral candidiasis in children with immune suppression: clinical appearance and therapeutic considerations. *ASDC Journal of Dentistry for Children*, 66 (3), 161–166.

Frattarelli, D.A., Galinkin, J.L., Green, T.P., Johnson, T.D., Neville, K.A., *et al.* (2014) Off-label use of drugs in children. *Pediatrics*, **133** (3), 563–567. doi:10.1542/peds.2013-4060.

Groll, A.H. & Tragiannidis, A. (2010) Update on antifungal agents for paediatric patients. *Clinical Microbiology and Infection*, 16 (9), 1343–1353. doi:10.1111/j.1469-0691.2010.03334.x.

Hibino, K., Wong, R.W., Hägg, U., & Samaranayake, L.P. (2009) The effects of orthodontic appliances on *Candida* in the human mouth. *International Journal of Paediatric Dentistry*, 19 (5), 301–308. doi:10.1111/j.1365-263X.2009.00988.x.

Holmstrup, P. & Axéll, T. (1990) Classification and clinical manifestations of oral yeast infections. *Acta Odontologica Scandinavica*, 48 (1), 57–59. doi:10.3109/00016359009012734.

Katakam, B.K., Kiran, G., & Kumar, U. (2016) A prospective study of herpes zoster in children. *Indian Journal of Dermatology*, 61 (5), 534–539. doi:10.4103/0019-5154.190121.

Lauritano, D., Moreo, G., Oberti, L., Lucchese, A., Di Stasio, D., *et al.* (2020) Oral manifestations in HIV-positive children: a systematic review. *Pathogens*, 9 (2), 88. doi:10.3390/pathogens9020088.

Letsinger, J.A., McCarty, M.A., & Jorizzo, J.L. (2005) Complex aphthosis: a large case series with evaluation algorithm and therapeutic ladder from topicals to thalidomide. *Journal of the American Academy of Dermatology*, 52 (3 Pt 1), 500–508. doi:10.1016/j.jaad.2004.10.863.

Leung, A.K. (1988) Gentian violet in the treatment of oral candidiasis. *Pediatric Infectious Diseases Journal*, 7 (4), 304–305.

Limeres, J., Feijoo, J.F., Baluja, F., Seoane, J.M., Diniz, M., & Diz, P. (2013, Feb). Oral self-injury: an update. *Dental Traumatology*, 29 (1), 8–14. doi:10.1111/j.1600-9657.2012.01121.x.

Mammas, I.N., Dalianis, T., Doukas, S.G., Zaravinos, A., Achtsidis, V., *et al.* (2019) Paediatric virology and human papillomaviruses: an update. *Experimental and Therapeutic Medicine*, 17 (6), 4337–4343. doi:10.3892/etm.2019.7516.

Mammas, I.N., Sourvinos, G., & Spandidos, D.A. (2009) Human papilloma virus (HPV) infection in children and adolescents. *European Journal of Pediatrics*, 168 (3), 267–273. doi:10.1007/s00431-008-0882-z.

Mustafa, M.B., Arduino, P.G., & Porter, S.R. (2009) Varicella zoster virus: review of its management. *Journal of Oral Pathology and*

Medicine, 38 (9), 673–688.
doi:10.1111/j.1600-0714.2009.00802.x.

Ooi, M.H., Wong, S.C., Lewthwaite, P., Cardosa, M.J., & Solomon, T. (2010) Clinical features, diagnosis, and management of enterovirus 71. *Lancet Neurology*, 9 (11), 1097–1105. doi:10.1016/S1474-4422(10)70209-X.

Padmanabhan, M.Y., Pandey, R.K., Aparna, R., & Radhakrishnan, V. (2010) Neonatal sublingual traumatic ulceration – case report & review of the literature. *Dental Traumatology*, 26 (6), 490–495.
doi:10.1111/j.1600-9657.2010.00926.x.

Pappas, P.G., Kauffman, C.A., Andes, D.R., Clancy, C.J., Marr, K.A., *et al.* (2016) Clinical practice guideline for the management of candidiasis: 2016 update by the Infectious Diseases Society of America. *Clinical and Infectious Diseases*, 62 (4), e1–e50. doi:10.1093/cid/civ933.

Park, K.K., Brodell, R.T., & Helms, S.E. (2011) Angular cheilitis, part 1: local etiologies. *Cutis*, 87 (6), 289–295.

Patel, S., Yeoman, C.M., & Murphy, R. (2005) Oral lichen planus in childhood: a report of three cases. *International Journal of Paediatric Dentistry*, 15 (2), 118–122. doi:10.1111/j.1365-263X.2005.00601.x.

Pinto, A., Haberland, C.M., & Baker, S. (2014) Pediatric soft tissue oral lesions. *Dental Clinics of North America*, 58 (2), 437–453. doi:10.1016/j.cden.2013.12.003.

Raborn, G.W., Martel, A.Y., Lassonde, M., Lewis, M.A., Boon, R., *et al.* (2002) Effective treatment of herpes simplex labialis with penciclovir cream: combined results of two trials. *Journal of the American Dental Association*, **133** (3), 303–309. doi:10.14219/jada.archive.2002.0169.

Rocha, V., Wagner, J.E., Jr., Sobocinski, K.A., Klein, J.P., Zhang, M.J., *et al.* (2000) Graft-versus-host disease in children who have received a cord-blood or bone marrow transplant from an HLA-identical sibling. Eurocord and International Bone Marrow Transplant Registry Working Committee on Alternative Donor and Stem Cell Sources. *New England Journal of Medicine*, 342 (25), 1846–1854.
doi:10.1056/NEJM200006223422501.

Rogers, R.S., 3rd., (1997) Recurrent aphthous stomatitis: clinical characteristics and associated systemic disorders. *Seminars in Cutaneous Medicine and Surgery*, 16 (4), 278–283. doi:10.1016/s1085-5629(97)80017-x.

Said, A.K., Leao, J.C., Fedele, S., & Porter, S.R. (2013) Focal epithelial hyperplasia – an update. *Journal of Oral Pathology and Medicine*, 42 (6), 435–442. doi:10.1111/jop.12009.

Sällberg, M. (2009) Oral viral infections of children. *Periodontology 2000*, 49, 87–95. doi:10.1111/j.1600-0757.2008.00277.x.

Samaranayake, L.P., Keung Leung, W., & Jin, L. (2009) Oral mucosal fungal infections. *Periodontology 2000*, 49, 39–59. doi:10.1111/j.1600-0757.2008.00291.x.

Samim, F., Auluck, A., Zed, C., & Williams, P.M. (2013) Erythema multiforme: a review of epidemiology, pathogenesis, clinical features, and treatment. *Dental Clinics of North America*, 57 (4), 583–596. doi:10.1016/j.cden.2013.07.001.

Santosh, A.B.R. & Muddana, K. (2020) Viral infections of oral cavity. *Journal of Family Medical Primary Care*, 9 (1), 36–42. doi:10.4103/jfmpc.jfmpc_807_19.

Scully, C. & Porter, S. (2008) Oral mucosal disease: recurrent aphthous stomatitis. *British Journal of Oral and Maxillofacial Surgery*, 46 (3), 198–206. doi:10.1016/j.bjoms.2007.07.201.

Singh, A., Verma, R., Murari, A., & Agrawal, A. (2014) Oral candidiasis: an overview. *Journal of Oral and Maxillofacial Pathology*, 18 (Suppl 1), S81–S85. doi:10.4103/0973-029x.141325.

Stoopler, E.T. & Al Zamel, G. (2014) How to manage a pediatric patient with oral ulcers. *Journal of the Canadian Dental Association*, 80, e9.

Summersgill, K.F., Smith, E.M., Levy, B.T., Allen, J.M., Haugen, T.H., & Turek, L.P. (2001) Human papillomavirus in the oral cavities of children and adolescents. *Oral Surgery, Oral Medicine, Oral Pathology, Oral Radiology,*

Endodontology, 91 (1), 62–69.
doi:10.1067/moe.2001.108797.

Syrjänen, S. (2018) Oral manifestations of human papillomavirus infections. *European Journal of Oral Science*, 126 (Suppl 1), 49–66. doi:10.1111/eos.12538.

Vila, T., Sultan, A.S., Montelongo-Jauregui, D., & Jabra-Rizk, M.A. (2020) Oral candidiasis: a disease of opportunity. *Journal of Fungi*, 6 (1). doi:10.3390/jof6010015.

Williams, D.W., Kuriyama, T., Silva, S., Malic, S., & Lewis, M.A. (2011) Candida biofilms and oral candidosis: treatment and prevention. *Periodontology 2000*, 55 (1), 250–265. doi:10.1111/j.1600-0757.2009.00338.x.

Index

Note: Page numbers in *italics* refer to figures. Page numbers in **bold** refer to tables.

Handbook of Clinical Techniques in Pediatric Dentistry, Second Edition. Edited by Jane A. Soxman.
© 2022 John Wiley & Sons, Inc. Published 2022 by John Wiley & Sons, Inc.